APPROACHING DEATH

IMPROVING CARE AT THE END OF LIFE

Committee on Care at the End of Life

Marilyn J. Field and Christine K. Cassel, *Editors*

Division of Health Care Services

INSTITUTE OF MEDICINE

NATIONAL ACADEMY PRESS
Washington, D.C. 1997

National Academy Press • 2101 Constitution Avenue, N.W. • Washington, D.C. 20418

NOTICE: The project that is the subject of this report was approved by the Governing Board of the National Research Council, whose members are drawn from the councils of the National Academy of Sciences, the National Academy of Engineering, and the Institute of Medicine. The members of the committee responsible for the report were chosen for their special competences and with regard for appropriate balance.

This report has been reviewed by a group other than the authors according to procedures approved by a Report Review Committee consisting of members of the National Academy of Sciences, the National Academy of Engineering, and the Institute of Medicine.

The Institute of Medicine was chartered in 1970 by the National Academy of Sciences to enlist distinguished members of the appropriate professions in the examination of policy matters pertaining to the health of the public. In this, the Institute acts under both the Academy's 1863 congressional charter responsibility to be an adviser to the federal government and its own initiative in identifying issues of medical care, research, and education. Dr. Kenneth I. Shine is president of the Institute of Medicine.

Support for this project was provided by the Project on Death in America of the Open Society Institute, the Greenwall Foundation, the Health Care Financing Administration, the Culpeper Foundation, and the Robert Wood Johnson Foundation. Additional support was provided by the Commonwealth Fund, the Archstone Foundation, and the Irvine Health Foundation. The views presented are those of the Institute of Medicine Committee on Care at the End of Life and are not necessarily those of the funding organizations.

Additional copies of this report are available for sale from: National Academy Press, Lock Box 285, 2101 Constitution Avenue, N.W., Washington, DC 20055. Call (800) 624-6242 or (202) 334-3313 (in the Washington metropolitan area), or visit the NAP on-line bookstore at http://www.nap.edu/nap/bookstore.

Call (202) 334-2352 for more information on the other activities of the Institute of Medicine, or visit the IOM home page at http://www.nas.edu/iom.

Library of Congress Cataloging-in-Publication Data

Approaching death : improving care at the end of life / Committee on
    Care at the End of Life, Division of Health Care Services, Institute
    of Medicine ; Marilyn J. Field and Christine K. Cassel, editors.
        p. cm.
        Includes bibliographical references (p.   ) and index.
        ISBN 0-309-06372-8 (cloth)
        1. Terminal care—United States. I. Field, Marilyn J. (Marilyn
Jane) II. Cassel, Christine K. III. Institute of Medicine (U.S.).
    Committee on Care at the End of Life.
    R726.8.A68 1997
    362.1′75′0973—dc21   97-21175

Printed in the United States of America

The serpent has been a symbol of long life, healing, and knowledge among almost all cultures and religions since the beginning of recorded history. The image adopted as a logotype by the Institute of Medicine is based on a relief carving from ancient Greece, now held by the Staatliche Museen in Berlin.

Front cover: Original photograph by Charlotte Hebeler; design and photo manipulation by Francesca Moghari.

Preface

After years of inattention, American society and American medicine are reexamining how we approach dying and death and how we care for people at the end of their lives. It may seem rather ironic that now, close to the year 2000, we are contemplating a reality as universal and certain as human mortality. Further, this is not the first time in this century that we have tried to rethink attitudes and practices as they relate to care at the end of life. In past years, critics and reformers have argued that medical technology has obscured humanistic compassion for dying people and those close to them. These voices have urged more humility about the reach of medicine and more compassion, empathy, and caring for people approaching death. Even though many important innovations, such as hospice programs and palliative medicine, have improved the care potentially available to dying patients, changes in attitudes and practices have been more limited than urged by reformers. Medical technology, meanwhile, has continued to advance, and the temptation remains great to ignore its limits and to evade the uncomfortable and emotionally challenging demands of facing these limits.

Dying, however, is part of life. This report argues that we can do much more to relieve suffering, respect personal dignity, and provide opportunities for people to find meaning in life's conclusion. We are heartened by the small but growing number of activities that are aimed at reaching these goals. Medical societies, health professions schools and certification organizations, charitable foundations, health systems, researchers, patient and community groups, and policymakers are all involved. When this Institute of Medicine (IOM) study was first contemplated more than four years ago, very little of this work had been initiated.

This study itself arose in response to a request that the IOM conduct a project to develop guidelines for identifying and limiting futile treatments. After extensive consultations revealed many concerns that such a focus would not prove successful, the IOM undertook a six-month study of the feasibility and probable contribution of an IOM study on care at the end of life (Appendix A). Following two meetings and a workshop for which several background papers were prepared, the planning committee appointed to consider the question strongly endorsed a full-scale study that would both generally examine issues related to dying, decisionmaking, and appropriate care and selectively focus on several narrower topics. The group concluded that although much is being done to improve the care of critically ill and dying patients, many questions remain to be persuasively answered—or, for that matter, asked—about what constitutes appropriate care for different kinds of patients and how choices about care for dying patients can best be made and implemented.

In response, the IOM embarked on an extended effort to raise funds for a broad study that would make recommendations for improving care at the end of life. In late 1995, sufficient funding had been secured to permit the study to begin. To undertake the study, the IOM appointed a 12-member committee of experts in medical and nursing care for chronically and severely ill patients, ethics, quality of care, health policy, health services research, law, economics, social services, and related fields. The committee's broad tasks were to

• assess the state of knowledge about the clinical, behavioral, legal, economic, and other important aspects of care for patients with life-threatening medical problems;
• evaluate methods for measuring outcomes, predicting survival and functional status, determining patient and family preferences, and assessing quality of care;
• identify factors that impede or promote high-quality care for patients approaching death; and
• propose steps that policymakers, practitioners, and others could take to improve the organization, delivery, financing, assessment, and quality of care for those with terminal illnesses and to increase agreement on what constitutes appropriate care.

Between January 1996 and January 1997 the committee met five times. It also conducted two public meetings, one in Washington, D.C., and another in Irvine, California. Of the nearly 100 groups contacted, thirty-six groups presented statements at these meetings (see the meeting agendas in

Appendix B), and another 11 groups submitted written statements. The committee also met with researchers from the National Institutes of Health and other organizations. In addition to learning from the papers commissioned for the planning study, committee and staff reviewed literature (often quite sparse) on the issues identified in its charge. In addition, committee members participated in a workshop organized by the George Washington University Center to Improve Care of the Dying that began a process of developing a "toolkit" of quality and outcomes measures for end-of-life care. The committee also commissioned supplemental work for discussions of the epidemiology of dying and the cost of care at the end of life. This report, thus, reflects a wide-ranging effort to understand what we know about care at the end of life and what we have yet to learn.

The importance of this topic is undeniable. Unlike research about individual diseases, research about dying has the potential to touch every family and every individual in some way. Even those who die suddenly and unexpectedly can expect their survivors to benefit from a better understanding of grief and bereavement. The work of this committee and a growing number of others thus can bring great benefit. That biomedical science is making enormous strides also creates reasons for optimism about opportunities to better understand the pathophysiology of physical and emotional symptoms and to develop new approaches to preventing and ameliorating these symptoms. Increasing understanding of genetics, human biology, and longevity should not lead to dreams of near immortality but, rather, give us greater respect for the cycle of human life.

Medicine and public health should continue to help people live long, healthy lives. When medicine can no longer promise an extension of life, people should not fear that their dying will be marked by neglect, care inconsistent with their wishes, or preventable pain and other distress. They should be able to expect the health care system to assure reliable, effective, and humane caregiving. If we can fulfill that expectation, then public trust will be strengthened. The memorable words of Sir William Osler that we must "care always" will be renewed as a fundamental and abiding value.

Christine K. Cassel, M.D.
Chair

Acknowledgments

Many individuals and groups assisted the study committee and staff in the development of this report. At the start, those who served on the feasibility study committee shaped the direction of the report in major ways, and the authors of several papers commissioned for that activity provided important insights and information. The members of that committee and the paper authors are listed in Appendix A (see also IOM, 1994). Two of the background papers are included in Appendices D and E.

Additional information and insights came from two public meetings, during which the committee heard from many organizations and individuals deeply involved with care of people with advanced progressive illnesses. Many participants made contributions beyond the public meetings to help us understand the difficult issues in end-of-life care. Appendix B includes the meeting agendas and participant lists and also cites the organizations that provided written testimony.

In addition, a workshop coordinated with Joan Teno, M.D. (then of the George Washington University's Center to Improve Care of the Dying, now at Brown University) was tremendously useful in understanding the array of potentially useful tools and instruments for measuring the quality of life and the quality of care for those approaching death. Information about the workshop is included in Appendix F.

Two very informative meetings were held with the following staff from the National Institutes of Health: Patricia Bryant, Ph.D., and Mitchell Max, M.D., of the National Institute of Dental Research; Bill Foster, M.D., Senior Staff Physician at NIH; Jack Killen, M.D., of the Division of AIDS in the National Institute of Allergy and Infectious Disease; June Lunney, Ph.D., R.N., of the National Institute of Nursing Research; Mary Schwarz McCabe, B.A., B.S.N., and Claudette Varricchio, D.S.N., of the National Cancer Institute; Emanuel Stadlan, M.D., of the National Institute on Neurological Disorders and Stroke; and Alan Trachtenberg, M.D., of the National Institute on Drug Abuse. In addition to these meetings, Drs. Max and Killen provided very helpful ideas about important biomedical research issues. Other valuable assistance in understanding research questions and priorities was provided by Kathryn Foley, M.D. and William Breitbart, M.D., of Memorial Sloan-Kettering Cancer Center, and Gary Bennett, Ph.D., of Allegheny University of the Health Sciences.

The staff of the George Washington University's Center to Improve Care for the Dying provided much assistance, including work in developing Appendix C. Anne Wilkinson, Ph.D., Elise Ayers, Ann Bolin, and Kristen Landrum made particular contributions. At Mt. Sinai Medical Center, the patience and cooperation of Helen Blakes and Sylvia Giamarino is very much appreciated.

Susan Tolle, M.D., Director of the Center for Ethics in Health Care at the Oregon Health Sciences University, and Betty Ward provided an opportunity to meet with many people participating in a series of Oregon initiatives to improve care at the end of life. A day-long conference involving clinicians and managers in long-term care offered insights into the challenges and opportunities to improve care in these settings. Among others sharing their experience and knowledge were Marian Hodges, M.D., of Sisters of Providence Hospitals; Paul Bascom, M.D., chair of OHSU University Hospitals' comfort care team, and several other team members: Michael Garland, D.Sc.Rel., Miles Edwards, M.D., and Ralph Crawshaw, M.D.

At the University of Virginia, Carlos Gomez, M.D., arranged a similarly useful visit that included opportunities to meet with community hospice, hospital, medical school, and other people involved in developing an inpatient hospice unit and in expanding the education of students and residents in end-of-life care. Among the many who were helpful to us were Victoria Todd, M.B.A., and Mary Jane Griffith, R.N., of the Hospice of the Piedmont; Elizabeth McGovern and John Herrmann from the Center for Hospice and Palliative Care; Carolyn Englehard, M.A.P.A., of the Virginia Health Policy Center; James Childress, Ph.D., and Marcia Finney, Ph.D.; and members of the Division of General Medicine including Drs. Daniel Becker, Munsey Wheby, Robert Carey, Margaret Reitmeyer, and Scott Robertson.

Linda Blank, Vice President, American Board of Internal Medicine, was helpful in innumerable ways based on her experience with the Board's work to improve residency education. David Joranson, M.S.S.W., and Aaron

Gilson, M.S., M.S.S.W., of the Pain and Policy Studies Group at the University of Wisconsin's Comprehensive Cancer Center, offered much guidance in understanding the legislative and policy barriers to good pain treatment. Chris Cody and John Mahoney of the National Hospice Organization responded time and again to requests for demographic and policy clarification. The committee also wishes to thank Knight Steel, M.D., Hackensack University; Susan Bloch, M.D., and J. Andrew Billings, M.D., Harvard University; Tom W. Smith, Ph.D., of the National Opinion Research Council; Ira Byock, M.D., Academy of Hospice and Palliative Care Physicians; Kathleen Lohr, Ph.D., Research Triangle Institute; Diane Meier, M.D., Mt. Sinai Medical Center (NYC); Daniel Sulmasy, M.D., Georgetown University; and James Lubitz, Ph.D., and Gerald Riley, Ph.D., of the Health Care Financing Administration.

The study's sponsors and project officers provided information and assistance on several occasions. We particularly thank William Stubing of the Greenwall Foundation, Mary Calloway of the Open Society Institute, Rosemarie Hakim of the Health Care Financing Administration, Linda Jacobs and Mary Ellen Bucci of the Culpeper Foundation, and Rosemary Gibson of the Robert Wood Johnson Foundation.

As usual, a number of people within the Institute of Medicine provided assistance to the study committee and study staff in many different ways. We would especially like to thank Molla Donaldson, Claudia Carl, Francesca Moghari, Sally Stanfield, Constance Pechura, Ph.D., Mike Edington, Mary Lee Schneiders, Luis Nuñez, and Dan Quinn.

Contents

TABLES, FIGURES, AND BOXES

Tables

Figures

Boxes

Summary

Dying is at once a fact of life and a profound mystery. Death comes to all, yet each person experiences it in ways that are only partly accessible to the physician or family member, the philosopher or researcher. In principle, humane care for those approaching death is a social obligation as well as a personal offering from those directly involved. In reality, both society and individuals often fall short of what is reasonably—if not simply—achievable. As a result, people have come both to fear a technologically overtreated and protracted death and to dread the prospect of abandonment and untreated physical and emotional distress.

A humane care system is one that people can trust to serve them well as they die, even if their needs and beliefs call for a departure from typical practices. It honors and protects those who are dying, conveys by word and action that dignity resides in people—not physical attributes—and helps people to preserve their integrity while coping with unavoidable physical insults and losses. Such reliably excellent and respectful care at the end of life is an attainable goal, but realizing it will require many changes in attitudes, policies, and actions. System changes—not just changes in individual beliefs and actions—are necessary.

A number of developments suggest that the time is right for action at all levels to improve care at the end of life and to assure people that they will be neither abandoned nor maltreated as they approach death. This Institute of Medicine report is intended to support such action by strengthening popular and professional understanding of what constitutes good care at the end of life and by encouraging a wider societal commitment to caring well for people as they die. More specifically, it is intended to stimulate health professionals and managers, researchers, policymakers, funders of health care, and the public at large to develop more constructive perspectives on dying and death and to improve the practices and policies under their control. To these ends, this report stresses several themes.

- Too many dying people suffer from pain and other distress that clinicians could prevent or relieve with existing knowledge and therapies.
- Significant organizational, economic, legal, and educational impediments to good care can be identified and, in varying degrees, remedied.
- Important gaps in scientific knowledge about the end of life need serious attention from biomedical, social science, and health services researchers.
- Strengthening accountability for the quality of care at the end of life will require better data and tools for evaluating the outcomes important to patients and families.

CONTEXT AND TRENDS

In the United States, death at home in the care of family has been widely superseded by a technological, professional, and institutional process of treatment for the dying. That process—its benefits notwithstanding—often isolates the final stage of life from the rest of living. Likewise, the mobility of Americans quite literally puts distance between many younger and older family members. Many adults, even in middle age, have not lived with or cared for someone who was dying.

Because Americans, on average, live much longer now than they did at the end of the nineteenth century, a much larger proportion of the population dies at an advanced age. More than 70 percent of those who die each year are age 65 or over, and those who die in old age tend to die of different causes than those who die young. For both younger and older people, the major causes of death and the typical experience of dying differ from 100 years ago. The dying process today tends to be more extended, in part because medical treatments can manage pneumonia, infections, kidney failure, and other immediate causes of death that come in the wake of cancer and other "slow killers."

The field of palliative care is one response to the changing profile of death in the twentieth century. It focuses on the prevention and relief of suffering through the meticulous management of symptoms from the early through the final stages of an illness; it attends closely to the emotional, spiritual, and practical needs of patients and those close to them. Other community, professional, and governmental responses include the development of hospice programs, bereavement support groups, and policies and programs that encourage communication about people's goals and preferences as they approach death.

The twenty-first century will bring new realities as well as continuing problems and opportunities in care at the end of life. It will undoubtedly deliver improvements in what medical science can do to prevent and relieve distress for those approaching death, but demographic, economic, and other trends will strain systems that already find it difficult to deliver what clinical knowledge currently allows—and what compassion should grant.

The next century will see the final demographic consequences of the post-World War II baby boom. The oldest members of the baby boom generation will reach age 65 in the year 2011, and the youngest members will do so nearly 20 years later. The elderly will constitute a larger proportion of the population than today, and the absolute numbers of dying patients will be substantially higher. Although health care and social service providers have a long lead time compared with the educators and communities who had to scramble to provide schooling for the baby boom generation, the difficulties that policymakers are already having with Social Security and Medicare do not bode well for the nation's ability to cope with the social, medical, economic, and other effects of an aging population.

Contrary to some popular thinking, however, the increase in overall personal health care spending is not explained by disproportionate growth in costs for end-of-life care. The small percentage of people who die each year do account for a significant proportion of health care expenditures, but the share of spending accounted for by this group does not appear to have changed much since the 1970s. Overall, increased health care spending is primarily accounted for by population growth, general inflation in the economy, and additional medical care inflation. One reason for the attention to the cost of care at the end of life is that such care is, in considerable measure, funded through Medicare, Medicaid, veterans, and other public programs.

Pressures to control public and private health care costs will continue and, indeed, will likely intensify with consequent restructuring of how health care is organized, delivered, and financed. More older people with advanced disease will be served by different kinds of managed care organizations. If effective quality monitoring and improvement methods are in place, the strengths and limitations of these varied arrangements will become clearer as their experience with end-of-life care grows. Possible problem areas include contracting, payment, and review mechanisms that limit access to clinicians and care teams experienced in palliative care; patient scheduling norms that limit time for careful patient-clinician communication; and marketing strategies that may discourage enrollment by seriously ill people.

CONCEPTS AND PRINCIPLES

Notions of "good" and "bad" deaths are threaded throughout discussions about dying and death. These concepts are not fixed in meaning but rather are shaped by people's experiences, spiritual beliefs, and culture and by changes in social mores, technology, and options for dying. Reflecting its members' personal and professional experiences and philosophical perspectives, the study committee that developed this report proposed that people should be able to expect and achieve a decent or good death—*one that is free from avoidable distress and suffering for patients, families, and caregivers; in general accord with patients' and families' wishes; and reasonably consistent with clinical, cultural, and ethical standards.* A bad death is characterized by needless suffering, disregard for patient or family wishes or values, and a sense among participants or observers that norms of decency have been offended.

The committee that prepared this report was guided by a set of working principles that reflect a combination of value judgments and empirical assumptions. Only the first of the following principles applies exclusively to care at the end of life.

Care for those approaching death is an integral and important part of health care. Everyone dies, and those at this stage of life deserve attention that is as thorough, active, and conscientious as that granted to those for whom cure or longer life is a realistic goal.

Care for those approaching death should involve and respect both patients and those close to them. Particularly for patients with a grim prognosis, clinicians need to consider patients in the context of their families and close relationships and to be sensitive to their culture, values, resources, and other characteristics.

Good care at the end of life depends on strong interpersonal skills, clinical knowledge, and technical proficiency, and it is informed by scientific evidence, values, and personal and professional experience. Clinical excellence is important because the frail condition of dying patients leaves little margin to rectify errors.

Changing individual behavior is difficult, but changing an organization or a culture is potentially a greater challenge—and often is a precondition for individual change. Deficiencies in care often reflect flaws in how the health care system functions, which means that correcting problems will require change at the system level.

The health care community has special responsibility for educating itself and others about the identification, management, and discussion of the last phase of fatal medical problems. Although health care professionals may not have a central presence in the lives of some people who are dying, many others draw heavily on physicians, nurses, social workers, and others for care—and caring. Thus, health care professionals are inescapably responsible for educating themselves and helping to educate the broader community about good care for dying patients and their families.

More and better research is needed to increase our understanding of the clinical, cultural, organizational, and other practices or perspectives that can improve care for those approaching death. The committee began—and concluded—its deliberations with the view that the knowledge base for good end-of-life care has enormous gaps and is neglected in the design and funding of biomedical, clinical, psychosocial, and health services research.

CARING AT THE END OF LIFE: DIMENSIONS AND DEFICIENCIES

Care for most dying patients involves several basic elements: (1) understanding the physical, psychological, spiritual, and practical dimensions of caregiving; (2) identifying and communicating diagnosis and prognosis; (3) establishing goals and plans; and (4) fitting palliative and other care to these goals. In looking at current systems and practices, the committee found much that was good, including clinical, organizational, and ethical practices of palliative medicine that are implemented through hospices, interdisciplinary care teams in varied settings, innovative educational programs, and nascent outcomes measurement and quality monitoring and improvement strategies.

Notwithstanding these positive features, the committee concluded that very serious problems remain. It identified four broad deficiencies in the current care of people with life-threatening and incurable illnesses.

First and most fundamentally, too many people suffer needlessly at the end of life, both from errors of omission (when caregivers fail to provide palliative and supportive care known to be effective) and from errors of commission (when caregivers do what is known to be ineffective or even harmful). Studies have repeatedly indicated that a significant proportion of dying patients and patients with advanced disease experience serious pain, despite the availability of effective pharmacological and other options for relieving most pain. Other symptoms are less well studied, but the information available to the committee suggested a similar pattern of inadequate care. In perverse counterpoint to the problem of undertreatment, the aggressive use of ineffectual and intrusive interventions may prolong and even dishonor the period of dying. Some of this care is knowingly accepted; some is provided counter to patients' wishes; much is probably provided and accepted with little knowledge or consideration of its probable benefits and burdens.

Second, legal, organizational, and economic obstacles conspire to obstruct reliably excellent care at the end of life. Outdated and scientifically flawed drug-prescribing laws, regulations, and interpretations by state medical boards continue to frustrate and intimidate physicians who wish to relieve their patients' pain. Addiction to opioids appropriately prescribed to relieve pain and other symptoms is virtually nonexistent, whereas underuse of these medications is a well-documented problem. Fragmented organizational structures often complicate coordination and continuity of care and impede the further development and application of palliative care strategies in patient care, professional education, and research. Medicare hospice benefits have made palliative services more available to a small segment of dying patients, but many more have illnesses that do not readily fit the traditional hospice model or government benefit requirements. Traditional financing mechanisms—including arrangements based on discounted fees—still provide incentives for the overuse of procedural services and the underprovision or poor coordination of the assessment, evaluation, management, and supportive services so important for people with serious chronic or progressive medical problems.

Third, the education and training of physicians and other health care professionals fail to provide them the attitudes, knowledge, and skills required to care well for the dying patient. Many deficiencies in practice stem from fundamental prior failures in professional education. Undergraduate, graduate, and continuing education do not sufficiently prepare health professionals to recognize the final phases of illnesses, understand and manage their own emotional reactions to death and dying, construct effective strategies for care, and communicate sensitively with patients and those close to them.

Fourth, current knowledge and understanding are insufficient to guide and support the consistent practice of evidence-based medicine at the end of life. Biomedical and clinical research have focused almost exclusively on the development of knowledge that contributes to the prevention, detection, or cure of disease and to the prolongation of life. Research on the end stages of diseases and the physiological bases of symptoms and symptom relief has had negligible support. Epidemiological and health services research has likewise not provided a strong base for understanding the degree to which people suffer symptoms (except, perhaps, cancer pain), experience death alone rather than in the company of those who care, comprehend diagnostic and prognostic information, and achieve a dying that is reasonably consistent with their preferences, palliative care principles, and community norms. Methods development is important to define and measure outcomes other than death (including patient and family perceptions) and to monitor and improve the quality of care for those approaching death.

More generally, this committee concluded that people in this country have not yet discovered how to talk realistically but comfortably about the end of life, nor have they learned how to value the period of dying as it is now experienced by most people. Except for the occasional newspaper feature or television documentary, the reality of dying as most often experienced in the United States has been largely shunned by the news, information, and entertainment media as distasteful or uninteresting. One result is an unhelpful combination of fear, misinformation, and oversimplification that contributes to a public perception of misery as inescapable, pain as unavoidable, and public spending as misdirected for people approaching death.

RECOMMENDATIONS AND FUTURE DIRECTIONS

Seven recommendations address different decisionmakers and different deficiencies in care at the end of life. Each applies generally to people approaching death including those for whom death is imminent and those with serious, eventually fatal illnesses who may live for some time. Each is intended to contribute to the achievement of a compassionate care system that dying people and those close to them can rely on for respectful and effective care.

RECOMMENDATION 1: People with advanced, potentially fatal illnesses and those close to them should be able to expect and receive reliable, skillful, and supportive care. Educating people about care at the end of life is a critical responsibility of physicians, hospitals, hospices, support groups, public programs, and media. Most patients and families need information not only about diagnosis and prognosis but also about what support and what outcomes they should reasonably be able to expect. They should, for example, not be allowed to believe that pain is inevitable or that supportive care is incompatible with continuing efforts to diagnose and treat. They should learn—before their last few days of life—that supportive services are available from hospices and elsewhere in the community and that those involved in their care will help arrange such services. Patient and family expectations and understanding will be aided by advance care planning that considers needs and goals, identifies appropriate surrogate decisionmakers, and avoids narrow preoccupation with written directives. To these ends, health care organizations and other relevant parties should adopt policies regarding information, education, and assistance related to end-of-life decisions and services. For those who seek to build public understanding of dying as a part of life and to generate public demand for better supportive services, one model can be found in the perspectives, spirit, and strategies that have guided efforts to promote effective prenatal care and develop mother and family-oriented arrangements for childbirth.

RECOMMENDATION 2: Physicians, nurses, social workers, and other health professionals must commit themselves to improving care for dying patients and to using existing knowledge effectively to prevent and relieve pain and other symptoms. Patients often depend on health care professionals to manage the varying physical and psychological symptoms that accompany advanced illness. To meet their obligations to their patients, practitioners must hold themselves responsible for using existing knowledge and available interventions to assess, prevent, and relieve physical and emotional distress. When they identify organizational and other impediments to good practice, practitioners have the responsibility as individuals and members of larger groups to advocate for system change.

RECOMMENDATION 3: Because many problems in care stem from system problems, policymakers, consumer groups, and purchasers of health care should work with health care practitioners, organizations, and researchers to

a. strengthen methods for measuring the quality of life and other outcomes of care for dying patients and those close to them;

b. develop better tools and strategies for improving the quality of care and holding health care organizations accountable for care at the end of life;

c. revise mechanisms for financing care so that they encourage rather than impede good end-of-life care and sustain rather than frustrate coordinated systems of excellent care; and

d. reform drug prescription laws, burdensome regulations, and state medical board policies and practices that impede effective use of opioids to relieve pain and suffering.

Although individuals must act to improve care at the end of life, systems of care must be changed to support such action. Better information systems and tools for measuring outcomes and evaluating care are critical to the creation of effective and accountable systems of care and to the effective functioning of both internal and external systems of quality monitoring and improvement. Policymakers and purchasers need to consider both the long-recognized deficiencies of traditional fee-for-service arrangements and the less thoroughly understood limitations of alternatives, including various kinds of capitated and per case payment methods. Particularly in need of attention are payment mechanisms that fail to reward excellent care and create incentives for under- or overtreatment of those approaching death.

State medical societies, licensing boards, legislative committees, and other groups should cooperate to review drug prescribing laws, regulations, board practices, and physician attitudes and practices to identify problem areas and then devise revisions in unduly burdensome statutes and regulations. Such regulatory change is not enough. It must be accompanied by education to increase knowledge and correct misperceptions about the appropriate medical use of opioids and about the biological mechanisms of opioid dependence, addiction, and pain management.

The committee identified characteristics of community care systems that would more effectively and reliably serve dying patients and their families. "Whole-community" approaches to end-of-life care would include a mix of programs, settings, personnel, procedures, and practices that extend beyond health care institutions and policies to involve entire communities. The goals would be to make effective palliative care available wherever and whenever the dying patient is cared for; help dying patients and their families to plan ahead and prepare for dying and death; and establish accountability for high quality care at the end of life. Box S.1 shows key features of a whole-community system for end-of-life care. A system with these components would reflect the understanding that there is not just one way to care for dying patients and that some flexibility is needed to respond to patients who do not comfortably fit the routines and standards that serve most patients well. Clearly, such a system represents an aspiration. The model implies cooperative effort involving public and private agencies on multiple levels—community, state, and national.

RECOMMENDATION 4: Educators and other health professionals should initiate changes in undergraduate, graduate, and continuing education to ensure that practitioners have relevant attitudes, knowledge, and skills to care well for dying patients. Dying is too important a part of life to be left to one or two required (but poorly attended) lectures, to be considered only in ethical and not clinical terms, or to be set aside on the grounds that medical educators are already swamped with competing demands for time and resources. Every health professional who deals directly with patients and families needs a basic grounding in competent and compassionate care for seriously ill and dying patients. For clinicians and others to be held truly accountable for their care of the dying, educators must be held accountable for what they teach and what they implicitly and explicitly honor as exemplary practice. Textbooks and other materials likewise need revision to reflect the reality that people die and that dying patients are not people for whom "nothing can be done." Box S.2 outlines the fundamental elements of professional preparation for skillful, compassionate, and respectful care at the end of life.

RECOMMENDATION 5: Palliative care should become, if not a medical specialty, at least a defined area of expertise, education, and re-

---

BOX S.1
A Whole-Community Model for Care at the End of Life

Programs and settings of care suited to the needs and circumstances of different kinds of dying patients

- Home hospice programs
- Other palliative care arrangements for patients that do not fit the home care model
  —Day programs in hospitals and nursing homes, similar to those developed by geriatricians
  —"Step-down" arrangements including nursing homes that permit a less intensive and less expensive level of inpatient care when appropriate
  —Specialized inpatient palliative care beds for those with severe symptoms that cannot be well managed elsewhere
  —Respite programs to relieve families of patients with a long dying trajectory (e.g., those with Alzheimers Disease) that imposes major physical and emotional burdens on families

Personnel, protocols, and other mechanisms that support high quality, efficient, timely, and coordinated care

- Practical and valid assessment instruments and practice guidelines for patient evaluation and management that can be applied at both the individual and organizational level
- Protocols for evaluating patient's need for referral or transfer to other individual or organizational caregivers
- Procedures for implementing patient transitions in ways that encourage continuity of care, respect patient and family preferences and comfort, and assure the transfer of necessary patient information
- Consulting and crisis teams that extend and intensify efforts to allow patients to remain home despite difficult medical problems or crises
- Ongoing professional education programs fitted to the varying needs of all clinicians who care for dying patients
- Performance monitoring and improvement programs intended to identify and correct problems and to improve the average quality of care

Public and private policies, practices, and attitudes that help organizations and individuals

- Provider payment, coverage, and oversight policies that, at a minimum, do not restrict access to appropriate, timely palliative care and, as a goal, promote it
- Support systems provided through workplaces, religious congregations, and other institutions to ease the emotional, financial, and practical burdens experienced by dying patients and their families
- Public education programs that aim to improve general awareness, to encourage advance care planning, and to provide specific information at the time of need about resources for physical, emotional, spiritual, and practical caring at the end of life

BOX S.2
Professional Preparation for End-of-Life Care

Scientific and clinical knowledge and skills, including:

- Learning the biological mechanisms of dying from major illnesses and injuries
- Understanding the pathophysiology of pain and other physical and emotional symptoms
- Developing appropriate expertise and skill in the pharmacology of symptom management
- Acquiring appropriate knowledge and skill in nonpharmacological symptom management
- Learning the proper application and limits of life-prolonging interventions
- Understanding tools for assessing patient symptoms, status, quality of life, and prognosis

Interpersonal skills and attitudes, including:

- Listening to patients, families, and other members of the health care team
- Conveying difficult news
- Understanding and managing patient and family responses to illness
- Providing information and guidance on prognosis and options
- Sharing decisionmaking and resolving conflicts
- Recognizing and understanding one's own feelings and anxieties about dying and death
- Cultivating empathy
- Developing sensitivity to religious, ethnic, and other differences

Ethical and professional principles, including:

- Doing good and avoiding harm
- Determining and respecting patient and family preferences
- Being alert to personal and organizational conflicts of interests
- Understanding societal/population interests and resources
- Weighing competing objectives or principles
- Acting as a role model of clinical proficiency, integrity, and compassion

Organizational skills, including:

- Developing and sustaining effective professional teamwork
- Understanding relevant rules and procedures set by health plans, hospitals, and others
- Learning how to protect patients from harmful rules and procedures
- Assessing and managing care options, settings, and transitions
- Mobilizing supportive resources (e.g., palliative care consultants, community-based assistance)
- Making effective use of existing financial resources and cultivating new funding sources

search. The objective is to create a cadre of palliative care experts whose numbers and talents are sufficient to (a) provide expert consultation and role models for colleagues, students, and other members of the health care team; (b) supply leadership for scientifically based and practically useful undergraduate, graduate, and continuing medical education; and (c) organize and conduct biomedical, clinical, behavioral, and health services research. More generally, palliative care must be redefined to include prevention as well as relief of symptoms.

RECOMMENDATION 6: The nation's research establishment should define and implement priorities for strengthening the knowledge base for end-of-life care. The research establishment includes the National Institutes of Health, other federal agencies (e.g., the Agency for Health Care Policy and Research, the Health Care Financing Administration, the National Center for Health Statistics), academic centers, researchers in many disciplines, pharmaceutical companies, and foundations supporting health research. One step is to take advantage of clinical trials by collecting more information on the quality of life of those who die while enrolled in experimental or treatment groups. A further step is to support more research on the physiological mechanisms and treatment of symptoms common during the end of life, including neuropsychiatric problems. Pain research appears to supply a good model for this enterprise to follow. To encourage change in the attitudes and understandings of the research establishment, the committee urges the National Institutes of Health and other public agencies to take the lead in organizing workshops, consensus conferences, and other projects that focus on what is and is not known about end-stage disease and symptom management and that propose an agenda for improvement. Demonstration projects to test new methods of financing and organizing care should be a priority for the Health Care Financing Administration. For the Agency for Health Care Policy and Research, the committee encourages support for the dissemination and replication of proven health care interventions and programs through clinical practice guidelines and other means.

RECOMMENDATION 7: A continuing public discussion is essential to develop a better understanding of the modern experience of dying, the options available to patients and families, and the obligations of communities to those approaching death. Individual conversations between practitioners and patients are important but cannot by themselves provide a more supportive environment for the attitudes and actions that make it possible for most people to die free from avoidable distress and to find the peace or meaning that is significant to them. Although efforts to reduce the entertainment and news media's emphasis on violent or sensational death and unrealistic medical rescue have not been notably successful, a modicum of balance has recently been provided by thoughtful analyses, public forums, and other coverage of the clinical, emotional, and practical issues involved in end-of-life care. Regardless of how the current, highly publicized policy debate over physician-assisted suicide is resolved, the goal of improving care for those approaching death and the barriers to achieving that goal should not be allowed to fade from public consciousness. Much of the responsibility for keeping the public discussion going will rest not with the media but with public officials, professional organizations, religious leaders, and community groups.

The committee agreed that it would not take a position on the legality or morality of physician-assisted suicide. It does, however, believe that the issue should not take precedence over those reforms to the health care system that would improve care for dying patients.

CONCLUSION

The analyses, conclusions, and recommendations presented here are offered with optimism that people, individually and together, can act to "approach" death constructively and reduce suffering at the end of life. This report identifies steps that can be taken to improve care at the end of life and to create a solid foundation for maintaining such improvements through difficult times. It also highlights the reasons for believing that professionals, policymakers, and the public are becoming more aware of what can and should be done and are ready to embrace change. These reasons range from the examples of well-known men and women facing death with grace to the more intense focus on deficiencies in care that has been stimulated by the debate over assisted suicide. In sum, the timing appears right to press for a vigorous societal commitment to improve care at the end of life. That commitment would motivate and sustain individual and collective efforts to create a humane care system that people can trust to serve them well as they die.

1

Introduction

With what strift and pains we came into the World we know not; but 'tis commonly no easie matter to get out of it.
Sir Thomas Brown, *Letter to a Friend*, c. 1680

In some respects, this century's scientific and medical advances have made living easier and dying harder. On the one hand, discoveries and innovations in public health, biomedical sciences, and clinical medicine have brought remarkable advances in our abilities to prevent, detect, and treat many illnesses and injuries. Killers such as smallpox, polio, diphtheria, and cholera have vanished or been greatly curbed by advances in sanitation, nutrition, and immunization. The infections that made childbirth so dangerous are now mostly avoidable. Especially in technologically developed countries such as the United States, many families cherish children who would have been lost to prematurity in decades past. Curative and rehabilitative treatments for previously disabling injuries and deadly diseases now allow many people to resume productive and satisfying lives.

On the other hand, many people have become fearful that the combination of old age and modern medicine will inflict on them a dying that is more protracted and, in some ways, more difficult than it would have been a few decades ago. In countries such as the United States, most people now die of chronic illnesses such as heart disease and cancer. The prevalence of chronic illness and death at an advanced age challenges health care delivery, financing, research, and education systems that were designed primarily for acute illness and injury rather than for serious chronic or progressive degenerative illness. The treatments that clinicians may see as rescuing people, if only briefly, from imminent death may sometimes be experienced by patients and families as a torment from which they need to be freed. News stories periodically appear that recount a daughter's or a husband's or a friend's grief and anger at being unable to save a loved one from being tethered to medical devices, violated by resuscitation maneuvers with little prospect of success, or maintained in the unknowable depths of catastrophic brain damage.

These news stories, even if not typical, may nonetheless significantly affect public anxieties. This is especially likely when the stories are presented in sensational or emotional terms that give the impression that poor care results from arrogance and callousness rather than from flaws in general systems of care or from uncertainties about the prognoses for gravely ill patients, the consequences of alternative treatments, the preferences of patients and families, and the applicable ethical and legal standards for care. In addition, the news and entertainment media may mislead and misinform through their frequent and persistent emphasis on violent or sudden death, death at a young age, and dramatic medical resuscitations that are, in real life, rarely successful (Baer, 1996; Diem et al., 1996). Television, in particular, is both saturated with spectacular death and largely uninterested in the everyday realities of dying as it is experienced by most people.

While an overtreated dying is feared, the opposite medical response— abandonment—is likewise frightening. Patients and those close to them may suffer physically and emotionally when physicians and nurses conclude that a patient is dying and then withdraw—passing by the hospital room on rounds, failing to follow up on the patient at home, and disregarding pain and other symptoms. Abandonment is also a societal problem when friends, neighbors, co-workers, and even family avoid people who are dying. As this report documents, the neglect of dying extends to medical curricula and research agendas that emphasize medicine's curative goals with little attention to the prevention and relief of distress and suffering for those people who, inevitably, will die of their illnesses or injuries. It is a dual perversity that interest in assisted suicide sometimes reflects anxiety about overly aggressive medical treatment, sometimes dread about abandonment, and sometimes fear that dying people may suffer simultaneously or sequentially from both misfortunes.

As will be described further in this report, the biomedical advances and health care practices that have institutionalized death and sometimes prolonged suffering and dying have not gone without notice or response by policymakers, clinicians, ethicists, and communities. For example, since the first U.S. hospice was founded in Connecticut in 1974, clinicians, patients, families, community volunteers, and policymakers have mobilized under the hospice banner to design and implement ways of reducing suffering and improving the quality of life for dying patients and those close to them. Within the health professions, the developing field of palliative medicine has helped focus biomedical and clinical research on the biological mechanisms of pain and other symptoms, the methods for assessing symptoms, and the means of preventing and relieving physical, psychological, and spiritual distress.

In the policy arena, by establishing limited Medicare coverage for hospice care, the government acknowledged the special needs of dying patients and those close to them. Legislators and judges have also attempted to give patients and their families more control over the way death occurs through policies that require informed consent to treatment, encourage planning in anticipation of death, and recognize patients' (and surrogates') right to stop medical interventions.

The time is right for further action at all levels to improve care for those approaching death and to assure the fearful that they will be neither abandoned nor maltreated. The intense debate over assisted suicide appears to be increasing public recognition of deficits in end-of-life care and consolidating agreement among proponents and opponents alike that people should not view suicide as their best option because they lack effective and compassionate care as they die.[1] As discussed further below, a small but growing number of initiatives are beginning to tackle a wide array of health care and other deficiencies that contribute to poor care at the end of life. In addition, a number of widely publicized books and stories have portrayed dying and death in ways that are realistic and positive but also sensitive to popular fears and concerns. On a more personal level, news reports on public figures such as Richard Nixon, Jacqueline Kennedy Onassis, and Joseph Cardinal Bernardin have portrayed older people with incurable illnesses preparing for and meeting death with grace and courage.

The goals of this Institute of Medicine (IOM) report are to extend understanding of what constitutes good care at the end of life and to promote a wider societal commitment to create and sustain systems of care that people can count on for spiritual, emotional, and other comfort as they die. More specifically, it is intended to stimulate health professionals and managers, researchers, policymakers, funders of health care, and the public at large to develop more constructive perspectives on dying and death and to change practices, policies, and attitudes that contribute to distress and suffering at the end of life.

This report focuses on health care-related aspects of dying including clinical and supportive services, financing of such services, and professional education. These are, of course, only a part—often a minor part—of the dying process as experienced by patients and those close to them. The support of family and friends, religious congregations, workplaces, and

---

[1]While this report was being prepared, two cases involving assisted suicide were argued before the U.S. Supreme Court. The Court ruled on June 30, 1997 (after this report was publicly released) that there is no general constitutional right to physician assistance in suicide. See Chapter 7 for further discussion.

other parts of the community may be more significant and more meaningful to many, if not most, of those approaching death.

THE NEED FOR CONSENSUS AND ACTION

The need for consensus and action to improve care for those approaching death is growing more urgent. Part of this urgency stems from demographic and social trends, including the nation's aging population, changing family structure, and growing ethnic and religious diversity. In addition, efforts to control health care costs and reduce government spending are putting pressure on Medicare, Medicaid, and Social Security programs that are especially important to those with serious chronic and advanced illnesses. These changes and developments can impose serious stress on those providing medical care, who often feel trapped by conflicting demands—from patients, families, colleagues, health care purchasers, health plan managers and stock owners, and government officials—for compassion, economy, and conformity with professional and legal standards of practice.

Care for dying patients is, in considerable measure, publicly funded, because almost three-quarters of those who die each year are age 65 or over and are covered by Medicare and, to a lesser extent, by the federal-state Medicaid program. Medicare and Medicaid also cover many younger people, for example, young adults and children dying of AIDS. In addition, care for some among the dying may be covered by programs for veterans, military personnel, and homeless people or others who lack public or private insurance. For those approaching death, therefore, government policies play a major role in determining what health care and related services are covered, how health care practitioners and institutions (including health plans) are paid, and how those serving beneficiaries are to be held accountable for the quality, cost, and accessibility of care. In addition, federal and state laws govern many other aspects of health care, including consent for services and protection from racial and other discrimination. Thus, improving care at the end of life requires supportive federal and state policies, including financing policies.

Efforts by public and private purchasers of health care to control costs have emphasized what is popularly described as managed care. As discussed further in Chapters 4 and 6, managed care has a variety of dimensions and meanings, which users of the term often do not specify precisely and which listeners may perceive in ways quite different from what the user had in mind. In process terms, managed care may refer to any one or a combination of several financial, organizational, legal, educational, or other techniques intended to influence whether, how, or from whom patients receive preventive, diagnostic, therapeutic, or other services. In organizational terms, managed care may refer to an entity that employs these techniques in one of several different formats. Beyond a general agreement that cost control has been the driving force behind the surge in managed care, health policy analysts and researchers disagree on what specific processes and formats should qualify for the managed care label.

One idealistic view of managed care (most often associated with cohesive, integrated health plans such as well-established, staff- or group-model health maintenance organizations) is that it will do more than traditional fee-for-service medicine to limit costs and to serve other valuable goals. These goals include preventing illness, encouraging patient responsibility, diminishing inappropriate treatment, improving continuity of care, coordinating care through primary care teams rather than relying on a collection of independent specialists, and making available services not traditionally covered by health insurance. If "preventing pain and other distressing symptoms" is substituted for "preventing illness" in the above description of managed care, then this idealistic image mirrors in many respects the ideal described above for the hospice movement and the field of palliative care.

Unfortunately, market competition, rapid growth, and continuing pressure to control costs and increase profits may encourage practices by some health plans and organizations that are seriously at odds with the ideal image of managed care. Such practices may include undertreating illnesses and symptoms, discouraging new or continued enrollment by sicker individuals, and failing to make timely referrals for specialized care. Both fee-for-service and managed care appear to fall short in rewarding care that ensures meticulous symptom evaluation and reevaluation, services and settings appropriate to patient needs, coordination of services, and counseling paced to what people can absorb and tolerate. Later chapters of this report explore these issues in more depth.

INITIATIVES TO IMPROVE CARE AT THE END OF LIFE

Since this study was originally conceived, several promising collaborative initiatives have gotten under way to improve the quality, accessibility, and affordability of care for dying patients and those close to them. The focus and scope of these initiatives is quite varied. Some involve one or more institutions within the same community whereas others extend to whole states; some are national in scope. Funding comes from diverse internal and external sources including government agencies and several private foundations such as the Open Society Institute's Project on Death in America, the Robert Wood Johnson Foundation, the Commonwealth Fund, the Greenwall Foundation, the Culpeper Foundation, and the Milbank Memorial Fund. A grantmakers group including these and other organizations is also meeting to encourage knowledge sharing, coordination, and identification of neglected issues.

The leaders in these initiatives range from community hospitals and hospices to regional health care systems to national organizations such as the American Medical Association and the Joint Commission on the Accreditation of Health Care Organizations. Objectives are likewise varied as illustrated below and in later chapters and Appendix C.

In Missoula, Montana, a broad coalition of community leaders and health care providers is undertaking a community-wide demonstration project to examine and improve the care and support available to dying people and those close to them (MDP, 1996). The effort crosses the spectrum of services and settings—including emergency medical services, long-term care, hospice, hospital, and home care. The initiative includes a research component as well as the demonstration aspect.

Across the country in New York City, the United Hospital Fund has organized a three-year, 12-hospital project that will investigate how care is delivered to dying patients and test innovative palliative care programs (UHF, 1997). Hospitals receiving planning grants from the Fund will review care patterns for common fatal illnesses, use focus groups of survivors to assess satisfaction with care, survey hospitals to assess the availability of palliative care services, and convene focus groups of health care professionals to assess their knowledge and attitudes. Follow-up grants for selected hospitals will support the implementation and evaluation of new palliative care strategies.

Supportive Care of the Dying: A Coalition for Compassionate Care involves six Catholic health care organizations around the nation in work to promote appropriate and compassionate care for people with life-threatening illness, and their families (Super, 1996). The coalition coordinates efforts to develop and test care models, practice guidelines, leadership and skills, and educational and mentoring programs in health systems. One stimulus for the coalition was Oregon voters' approval of physician-assisted suicide in 1994, which demonstrated public concern about how modern medicine cares for the dying. An important element of the initiative is the convening of 50 focus groups around the nation to develop a better understanding of people's needs and expectations.

The Oregon vote (which was under judicial challenge while this report was being drafted) also prompted other efforts within that state to improve care at the end of life (Lee and Tolle, 1996). The Oregon Health Sciences University, for example, has helped organize hospitals, nursing homes, emergency medical personnel, state regulators, and others in a statewide effort to create practical, reliable procedures for seeing that patient preferences about end-of-life care are known and honored.

Researchers at George Washington University have organized a Center to Improve Care of the Dying. They have, among other projects, been working to improve the definition and measurement of outcomes relevant to people approaching death and those caring for them and to develop ways for managers and clinicians to use outcomes measures to improve care in hospices, nursing homes, and other settings (see Appendix E).

Improved end-of-life care has also been identified as a topic for the Breakthrough Series of the Institute for Healthcare Improvement (IHI). This activity uses intensive training and rapid cycles of innovation and evaluation to achieve so-called "breakthrough" improvements in participating programs. Projects have ranged from patient waiting times (e.g., for surgery, emergency treatment, office visits) to cesarean section rates (IHI, 1997). The series on care at the end of life will focus on pain management and palliative care, advance care planning, transfers among care settings, and family support.

Recognizing the deficits in the knowledge and practice of established physicians in caring for dying patients and those close to them, the American Medical Association has begun a comprehensive, collaborative educational strategy directed at established clinicians (*American Medical News*, 1997). It has solicited participation and information from a broad range of organizations, such as the American Board of Internal Medicine, the American Academy of Hospice and Palliative Medicine, the Picker Institute, the Supportive Care of the Dying Coalition, and many others. A major element of this initiative is a program to train initial groups of physicians who will then return to their communities to teach others. Various other projects are also seeking to redesign undergraduate, graduate, and continuing education in the health professions to help clinicians do better throughout their careers in recognizing, respecting, and meeting the needs of those they cannot cure.

Some organizations, including private foundations are attempting to enlist the mass media in public education about the nature of dying and the ways people can be helped to have a death free from avoidable distress and consistent with their wishes. Journalists, television producers, and others involved in mass communications are also being encouraged to present a less skewed portrayal of death with less emphasis on heroic but implausible resuscitations and violent but impersonal deaths that have few lasting effects on survivors.

A few initiatives are designed to shape Medicare policies related to care of those with serious and eventually fatal illnesses. One, for example, would direct the Health Care Financing Administration to undertake a demonstration and evaluation program in coordinated end-of-life care that would test a range of innovations and focus on capitated models of care (Lynn, 1996b). Others would change how hospice eligibility is determined. In addition, one initiative would require the Secretary of the Department of Health and Human Services to report to Congress annually on the state of affairs regarding care at the end of life.

OVERVIEW OF REPORT

The origins, approach, and purposes of this study are described in the Preface and in the report of a small group that planned this study (IOM, 1994a). The Institute of Medicine committee appointed to undertake the study prepared this report with the objectives of stimulating discussion, encouraging consensus on how care for those approaching death can be improved, and galvanizing action to implement that consensus. The target audiences include clinicians of all kinds, professional organizations, health professions educators, state and federal policymakers, managed care executives, public and private purchasers of health care, certifying and accrediting groups, organizations representing patients and families, and the public at large. This document, which was reviewed in accordance with the procedures required by the National Research Council, constitutes the final report of the committee. The nine following chapters examine

- the way people die—when, why, where, and how (Chapter 2);
- the elements of good care at the end of life (Chapter 3);
- the factors that make it easier or harder to care well for those who are dying including organizational structures and procedures (Chapter 4), quality assessment and improvement strategies (Chapter 5), financing arrangements (Chapter 6), laws (Chapter 7), and health professions educational programs (Chapter 8);
- the role that biomedical, health services, and other research can play in creating a stronger knowledge base for good end-of-life care (Chapter 9); and
- the steps that clinicians, policymakers, health care administrators, and others can take to correct deficiencies, improve performance, and generally help people have a better dying (Chapter 10).

Because health care and supportive systems are so closely connected to local and national policies, structures, and practices, the focus here is on the United States. Nonetheless, the committee tried to learn from the experience of other countries and to develop a report that would be useful beyond this nation's boundaries.

The committee also recognized that uncertainties and disagreements about appropriate care for those with life-threatening medical problems often focus on those at the extremes of life's range—the very young and the very old. The clinical situations characterizing these groups may also represent extreme points—catastrophic physiological deficits for the neonate and long-term deterioration and multiple organ failure for the very old person. Difficult decisions and troubling questions about care for those approaching death are not, however, limited to certain age groups, clinical problems, settings of care, treatment strategies, or decisionmakers (e.g., health professionals, patients, or families).

Because most of those who die are older adults, the discussion emphasizes but is not restricted to this group. Moreover, regardless of age, the process of dying varies considerably across individuals, even for individuals with the same diagnosis. The implications of this variation for the care of dying patients—including adults and children, mentally competent and otherwise, severely symptomatic and relatively comfortable—are considered throughout this report.

GUIDING PRINCIPLES

As the study committee discussed its charge and its approach, it recognized that it was being guided—sometimes explicitly, sometimes implicitly—by a set of working principles. Most reflect a combination of value statements and empirical assumptions. Below are some of the key precepts, and others are identified later in the report. Only the first of the following principles applies exclusively to care at the end of life.

Care for those approaching death is an integral and important part of health care. Everyone dies, and those at this last stage of life deserve attention that is as thorough, active, and conscientious as that provided to those for whom disease prevention, diagnosis, cure, or rehabilitation are still dominant goals. Individual and system failures to care humanely for dying patients—including failures to use existing knowledge to prevent and relieve distress—should be viewed as clinical and ethical failures.

Care for those approaching death should involve and respect both patients and those close to them. As for all patients, clinicians need to consider dying patients in the context of their families and close relationships and be sensitive to their culture, values, resources, and other characteristics. Although this report often refers to patients and those close to them, it also uses the term *family* in a general sense to include not only the traditional family (e.g., spouse, children, parents, siblings) but also others such as lovers, friends, and godparents who are significant and close to patients in an emotional, spiritual, or sometimes fiduciary sense.

Good care at the end of life depends on clinicians with strong interpersonal skills, clinical knowledge, technical proficiency, and respect for individuals, and it should be informed by scientific evidence, values, and personal and professional experience. Clinical excellence is important because the frail condition of dying patients leaves little margin to rectify errors. Scientific and clinical knowledge are important, but so are compassion, communication skills, experience, and thoughtful reflection on the meaning of that experience.

The health care community has special responsibility for educating itself and others about the identification, management, and discussion of the last phase of fatal medical problems. The "medical model" often acknowledges inadequately the emotional and spiritual aspects of life's ending. Still, dying is also a biological process that can be—in varying degrees depending on the circumstances—managed by teams of physicians, nurses, pharmacists, therapists, and others prepared to relieve distress, offer information and guidance, and provide support to dying patients and those close to them. Physicians and often nurses judge when death is imminent and thus signal that people should prepare for it, and for most people, physicians legally certify death. Given their central, if not always adequately performed, roles in care at the end of life, health care professionals are inescapably responsible for educating themselves and the broader community about good care for dying patients and their families.

More and better research is needed to increase our understanding of clinical, cultural, organizational, and other practices or perspectives that can improve care for those approaching death. The committee began—and concluded—its deliberations with the view that the knowledge base for good end-of-life care has enormous gaps and is neglected in design and funding of biomedical, clinical, psychosocial, and health services research. Such research is, however, particularly sensitive and in need of more than additional resources and data. Asking the right questions and answering them in ethically acceptable ways are critical.

Changing individual behavior is difficult, but changing a culture or an organization is potentially a greater challenge—and often is a precondition for individual change. Powerful statements about the importance of compassionate care, effective symptom management, advance planning, and similar matters are not enough to improve care of the dying. Making values and policies work organizationally, financially, politically, legally, and otherwise requires a combination of good practical judgment by policymakers and good mechanisms to hold organizations responsible for their performance.

CONCEPTS AND DEFINITIONS

During its work, the committee considered how it would define several key concepts, many of which are loaded with emotional and moral meanings and marked by disagreements. The discussion below covers some of these concepts, including those of "bad" and "good" deaths. Other concepts such as accountability, advance care planning, and managed care are defined elsewhere in the report. In general, the committee found that the "language of dying" was neither as clear nor as specific as it might usefully be. The discussion below attempts to clarify some concepts, but the committee does not suggest that the experience and meaning of dying can be reduced to a glossary of terms.

Good and Bad Deaths

Because notions of bad and good deaths are threaded throughout discussions about dying and death, some consideration of their meanings is appropriate—with the caveat that the concepts are not fixed in meaning but rather shaped by people's personal experiences, spiritual beliefs, and cultural backgrounds. The concepts are also somewhat fluid in response to changes in social mores, technology, and options for dying.

In reflecting upon members' professional and personal experiences, the committee suggested that a *decent or good death* is one that is: free from avoidable distress and suffering for patients, families, and caregivers; in general accord with patients' and families' wishes; and reasonably consistent with clinical, cultural, and ethical standards. A *bad death*, in turn, is characterized by needless suffering, dishonoring of patient or family wishes or values, and a sense among participants or observers that norms of decency have been offended. Bad deaths include those resulting from or accompanied by neglect, violence, or unwanted and senseless medical treatments.

Some would add other elements to the characteristics of a good death, for example, that it comes with reasonable warning, occurs in the company of loved ones, and provides the opportunity for people to reconcile with families and friends and achieve the kind of meaning, peace, or transcendence that is relevant and significant for them and those close to them (Gavrin and Chapman, 1995; Samarel, 1995; Jennings, 1996; Byock, 1997a, 1997b). Some people, however, clearly view sudden death as preferable, even if it deprives them of the chance to resolve their lives with meaning, to say goodbye to loved ones, and to settle financial and legal matters.

Further, although the more expansive vision of a good death is intended to encourage a sensitive regard for dying patients and a more positive view of how life can be lived in the face of death, such a vision also carries some potential risks. It may expose some patients and families to feelings of guilt and anger because conflicts were not resolved or reconciliations achieved or spiritual serenity reached. It may also reflect values of the dominant culture that are not shared by all, and it may induce some naive caregivers to try subtly or not so subtly to impose their values on dying patients and families. A humane care system is one that people can trust to serve them well as they die, even if their needs and beliefs call for departures from routine practices or idealized expectations of caregivers.

Another concept, that of a *dignified death*, also presents some perplexing questions (see, e.g., the introductory discussion in Nuland, 1994; also,

Madan, 1992; Quill, 1993, 1995; Byock, 1997b; Hennezel, 1997). To those who particularly stress autonomy, the phrase death with dignity has become a shorthand way to refer to laws and practices that "permit a competent terminally ill adult the right to request and receive physician aid-in-dying under carefully defined circumstances" (Humphrey, 1991, p. 177). To others it may imply a dying accompanied by respectful and skillful caregiving. To still others, a dignified death may suggest a death that is largely free from dependency or physiological affronts that are not usually perceived as dignified. Such affronts, which even superlative patient care may not always prevent, include pain, incontinence, vomiting, delirium, or traumatic but sometimes appropriate medical interventions. Given this conflict with the everyday meaning of dignity, the concept of a dignified death may unwittingly romanticize death, and its incautious use may produce distress or anger by creating expectations that professional and other caregivers cannot always fulfill for all patients, given the nature of their disease. A worthy and more achievable goal is death dignified by care that honors and protects—indeed cherishes—those who are dying, that conveys by word and action that dignity resides in people, not physical attributes, and that helps people to preserve their integrity while coping with unavoidable physical insults and losses.

Quality of Life, Quality of Dying, Quality of Care

Most people wish for a long, satisfying life, that is, they value both how long they live *and* how well they live. In response, the concept of health-related *quality of life* has emerged to emphasize health as perceived and valued by people for themselves (or, in some cases, for those close to them) rather than as seen by experts (see, e.g., Patrick and Erickson, 1993; Cohen, Mount, et al., 1995; Gold et al., 1996). Going well beyond traditional mortality and morbidity measures, health-related quality-of-life outcomes include physical, mental, social, and role functioning; sense of well-being; freedom from bodily pain; satisfaction with health care; and an overall sense of general health.

The concept of *quality of dying*, which is less fully developed, focuses on a person's experience of living while terminally ill or imminently dying (Wallston et al., 1988). It, too, focuses on outcomes broadly defined, but does so within the special world of the dying patient, for whom some physical outcomes become less realistic while other outcomes (e.g., spiritual well-being or sense of peace) may become more meaningful.

Quality of care stresses the link between the structure and processes of health care and outcomes for individuals and populations. High-quality care should contribute to the quality of living and the quality of dying but is not synonymous with them. Chapter 5 considers these concepts further.

Pain, Symptoms, and Suffering

Pain and *suffering* are terms that are often used interchangeably, but it is worth distinguishing between the two. Physical pain may be defined as "an unpleasant sensory and emotional experience associated with actual or potential tissue damage, or described in terms of such damage, or both" (International Association for the Study of Pain, 1979). This experience may include a range of physical and mental sensations (e.g., aching, burning, numbness, tightness) that vary in severity, persistence, source, and management. For pain and many other symptoms, assessment depends largely on patients' reports rather than on laboratory or other test results. Although some symptoms (e.g., vomiting, incontinence) are observable, patients' reports on their level of distress—how much the symptoms bother them—are still essential.

Suffering is a more expansive concept than pain. It goes beyond unpleasant sensations or distressing symptoms to encompass the anguish, terror, and hopelessness that dying patients may experience. A dying person who experiences few if any physical symptoms may suffer greatly if he or she feels that life has lost any meaning.

Cassell has suggested that a symptom or feeling becomes suffering when people perceive it as a "threat to their continued existence—not merely to their lives but their integrity as persons" (Cassell, 1991, p. 36). Such perceptions may have significant emotional and spiritual dimensions related to self-image, family relationships, past experiences, caregiver attitudes, and other circumstances of a patient's life (Byock, 1997a). Perceived helplessness and exhaustion of coping resources are key elements of suffering (Gavrin and Chapman, 1995). Ultimately, however, suffering is "a personal matter—something whose presence and extent can only be known to the sufferer" but which cannot be ignored (Cassell, 1991, p. 35).

The concept and meaning of suffering has a prominent and revered position in many religions and philosophies. The committee recognized that some people may esteem suffering and even reject efforts to alleviate the physical symptoms that may contribute to suffering. It believes, however, that those caring for dying patients have a responsibility, first, to explain to people that pain and other distress can often be relieved and, second, to consider whether the patient would benefit from an exploration with a chaplain or other counselor of the nature and significance of suffering.

The End of Life, Dying, and Death

What is meant by "the end of life?" This phrase as used in this report does not imply only old age or the concluding phase of a normal life span, although that is one common meaning of the phrase and is the focus of much of this report. Life's ending can come at any age and time, and death at a young age is a special sorrow. Although people can, in some respects, be considered to be approaching death from the moment they are born, the committee used the phrase *approaching death* partly to be more explicit and partly to take advantage of the idea that death is approached not just by those who are dying but—with varying degrees of intimacy and openness—by families, friends, caregivers, and communities.

In one formulation, "people are considered to be dying when they have progressive illness that is expected to end in death and for which there is no treatment that can substantially alter the outcome" (AGS, 1997). *Dying,* however, is not a precise descriptive or diagnostic term (Pollack et al., 1994; Thibault, 1994; Lynn et al., 1996). It was the committee's sense that those referred to as dying are often thought to be likely to die within a few days to several months but that those described as having an incurable, terminal, or fatal illness also include people with advanced progressive illnesses whose deaths are less predictable and might not come for years. This report tends to focus on those expected to die within days or months; much of the discussion also applies to care for all those with life-threatening illness.

The definition of *death* was not itself a central concern of the committee, because many—probably most—significant decisions about care for dying individuals do not hinge on precise determinations of death. Nonetheless, the committee recognized the uneasiness and controversies created by technologies that make possible the "artificial" prolongation of cardiac and respiratory functions (the traditional markers of life) long after cognition and consciousness and other brain functions are irretrievably lost. Likewise, the committee recognized that some people may fear being declared dead prematurely and that trust in those providing care at the end of life may be compromised by controversies about modifying the determination of death to expand the availability of organs for transplantation. Scientists, philosophers, clinicians, theologians, policymakers, and others have sought a scientific, moral, and political consensus on when death can be declared. Most rely on some conception of brain death.[2]

---

[2]A widely accepted statement defines death for legal purposes as the irreversible cessation of circulatory and respiratory function or the irreversible cessation of all functions of the entire brain, including the brain stem (President's Commission, 1981, p. 2; see also Morrison, 1971; Veatch, 1976, 1993; Pallis, 1983; Youngner et al., 1989, 1993; Bernat, 1992; Halevy and Brody, 1993; Lynn and Cranford, 1996). Some view this definition as conceptually inadequate on clinical or religious grounds, and some criticize the entire-brain criterion as impeding the contribution of organs suitable for transplantation. An alternative formulation argues that death is not an event but a process in which "different aspects of brain functioning cease at many different times" and that different criteria for death may be appropriate depending on the circumstances (Halevy and Brody, 1993, p. 523; see also Morrison, 1971). It is possible to accept the process argument and still conclude that a single socially, legally, and scientifically acceptable criterion for declaring death is desirable for practical reasons.

By not examining the issues in defining death, the committee did not discount the importance of continued efforts to understand the physical processes of death, to develop scientifically based and socially acceptable criteria that are feasible to use in declaring death, and to design processes that support clinicians in properly applying the criteria.[3] The committee did not, however, want such efforts and the controversies surrounding them to distract attention from the much more common deficiencies in care for those approaching death and from strategies that would improve end-of-life care.

The Trajectory of Dying

The concept of a *trajectory of dying* has been used to illuminate similarities and differences in patient experiences as they approach death (Glaser and Strauss, 1965, 1968; Pattison, 1977; McCormick and Conley, 1995). As described by Glaser and Strauss, "the dying trajectory of each patient has at least two outstanding [and variable] properties . . . duration and shape" (p. 6). Figure 1.1 offers greatly simplified examples of three possible trajectories toward death.

Some people die suddenly and unexpectedly (Figure 1.1A); others have forewarning. Those who die suddenly, for example, in an accident or of a massive heart attack, are not the focus here, although support for bereaved survivors is an important role for clinicians and others. Among those with forewarning of death, some may steadily and fairly predictably decline, as many cancer patients do (Figure 1.1B). Other people may have fairly long periods of chronic illness punctuated by crises, one of which may prove fatal—although an entirely different problem may intervene to cause death (Figure 1.1C). These patients may understand that they have a progressive disease that will likely kill them, but they nonetheless may not see themselves—or be seen by their families and friends—as dying.

Those with forewarning of death may be further differentiated between those thought to be imminently dying (i.e., likely to die within minutes to days) and those who are terminally ill but not thought to be "actively" dying (i.e., having a life expectancy of days to months, sometimes years). This latter group may have a period of "chronic living-dying" between diagnosis of an incurable illness and imminent death (McCormick and Conley, 1995). During this period, people may continue many ordinary activities of daily life while coping with the prospect of death and preparing

---

[3]As this study was being readied for release, the IOM was exploring a study of ethical, scientific, and clinical issues raised by medical interventions at the end of life that are undertaken to preserve organs for use in organ transplantation.

A. Sudden Death from an Unexpected Cause

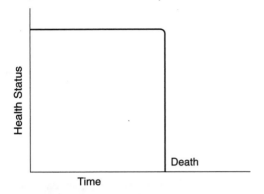

B. Steady Decline from a Progressive Disease with a "Terminal" Phase

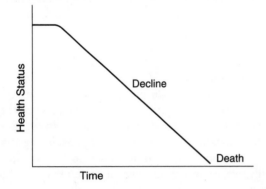

C. Advanced Illness Marked by Slow Decline with Periodic Crises and "Sudden" Death

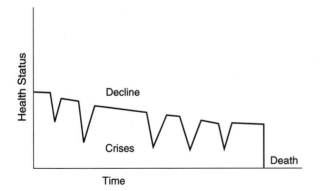

FIGURE 1.1 Prototypical death trajectories.

for it. Many pediatric patients, for example, spend years—and with better treatments, even decades—with illnesses such as cystic fibrosis, complex congenital malformations, and neurodegenerative disorders. Although families hope for a cure to emerge from scientific research, premature death (i.e., less than normal life expectancy) is a likely prospect. It may occur suddenly, for example, from a superimposed viral illness, or it may come after an extended but clearly evident physical decline. Chapters 3 and 4 further consider variations in the dying process and the implications for care at the end of life.

Diagnosis and Prognosis

The diagnosis of incurable, progressive disease that is expected to prove fatal is among the most difficult and sobering judgments that physicians make. Such a determination generally signals the need for patients, families, and clinicians to reconsider clinical and personal priorities. It is also currently important because Medicare coverage for hospice services, which are designed specifically for dying patients, requires a determination that a beneficiary has a terminal illness and, perhaps more intellectually daunting, has a life expectancy of six months or less.

Moving from a clinical diagnosis of a terminal or incurable illness expected to end in death to a prognosis—a prediction of the course of the illness and remaining life expectancy—is an exercise in uncertainty. (See Appendix D and Chapter 3 for further discussion.) One approach to prognosis uses explicit clinical criteria and formulas to generate a calculated probability that a person will live some defined period of time (e.g., a 50 percent probability of living six months) (McClish and Powell, 1989; Lynn et al., 1996). Even very near the actual time of death, however, prognosis is often imprecise. Some will die more quickly than expected; others will die more slowly.

Uncertainty about prognosis and methods for establishing it may have significant policy as well as personal implications. For example, "the Medicare hospice benefit, notably, manages to give a date" but not an expected rate or probability of surviving for six months (Lynn et al., 1996, p. 315). When insurance or other benefits are contingent on the accuracy of prognoses, physicians' judgments may be reviewed or even "audited" by hospice personnel or government officials who may not understand the uncertainty inherent in projecting survival. (See Chapter 6.)

Hospice and Palliative Care

As will be discussed throughout this report, hospice and palliative care are responses to perceived inadequacies in the prevention and relief of symptoms and distress in people approaching death. The term *hospice* has at least three somewhat different uses that can be confusing and even misleading. First, a hospice may be a discrete site of care in the form of an inpatient hospital or nursing home unit or a freestanding facility. Most care for hospice patients in the United States is, however, provided in the home by family members. Second, a hospice may be an organization or program that provides, arranges, and advises on a wide range of medical and supportive services for dying patients and their families and friends. This meaning is most common in this report. For example, when patients are described as entering hospice care, it means they are affiliating with a hospice program (and, often, qualifying for insurance coverage for care provided by such a program). Less than 20 percent of those who die in the United States are enrolled in hospice programs. The third and most culturally sweeping meaning of hospice encompasses an approach to care for dying patients based on clinical, social, and metaphysical or spiritual principles.

When this report refers to an approach to care rather than to hospice programs or organizations, it generally uses the term *palliative care*. In a broad sense, palliative care seeks to prevent, relieve, reduce, or soothe the symptoms of disease or disorder without effecting a cure (see, e.g., *Random House Dictionary,* 1983; *American Heritage Dictionary,* 1992; *Stedman's Medical Dictionary,* 1995.)[4] Palliative care in this broad sense is *not* restricted to those who are dying or those enrolled in hospice programs. For example, palliation of symptoms may be an important adjunct to life-prolonging therapies, both because the prevention or relief of pain and other symptoms is important for a patient's quality of life and because it may also allow people to begin and complete difficult treatment regimens that they might otherwise not tolerate or follow successfully (MacDonald, 1991). Palliative care, broadly conceived, is also important to those who live with chronic pain or other symptoms.

As an area of academic, scientific, and clinical specialization or empha-

---

[4]The committee consulted several definitions of palliative care. Many follow that offered by the World Health Organization: "the active total care of patients whose disease is not responsive to curative treatment . . . [when] control of pain, of other symptoms, and of psychological, social and spiritual problems is paramount" (WHO, 1990, p. 11). Thus, Foley speaks of the active total care of patients whose disease is not responsive to curative treatment (Foley, 1994). Another source refers to the "appropriate medical care of patients with advanced and progressive disease for whom the focus of care is quality of life and in whom prognosis is limited (although sometimes it may be several years)" (Association of Palliative Medicine of Great Britain and Ireland, cited in ABIM, 1996a). Similarly, the definition prepared in Great Britain in 1987 when palliative care was first recognized as a specialty describes palliative medicine as the "study and management of patients with active, aggressive, far-advanced disease for which prognosis is limited and the focus of care is quality of life" (Doyle et al., 1993, p. 3).

sis, the field of palliative medicine focuses on patients with life-threatening medical problems for which cure is not seen as possible.[5,6] Instead, it focuses on the prevention and relief of suffering through the meticulous management of symptoms from the early through the final stages of an illness; it attends closely to the emotional, spiritual, and practical needs and goals of patients and those close to them. These goals underscore two important realities: first, that a lot more happens to most dying people than the specific event of their death and, second, that helping people live well while dying requires sophisticated strategies and tools for measuring and monitoring symptoms, functional status, emotional well-being, and burdens associated with terminal illness and treatment. Thus, good palliative care is more than symptom management or management of patients with cancer, although both figure prominently in its practice. A fuller description of the dimensions of palliative care is presented in Chapters 3 and 4.

CONCLUSION

This IOM study arose in an environment of growing awareness of deficiencies in care at the end of life and growing conviction that steps to improve care were essential. In the years since the study was first contemplated, the environment seems to have become more favorable to positive change and more open to discussion of the dying process. Even the contentious and often bitter debate over the legality or morality of physician-assisted suicide has had positive benefits in forging agreement that deficiencies in care for dying patients may contribute to demands for assisted suicide and that such deficiencies need to be remedied.

When he was approaching death, Joseph Cardinal Bernadin reflected, "As you enter the dying process, that process prepares you for death as you slow down. . . . So when I talk about being at peace, I'm talking not only about peace at the level of faith, but also humanly speaking. Before too long, I'm going to go, and I think I will be ready for it" (Bernardin, 1996, p. 115). Communities, too, need to be ready, that is, prepared to support people through the dying process. The rest of this report examines how individual and collective changes in attitudes, knowledge, policies, and practices can create and sustain such readiness.

---

[5]The association between palliative care and end-of-life care was strengthened when the term was used as a substitute for hospice care by Dr. Balfour Mount, who founded the first palliative care program in Canada in 1974 (MacDonald, 1996). Dr. Mount was advised by French Canadian colleagues that, in translation, *hospice* implied a passive rather than active and positive model of care.

[6]Terms such as *comfort care* or *supportive care* are sometimes used as synonyms by those who believe that they are more understandable to dying patients and their families than palliative care.

2

A Profile of Death
and Dying in America

*To die of old age is a death rare, extraordinary, and singular
. . . a privilege rarely seen.*

Montaigne, *Of Age*, 1575

Death is not what it used to be.[1] For most of human history, medicine could do little to prevent or cure illness or extend life, and living to an old age required considerable good fortune. Dying—like being born—was generally a family, communal, and religious event, not a medical one. Because many deaths occurred at home, people were likely to care for dying relatives and, thus, to have a fairly personal and direct experience with dying and death.

In the United States, death at home in the care of family has been widely superseded by an institutional, professional, and technological process of dying. That process—its positive aspects notwithstanding—has distanced the final stage of life from the rest of living. Additionally, the mobility of Americans quite literally puts distance between many younger and older family members. Adults, even into middle age, may never have lived near or cared for someone who was dying. "A long-distance phone call announcing the passing of grandpa or grandma takes the place of the intimate, firsthand experience of a loved one's death" (DeSpelder and Strickland, 1996, p. 19). For many, the most common images of death are those presented in the news and entertainment media, which tend to focus

---

[1]The discussion in the first and last sections of this chapter draws generally on Choron, 1963; Brim et al., 1970; Aries, 1974, 1981; Fox, 1977; Reiser, 1978; Starr, 1982; Katz, 1984; Callahan, 1995; Hahn, 1995; Howell, 1995; Laqueuer, 1995; and DeSpelder and Strickland, 1996.

on the sensational, violent, or sentimental and which often depict death as an event without much social or personal context.

This chapter provides a brief epidemiological profile of dying and death in the United States, an overview of research on attitudes toward dying and death, and a short concluding reflection on cultural characteristics that influence attitudes and practices related to the end of life. Although the shifts in the rates and causes of death over time are, in considerable measure, the result of nonmedical factors such as better public health measures and economic development, they also reflect—and, in turn, shape—the technological capacities and organizational characteristics of health care including its continued emphasis on acute rather than chronic illnesses. Understanding when, why, where, and how people die and what they think about death and dying can help policymakers ask better questions about whether health care and supportive services are appropriately organized and distributed to fit the needs of dying patients and their families.

The discussion below shows that Americans, on average, live much longer now than they did at the end of the nineteenth century and that death in infancy has moved from routine to rare. Those who die in old age tend to die of different causes than those who die young, and for both younger and older people, the major causes of death and the typical experience of dying differ from 100 years ago.

The dying process today tends to be more extended, in part, because medical treatments can control pneumonia, kidney failure, and other immediate causes of death that accompany cancer, heart disease, and other "slow killers." Because death from these conditions can often be postponed, questions about life-prolonging treatment become central issues for patients, families, and clinicians. In the process, the tasks of preparing for death and caring well for those who are dying can be neglected, and opportunities for spiritual growth or completion of important relationships can be missed.

By arguing for changes in attitudes and practices related to dying and death, the committee does not endorse a romantic view of the past. In earlier ages, familiarity with death did not necessarily translate into kind treatment of the dying, particularly for those marked by disfiguring conditions. Likewise, familiarity did not banish fear, shame, or other difficult emotions in the face of death.

WHEN PEOPLE DIE: THE AGING OF AMERICA

Although less than 1 percent of Americans will die this year, the total number of deaths will be well over 2 million. In 1995, estimated deaths in the United States were 2,312,180 (Rosenberg et al., 1996), up from 1,989,841 in 1980 (NCHS, 1985) and 2,148,463 in 1990 (NCHS, 1994). To put this number in some perspective, 1995 estimated births in the United

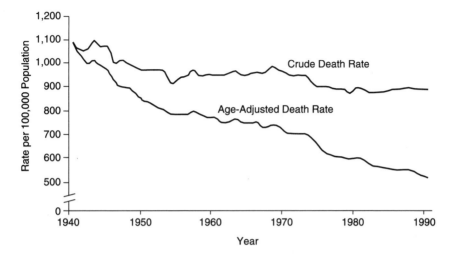

FIGURE 2.1 Crude and age-adjusted death rates: United States, 1940–1990.
Source: Singh et al., 1996.

States numbered 3,900,089—the lowest level in almost two decades
(Rosenberg et al., 1996).

Further perspective is provided by an examination of trends in death
rates over time. In 1900, the crude death rate was about 1,720 per 100,000
population (U.S. Department of Commerce, 1975) compared with a rate of
880.0 per 100,000 in 1995 (Rosenberg et al., 1996). Between 1940 and
1995, the age-adjusted mortality rate, which takes the aging population
into consideration, fell relatively steadily, from 1,076.1 deaths per 100,000
resident population in 1940, to 585.5 deaths per 100,000 resident population in 1980 (Singh et al., 1996), and to 503.7 in 1995 (Rosenberg et al.,
1996) (see Figure 2.1).

The typical American can now expect to live a lengthy life and die at an
old age. In 1900, average life expectancy at birth was less than 50 years
(Figure 2.2).[2] In 1995, the estimated life expectancy reached 75.8 years,
matching the all-time high attained in 1992. Women may now expect to
live nearly 79 years and men, almost 73 years (Rosenberg et al., 1996).
Among those who reach age 75, women may expect to live, on average,
11.9 additional years, while men can expect to live 9.7 years longer.

---

[2]A more likely reflection of "normal" conditions during the first half of the nineteenth
century was seen during the 1918 influenza epidemic, when life expectancy in the United
States fell to just below 40 years (Brim et al., 1970, p. 8). In 1900, mortality statistics were
based on 10 "death-registration" states, mainly in the northeastern United States, and the
District of Columbia. Not until 1933 did all states contribute data (Brim et al., 1970).

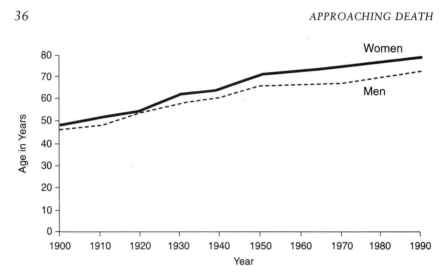

FIGURE 2.2 Life expectancy at birth by gender, 1900–1990. Source: Robert Wood Johnson Foundation, Chronic Care in America: A 21st Century Challenge. Princeton, N.J.; August 1996.

The decline in death rates and the increase in life expectancy coexist, however, with significant racial differences. In 1995, black males had an age-adjusted death rate (1,006.9 per 100,000 resident population) almost twice that of white males (611.2). Black females had an age-adjusted death rate (566.2 per 100,000 resident population) more than one and one-half times that of white females (365.6) (Rosenberg et al., 1996). Similarly, estimates based on 1995 data show that an average black woman could expect to live 74.0 years compared to 79.6 for white women. For black men, estimated life expectancy at birth was 65.4 years compared to 73.4 for whites.

The increase in life expectancy has come primarily from reduction in child—especially infant—mortality. In 1900, the death rate for newborns and infants under the age of 1 was 162.4 per 1,000. This rate fell steeply once a child reached the age of 1 and was only matched by those people who survived beyond the age of 85. By 1970, the infant mortality rate had fallen to 21.4 per 1,000, and all adults age 65 and over died at a greater rate than that (U.S. Department of Commerce, 1975). Estimates for 1995 indicate that less than 2 percent of deaths involved people under 15 years of age, whereas 73 percent involved those age 65 and over (49 percent in the 65 to 84 age group and the other 24 percent in the 85 and older group (Rosenberg et al., 1996).

As a result of changing mortality patterns, those age 65 and over constitute an increasingly large number and proportion of the U.S. population. In 1994, this age group accounted for approximately 1 in 8 persons (13 percent) of the population; in 2030, when the large baby boom cohort has entered old age, 1 in 5 persons (20 percent) is expected to be in this age group (Hobbs and Damon, 1996). These demographics explain this report's emphasis on older people.

WHY PEOPLE DIE: CAUSES OF DEATH

A century ago, communicable diseases—in particular, influenza, tuberculosis, and diphtheria—were leading causes of death in the United States. Heart disease, stroke, and cancer ranked fourth, fifth, and ninth (Brim et al., 1970). Today and for many years previous in the United States (and economically advanced nations generally), the three leading causes of death for the population as a whole have been heart disease, cancer, and stroke. Preliminary data for 1995 estimate that these causes—which disproportionately affect older people—accounted for 62 percent of all deaths and 67 percent of deaths for those age 65 and older (Rosenberg et al., 1996, p. 31). For children, however, causes of death are quite different (Rosenberg et al., 1996). For children ages 1 to 14, the leading causes of death are unintentional injuries, cancer, congenital abnormalities, and homicide.

Consistent with data on death rates and life expectancy, data on causes of death by race and age offer a grim picture of the racial and social disparities that characterize life in America for certain groups. For all black males in 1993, homicide, HIV infection, and unintentional injuries preceded stroke as the third, fourth, and fifth leading causes of death (PHS, 1996). After heart disease and cancer, Hispanic males were most likely to die from unintentional injuries and HIV infection. Suicide was among the ten leading causes of death for American Indian or Alaskan Native and Asian or Pacific Islander women but not for white, black, or Hispanic women.

As Table 2.1 shows, in 1995, among white infants, the leading cause of infant mortality was congenital anomalies (165.2 deaths per 100,000 live births); among black infants, it was the second leading cause but the actual death rate (199.1) was considerably higher than for whites. Disorders relating to short gestation and unspecified low birth weight were the leading cause of death for black infants and the third most important for white infants, but these rankings do not reveal the disparity in actual death rates of 292.0 and 64.6 respectively (Rosenberg et al., 1996).

Those who die from chronic illness—and their survivors—will look to care systems for somewhat different kinds of physical, emotional, spiritual, and practical support than those who experience violent or premature death. The committee focused on the former group but recognized the need for systems able to care reliably and well for people with different problems and needs.

TABLE 2.1 Infant Mortality Rates for the Ten Leading Causes of Infant Death, by Race: United States, January 1995

Rank	Cause of Death	Rate
White		
	All causes	628.5
1	Congenital anomalies	165.2
2	Sudden infant death syndrome	69.5
3	Disorders relating to short gestation and unspecified low birthweight	64.6
4	Respiratory distress syndrome	30.4
5	Newborn affected by maternal complications of pregnancy	25.2
6	Newborn affected by complications of placenta, cord, and membranes	21.7
7	Infections specific to the perinatal period	16.8
8	Accidents and adverse effects	16.6
9	Intrauterine hypoxia and birth asphyxia	11.1
10	Pneumonia and influenza	9.5
	All other causes	198.0
Black		
	All causes	1,477.6
1	Disorders relating to short gestation and unspecified low birth weight	292.0
2	Congenital anomalies	199.1
3	Sudden infant death syndrome	167.7
4	Respiratory distress syndrome	79.2
5	Newborn affected by maternal complications of pregnancy	71.2
6	Newborn affected by complications of placenta, cord, and membranes	44.1
7	Accidents and adverse effects	36.4
8	Infections specific to the perinatal period	36.1
9	Pneumonia and influenza	25.2
10	Intrauterine hypoxia and birth asphyxia	18.9
	All other causes	507.6

NOTE: Data based on continuous file of records received from states. Rates per 100,000 live births. Figures are based on weighted data rounded to nearest individual, so categories may not add to totals.

SOURCE: Rosenberg et al., 1996.

WHERE PEOPLE DIE:
DEATH IN INSTITUTIONS AND RESIDENCES

Over the last century, death has moved out of homes and into institutions. In 1949, national statistics revealed that 49.5 percent of deaths occurred in institutions (39.5 percent in general hospitals and the rest in psychiatric and other kinds of hospitals and nursing homes); by 1958, the comparable figure had risen to 60.9 percent (47.6 percent for general hospitals) (Brim et al., 1970). Final mortality statistics for 1980 indicated that 74 percent of deaths occurred in institutions (60.5 percent in hospitals and 13.5 percent in other institutions) (Brock and Foley, 1996, p. 5).

In the early and mid-1980s, two developments provided some incentives for change in this pattern. First, Medicare began to cover hospice care in 1983 (Hoyer, 1996), and private insurance coverage for hospice also began to spread. Second, and more broadly, starting in 1983, Medicare phased in a new prospective, per-case method of paying hospitals to encourage reduced use of inpatient hospital care. Inpatient hospital deaths for Medicare beneficiaries showed a modest decline (McMillan et al., 1990). Nursing home death rates increased, particularly for the oldest old (Sager et al., 1989; Brock and Foley, 1996). Although deaths in residences were not identified as a separate category in national reporting of vital statistics until 1989, McMillan et al. (1990) interpreted less specific data as indicating a particular increase in the percentage of cancer deaths occurring at home.

For 1992, U.S. mortality statistics showed about 57 percent of deaths occurring in hospitals (excluding those declared dead on arrival), 17 percent in nursing homes, 20 percent in residences, and 6 percent elsewhere (including those declared dead on arrival at the hospital). Of the deaths in hospitals, approximately 84 percent occurred in inpatient units with most of the rest taking place in emergency departments or outpatient clinics.

Site of death varies by age. For example, in 1980, 8 percent of those age 65 to 74 died in institutions other than hospitals or medical centers (mainly nursing homes) compared to 34 percent of those in the 85 and over age group (Riley et al., 1987). Unfortunately, data on the site of death, although improving, are still incomplete, and more detailed data (e.g., by age) are not routinely published.

Patterns for site of death also vary considerably across the nation. Medicare data for 1990 suggest that most of the Pacific Coast and Mountain states had less than 40 percent of beneficiary deaths occurring in hospitals. Data from Oregon indicate that deaths in that state are almost evenly distributed across hospitals, nursing homes, and homes (with a small additional percentage accounted for, e.g., by people declared dead at the site of an accident) (Tolle, 1996a). In contrast, Medicare data show that from Texas and Oklahoma through the South, Middle Atlantic states, and

New England states, the figure for hospital deaths was above 40 percent or even 50 percent in many areas (Pritchard et al., 1994). Nonetheless, it seems reasonable to expect that, in the future, deaths will occur more often outside the hospital than in the immediate past. Delivery systems and financing practices designed for inpatient care will need to be reevaluated to see how well they fit the circumstances and needs of patients dying at home or in nursing homes.

Data on site of death tell only a part of the story about the end of life. Relatively little is known about where dying patients spend their last few months. For example, the statistics reported above do not capture the experience of many older patients who live in nursing homes and are then transferred to hospitals on the day they die. In 1985, according to the Survey of the Last Days of Life (SLDOL)(which was limited to one part of Connecticut), 33 percent of women aged 65 to 74 but only 17 percent of those aged 85 and over died in the hospital after being transferred there from a private residence in the community within the last three months of their lives (Brock and Foley, 1996) (see Table 2.2). Among those in the 85 and over group, 21 percent of men and 35 percent of women spent their entire final three months in a nursing home and died there; about 8 percent of men and 9 percent of women died after being transferred from a nursing home to a hospital. The issue of patient transfers and the quality of end-of-life care are considered further in Chapter 4.

To say simply that someone spent their last days at home or in the hospital says little about the environment in which they died. A hospice unit within a hospital, for instance, may provide more support and comfort for the dying patient and the family than an intensive care unit. For those dying at home, hospice personnel are more intensively trained than other home care personnel to provide physical, psychological, spiritual, and practical care. In addition, for those who qualify for the hospice benefit, additional services are available (e.g., respite care for families) that are not normally covered by Medicare.

In 1993, the reported number of patients served by hospice was 256,900, indicating that only about 11 percent of the nearly 2.27 million people who died received hospice services (Christakis, 1996). More recent data from the National Hospice Organization estimated the number of those served by hospices in 1995 at 390,000, about 17 percent of the 2.31 million deaths that year (NHO, 1996a).

Although beneficiaries must have a life expectancy of six months or less to qualify for the Medicare hospice benefit, most patients spend much less time under hospice care. An analysis of a sample of Medicare beneficiaries admitted to hospice found a median length of survival after admission of 36 days (Christakis and Escarce, 1996). Notably longer median stays were found for patients with dementia (74 days) and chronic obstructive pulmo-

TABLE 2.2 Percentage Distribution for Locations Lived During the Last 90 Days of Life, According to Age and Sex (Survey of the Last Days of Life)

Locations Lived	Age of Men (no.)			Age of Women (no.)		
	65–74 (297)	75–84 (183)	≥85 (119)	65–74 (300)	75–84 (141)	≥85 (187)
C-H	33.7%	29.5%	20.2%	33.3%	19.9%	17.1%
C	30.0	19.5	14.3	21.7	20.6	15.0
I	3.4	12.0	21.0	6.7	15.6	35.3
C-H-C-H	10.4	7.7	2.5	10.0	4.3	4.3
I-H	1.7	3.8	7.6	2.7	9.2	8.6
C-H-C	6.1	4.9	5.9	4.7	8.5	4.3
C-H-I	0.3	3.3	6.7	1.7	4.3	3.7
I-H-I	0.7	0.0	1.7	0.7	2.8	3.7
H	1.0	1.1	0.8	1.7	3.6	0.0
Other Paths	12.7	8.2	19.3	16.8	11.2	8.0

NOTE: C = community, H = hospital, I = institution.

SOURCE: Brock and Foley, 1996.

nary disease (76.5 days), but these patients comprised less than 5 percent of the sample. Similar proportions of patients died within 7 days of admission (15.6 percent) or more than 180 days after admission (14.9 percent), and about 8 percent lived more than a year.[3]

---

[3]Many important questions have yet to be answered about hospice care including: which patients are appropriate for hospice referral and at what point in their illness; what the cost implications are of earlier referral; and what financial, cultural, or other factors affect the use of hospice services. Chapter 6 urges caution in government actions to penalize hospices caring for patients who outlive their six month prognoses. A recent story in the Boston Globe about a woman who lived more than a year longer than expected under hospice care illuminated the uncertainty of predicting the time of death (Foreman, 1996).

HOW PEOPLE DIE:
SYMPTOMS OF IMPENDING DEATH

Detailed studies of the experience of dying are fairly limited, but the available data indicate both a considerable degree of commonality in the dying process and enough variability that no uniform model of caregiving or preparing for death will suffice. Common physiological signs of imminent death (i.e., death likely to occur within a few hours or days) include: "hypersomnolence, disorientation, irregular breathing, excessive secretions, visual and auditory hallucinations, decreased clarity of sight, decreased urine production, mottled skin, cool extremities, and truncal warmth" (Gavrin and Chapman, 1995, p. 269; also, many hospice publications). Some of these signs (e.g., disorientation, irregular breathing, hallucinations) may be distressing to families and perhaps to patients, whereas others (e.g., truncal warmth) may not.

The SLDOL study mentioned earlier reported that on the last day of life, three out of four elderly patients were nonambulatory, and 40 percent had difficulty recognizing family (Brock and Foley, 1996). Fifty-five percent were unable to eat, 44 percent were short of breath, and 33 percent reported some pain. The study also reported that 53 percent of patients were perceived to be in good or excellent health one year before their death with this number falling to 24 percent one month before death and to 11 percent the day before death. Unlimited mobility fell from 59 percent one year before death, to 30 percent one month before, and then to 13 percent on the day before death. Cognitive function declined at a slower rate than did physical function. One year prior to death, 87 percent of decedents had no difficulty with cognitive ability, as did 78 percent at the one-month mark, and 51 percent the day before death.

A patient's cognitive abilities may have a significant effect on caregivers, including their inclination to deny impending death or to become more emotionally distant. Figure 2.3 depicts rates of consciousness and ability to communicate in the three days before death as reported by family members in a large study of severely ill hospitalized patients (Lynn et al., 1996). A study of advanced cancer patients found that in the week before death, approximately half volunteered that they felt fatigued or mentally hazy/confused (Coyle et al., 1990). Generalized weakness, pain, shortness of breath, and anxiety were reported by more than a quarter of these patients.[4]

---

[4]Although the patient population must have been quite different with respect to diagnoses, treatments, and other characteristics and the data collection process was different, this pattern shows some similarities to what physician William Osler reported early in the twentieth century. Based on an examination of about 500 death bed records, he determined that the records showed physical or emotional distress in about 20 percent of patients, but for the majority "no sign one or the other; like their birth, their death was a sleep and a forgetting" (Osler, 1905, p. 19).

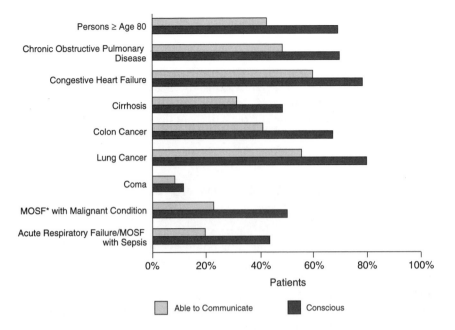

FIGURE 2.3 Rates of consciousness and ability to communicate (in patients 3 days before death, by medical condition, as reported by family members). *MOSF, multiple organ system failure. Source: Adapted from Lynn, J., Teno, J.M., Phillips, R.S., et al. Perceptions by family members of the dying experience of older and seriously ill patients. Annals of Internal Medicine 126(2): 97–106, 1997.

In addition to the nature of their disease, age affects people's experience of dying. Prior to death, according to data from the established Populations for Epidemiologic Studies of the Elderly, those dying at older ages experience more disability than those dying at younger ages (Guralnick et al., 1991).[5] With the aging of the large baby boom generation, it is evident that these high disability rates "can have grave implications for the total population burden of morbidity and disability in future years" (Guralnick et al., 1991, p. 447).

The impact of age and disability will differ somewhat depending on trends in chronic disability among older people. The compression of mor-

---

[5]For the sake of clarity in understanding changes in functional status and disease prior to death, the analysis was limited to those for whom interview data was available for three consecutive years.

bidity hypothesis posits that an increase in healthier life styles means that people will have relatively less disability before they die and, thus, that increasing life spans will mean less disability than would otherwise be expected. Evidence on this hypothesis has been mixed (see, e.g., Leibson et al., 1992; Leigh and Fries, 1994; Moons and Mackenbach, 1994; Tu and Chen, 1994). A recent analysis, however, reported declines in the prevalence of chronic disability among the elderly in the United States with recent declines (1989–1994) greater than in earlier years (1982–1989) (Manton et al., 1997).

ATTITUDES TOWARD DYING AND DEATH

Reliable and valid research on American attitudes toward dying and death is surprisingly limited. In part, this reflects conceptual and methodological difficulties, for example, imagining hypothetical and—given current life expectancy—often far-distant situations (e.g., being incurably ill or comatose). The most intensive studies often rely on small, opportunistic samples, especially college students, but more methodologically rigorous surveys rarely focus on dying and death. One consequence is that it may difficult to assess how current initiatives to change perspectives and practices in end-of-life care actually affect attitudes.

Much of the social science literature on attitudes, particularly that generated in the 1970s and 1980s, has focused on the psychological construct of "death anxiety" (variously and confusingly viewed as a realistic fear of a real threat *or* as a neurotic over-reaction to the general prospect of death). In addition to reliance on small unrepresentative samples, critics have identified numerous conceptual methodological problems in such research (see generally the review by Neimeyer and van Brunt, 1995). For example, simple scales assume a single dimension of anxiety whereas fears or concerns about death appear to involve multiple dimensions including fears of pain and suffering, fears of the unknown, and concerns about the death of significant others. The growing interest in measures of quality of life has brought new perspectives to the field and an interest in identifying and improving the more rigorous instruments, such as the Death Attitude Profile-Revised (Wong et al., 1994; see also Thorson and Powell, 1994 and Chapter 5 of this report).

Broader public opinion polls have rarely dealt with anxieties about death. A 1995 poll sponsored by the American Association of Retired Persons (AARP) found that a substantial majority of those surveyed reported that thinking about death did not bother them (with 68 percent of those 18 to 64 and 76 percent of those 65 and over agreeing)(AARP, 1995). An earlier Gallup Poll indicated that most Americans rarely think about death (Gallup and Newport, 1991), which some might interpret as reflecting death anxiety or denial. However, despite characterizations of the United States as a "death-denying society," direct evidence for this thesis is "remarkably sparse" (Neimeyer and van Brunt, 1995, p. 52). Moreover, some evidence suggests that education aimed at altering attitudes may sometimes arouse death anxiety rather than dampen it (McClam, 1980; Testa, 1981; Rigdon and Epting, 1985; Durlak and Riesenberg, 1991; Durlak, 1994).

Public opinion research has tended to focus on specific issues such as attitudes about assisted suicide, hospice, or advance directives. Since 1977, 13 surveys conducted by the National Opinion Research Center (NORC) have asked whether doctors should be legally allowed to painlessly end a patient's life if the patient and family request it. During this period, the percentage of respondents agreeing has risen from approximately 60 percent to about 70 percent. The 1996 poll showed that support was highest among younger people (over 75 percent in the 18 to 34 age group) and lowest among older people (about 60 percent in those age 65 and over). On the issue of whether a person has the right to end his or her own life (in an unspecified fashion) because of incurable illness, NORC surveys report a shift from majority disagreement in the 1970s and early 1980s to majority agreement in recent years (64 percent in 1996).

The NORC findings are generally consistent with other research (Harvard School of Public Health/Boston *Globe* Poll, 1991; Blendon et al., 1992; Foreman, 1996). A Gallup Poll taken in late summer 1996, however, reported that only 50 percent of those surveyed believed physician-assisted suicide should be legal (NHO, 1996b). This compared to 75 percent of those in an April 1996 Gallup Poll who responded positively to a question that was similar to the NORC question in not using the term suicide (Foreman, 1996). The late summer survey showed that women were less likely to believe that physician-assisted suicide should be legal and less likely to predict that they would avail themselves of that option should they become terminally ill.

Patient preferences regarding end-of-life care have been a particular interest of researchers, clinicians, and policymakers as reflected in the considerable literature on advance directives and similar measures, which is discussed in Chapter 3. When questioned about who people would want to make final choices about their care if they were seriously ill, a 1994 Louis Harris Poll reported that 67 percent of the national sample said that they wanted to make the decisions, but 28 percent wanted their doctor to decide (Medica Foundation, 1994).

Two Gallup Polls, one in 1992 and another in 1996, found 9 out of 10 respondents reporting that they would prefer to be cared for at home if they were terminally ill with six months or less to live (Seidlitz et al., 1995; Foreman, 1996; NHO, 1996b). These results are consistent with smaller studies (Townsend et al., 1990; McCormick et al., 1991). Although a majority of patients in both Gallup surveys expressed interest in a comprehensive program of end-of-life care at home, not all of those who were interested identified the term "hospice" with such a program. In the 1996 survey, 70 percent of respondents reported that they would seek hospice care, and 62 percent said they would still seek curative care. The latter figure indicates that people do not necessarily wish to forego curative efforts when they accept comprehensive palliative care.

Other research suggests that younger people express more willingness to forego resuscitation or ventilator support than do older people when they are asked hypothetical questions about preferences in the event of terminal illness (Gallup and Newport, 1991). A small study of patients seen at a Veterans Affairs medical center found that almost half said they would accept intubation and ventilator support even if the outcome would be persistent mental deficits (Mazur and Merz, 1996). In one exploratory study investigating patient views of states worse than death, coma, severe dementia, and loss of such functions as the ability to feed oneself were cited as possibly worse than death, but the stability of such views is unknown (Pearlman et al., 1993).

Surveys tend to highlight "mainstream" attitudes, or at least those attitudes easily tapped by pollsters, but there really is no "one" American attitude toward death and dying (Koenig and Gates-Williams, 1995; see also Appendix D). For example, studies of attitudes about advance directives and preferences for end-of-life care tend to show that whites are more favorably inclined to advance directives than African Americans and more likely to indicate that they would forego life-sustaining therapy (Caralis et al., 1993; Garrett et al., 1993; Steinberg et al., 1996). In a study of cancer patients (not necessarily terminally ill), researchers found cultural differences in views on family roles, information disclosure, expression of pain, and attitudes toward illness (Die Trill and Holland, 1993). In a study of 800 elderly patients, the University of Southern California found that the family dynamics in immigrant Korean or Mexican families allowed for less patient autonomy than in black or white families that had not recently immigrated (Blackhall et al., 1995; see also Mydans, 1995). The immigrant families were far more likely to believe that the truth about terminal diagnoses should be withheld from patients. Families, and not patients, were considered the proper decisionmakers in end-of-life care.

CONCLUSION

Dying is a both a biological process and a psychological and social experience that occurs in a cultural context. Trying to characterize briefly the distinctive aspects of the dominant American culture that influence attitudes toward death and dying is a task fraught with the risk of oversimplification, overstatement, or even caricature. The dominant culture—as expressed in the news and entertainment media, the professions, and other prominent social institutions—tends to be loosely described as Western (or European-American) and Judeo-Christian. The United States is, however, far from a cultural monolith. As described above, important cultural differences in attitudes and practices regarding end-of-life care exist within the United States, and these are often divided along racial, ethnic, and religious boundaries (Koenig and Gates-Williams, 1995; see also Appendix E). Nonetheless, the committee's experience with various health care systems and its review of comparative analyses points to the influence on end-of-life care of an actively interventionist medical profession, a deeply ingrained public philosophy of individualism, and a general American unwillingness to accept limits—including aging and death.

The interventionist bent of U.S. medicine, apparent in clinical practice and medical literature, has been widely noted (see, for example, Fuchs, 1974; Sontag, 1978; Aaron and Schwartz, 1984; Schroeder, 1984; Payer, 1988; McPherson, 1989; Aaron, 1991; Jecker, 1991; Jecker and Emanuel, 1995).[6] Even a century ago, physician Oliver Wendell Holmes, Sr., was asking, "how could a people which has a revolution once in four years, which has contrived the Bowie knife and revolver . . . be content with any but 'heroic' practice?" (cited in Davies et al., 1983, p. 912).

The United States generally has high rates of surgery, diagnostic tests, and other procedures compared to other countries, even with neighboring Canada (see, e.g., Bunker, 1970; Notzon et al., 1987; McPherson, 1989; Aaron and Schwartz, 1990; Tu et al., 1997). Overall, a "technological imperative" (Fuchs, 1974) seems to characterize medical practice, including care of the dying. The result of this medical activism, some argue, can be tragic. Callahan has, for example, described "an unwillingness to let nature take its course" that often leads to an impersonal and unwittingly cruel "death in a technologic cocoon" (Callahan, 1995, p. 228). One study of physicians and nurses reported that nearly half of those interviewed admitted to having acted contrary to their consciences, mostly by providing overly burdensome treatment (Solomon et al., 1993).

The individualist strain in U.S. society seems to have become more evident in health care in recent decades and may, in some measure, be a response to excessive medical intervention. Traditionally, physicians have

---

[6]This activist mentality is sardonically depicted in Samuel Shem's novel *The House of God*, in which one of his characters declares "I deliver medical care, which . . . means not doing nothing but doing something. In fact, doing everything you can, see?" (Shem, 1978, p. 76). This novel reveals how literature can—sometimes with dark humor—capture and illuminate a cultural moment and why the humanities have found a place in health professions' curricula.

been guided primarily by the principle of beneficence (doing good on some-one else's behalf) rather than by the principle of autonomy (generally acting in accord with the wishes of informed patients) (see, e.g., President's Commission, 1983; Katz, 1984; Englehardt, 1986; Jonsen and Toulmin, 1988; Pellegrino and Thomasma, 1988; Kapp, 1989; Childress, 1990; Emanuel and Emanuel, 1992; Pellegrino, 1993; Beauchamp and Childress, 1994). Critics of this emphasis on beneficence characterize it as paternalistic, with too little regard for patients' concerns and values. The more recent ascendence of the principle of autonomy shows itself in the attention paid to issues such as patient preferences, informed consent, and physician-assisted suicide.

The stress on autonomy has, in turn, been criticized for sometimes being contrary to individual patient welfare and for being inimical to collective well-being (see, e.g., McCullough, 1988; Etzioni, 1991; Agich, 1995). For example, in contrasting the highly individualistic United States with the more community-minded Canada and Western Europe, observers repeatedly cite the lack of a "social contract" in the United States that would provide a basic level of health care (or, at least, insurance coverage) for all residents. In the United States, these critics argue, people may have the theoretical right to make their own medical choices, but many do not have the financial access to minimal care necessary for implementation of those choices. Moreover, a preoccupation with autonomy may encourage inattention to patients' concerns about their families (Doukas and Gorenflo, 1993). For example, in one public opinion poll, the most frequently expressed fear about death was the fear of being a burden to one's family (Foreman, 1996).

As noted earlier, some critiques characterize American culture as one that, in addition to being strongly individualistic, also is "death denying" and regards "death as a kind of accident, a contingent event that greater prevention, proven technology, and further research could do away with" (Callahan, 1995, p. 227). Although research support is limited, a cursory glance at bookstore shelves, magazine articles, advertisements for plastic surgery and miraculous herbal remedies, and similar sources would suggest that Americans are, at the very least, not very sanguine about aging (illustrated by, e.g., the cover article, "How Science Is Searching for Ways to Keep Us Forever Young," in the November 25, 1996 issue of *Time* magazine and also by books such as *Stop Aging Now!* [Carper, 1995] and *Stay Young the Melatonin Way* [Bock and Boyette, 1995]). Other critiques have suggested that Americans do not deal very well with dying and death and suffer much avoidable angst and expense as a result (see, e.g., Kübler-Ross, 1969; Veatch, 1979). A more sanguine view is that people in the United States are not so much death-denying as focused on the notion "of bringing to bear every possible resource to prolong active and healthy life" and of accepting death only when "it is felt to be inevitable" and, then, trying "to mitigate its connections with suffering" (Parsons, 1963, p. 61).

The next chapter considers dimensions of caring at the end of life and ways of mitigating suffering. Each dimension involves patients, families, and clinicians in decisions that are often painful to make and difficult to implement. The nature and range of these decisions reflect the consequences of a century's worth of changes that have altered when, why, where, and how people die and intensified the need for better support for dying patients and those close to them.

3

Caring at the End of Life

When you come into my room . . .
Sit at my "mourning bench" if you are my physician
listen to me, talk truthfully to me
Steven Schmidt, *When You Come into My Room,* 1996

The twentieth century has seen birth and death—and much that happens in between—become events for institutional management. For most Americans, physicians direct and hospitals regulate many details of life's beginning and ending, sometimes excessively so. Technical and technological responses to illness can leave little time or thought for talking with patients, listening to their concerns, caring for them as people not diseases, and sitting at their "mourning bench," in the poetic words of Steven Schmidt, a sufferer from Crohn's disease (Schmidt, 1996).

The aggressively technical treatment of many kinds of health problems has been questioned, moderated, and sometimes spurned as its limits—not just its benefits—have been increasingly recognized. (See, for example, Wennberg and Gittelsohn, 1973, 1982; Illich, 1976; Reiser, 1978, 1993; Starr, 1982; Brook et al., 1986; Chassin et al., 1986; Blendon, 1988; Roper et al., 1988; Ware et al., 1988; Wennberg et al., 1988; Stevens, 1989; Cassell, 1991; Rothman, 1991; Gerteis et al., 1993; and Nelson and Nelson, 1995.) Attempts to mitigate the negative consequences of advanced technologies and narrow medical approaches to human problems have sometimes been based on the results of research or systematically defined professional consensus; other times, their basis has been primarily ethical or philosophical. Such attempts involve an acknowledgement that death brings losses but also a declaration that people can grow emotionally and spiritually as death approaches (see, e.g., Bernard and Schneider, 1996; Byock, 1997a; de Hennezel, 1997).

At life's beginning, birthing centers, selective use of medications and

50

surgical procedures, home birthing, renewed use of midwives, and child-birth education classes represent some responses to medical overreaching. At life's end, hospice and the recognition of a patient's right to refuse treatment likewise are indicative of medicine's need to recognize its limits. More general initiatives to change the nature of caregiving, which have been diverse and occasionally controversial, also may influence care at the end of life. Such initiatives include efforts to

- employ less invasive or disabling care options such as lumpectomy for certain breast cancers and "watchful waiting" for benign prostatic hypertrophy (see, e.g., Brook et al., 1986; Barry et al., 1988; Wennberg et al., 1988; Jackson, 1990);
- recognize the value of the caring function of medicine in addition to the curing and life-prolonging functions (see, e.g., Wheeler, 1990; Cassell, 1991; Gerteis et al., 1993);
- design friendlier environments of care as exemplified in warmer and more welcoming physical spaces, reduced noise levels, and displays of photographs and other personal items in patient or resident rooms (see, e.g., Gerteis et al., 1993);
- strengthen the quantity and quality of communication with patients and families, respond to requests for patient education, and recognize cultural differences (see, e.g., Greenfield et al., 1985; Koenig and Gates-Williams, 1995; Nelson and Nelson, 1995);
- develop instruments for assessing patient outcomes and perceptions of their care as a basis for establishing more accountability for clinician and system performance (see, e.g., Ware et al., 1988; Berwick et al., 1990; Gold and Wooldridge, 1995; and Chapter 5 of this report); and
- incorporate and welcome the contributions of many different health care personnel and of supportive services such as music and art therapy and other psychological approaches (see, e.g., Hurney, 1990; Sourkes, 1991; Connell, 1992; Larsson and Starrin, 1992; Breslow, 1993; Skaife, 1993).

The number and variety of these initiatives reinforce the basic messages that people—not diseases or technologies—are the central concern of health care and that people are much more than their illnesses. These initiatives likewise reinforce—and indeed have shaped and been shaped by—efforts to improve care for those approaching death and to establish palliative care as a legitimate clinical field. One practical challenge to those responsible for activating major changes in health care delivery is to distinguish intellectual or ideological fads from more enduring strategies and shifts in values.

This chapter focuses primarily on the patient, those close to the patient, and those directing and providing end-of-life care. It emphasizes that the experience and fear of unrelieved symptoms are fundamentally important in their own right, as are concerns about loss of control and abandonment. The discussion attempts to provide a broad perspective on strategies for helping people live well while dying, but it does not attempt to serve either as a palliative care text or as more than an overview of the sources of support and comfort that lie outside the health care system. It also acknowledges that, particularly for those dying at home, professional caregivers may not have a substantial presence and that some may find medical care intrusive, especially if caregivers are not alert to patient and family wishes. Still, many patients and those close to them welcome an attentive medical presence, and for some, the absence of supportive and effective medical care may lead to despair and thoughts of suicide.

DIFFERENCES IN DYING PATHWAYS:
ILLUSTRATIVE CASES

Over 300 years ago, the playwright John Webster wrote in *The Duchess of Malfi*, "I know death hath ten thousand several doors for men to take their exits." The doors to death remain many and varied, although, as Chapter 2 described, today's most common patterns of death differ in key ways from the past. This section supplements the definitional and statistical discussions presented in Chapters 1 and 2 with a more qualitative consideration of how people may die and how care for dying patients may need to be adjusted to their circumstances.

Figure 1.1 depicted three prototypical trajectories of dying: sudden and unexpected; steady decline; and slow decline marked by periodic crises, one of which brings death. In addition to those people who are recognized as incurably ill with a clearly defined disease such as cancer or amyotrophic lateral sclerosis, two other groups are of interest. One consists of very old people who are functioning reasonably well but who are frail and have limited reserves to face an acute illness such as influenza or an injury such as a broken hip. Although these people initially may be expected to recover from the acute problem and their dying would not have been seen as likely in advance, a relatively minor event can precipitate a catastrophic cascade of complications that lead to death. The other group likewise consists of very old people whose organ systems are slowly deteriorating and who seem to just "wear out." That is, they have gradually diminishing cardiac function combined with osteoarthritis or some other condition that limits stair climbing, then housekeeping, and then other self-care tasks. Alzheimer's disease may develop, or stroke or renal failure, and pneumonia or other infections may become more frequent with flagging immune response. Whatever organ system is most relentlessly failing may be labeled the primary cause of death, but this is in the context of other less obviously failing organ systems.

Patients' experiences while dying are differently shaped by the nature of their illness; by patient, family, and others' reactions to it; and by the care provided for their physical, psychological, spiritual, and practical needs. To convey this variety of patient circumstances and needs, the committee composed a series of vignettes or synthetic case histories. The cases were selected to illustrate that the dying process for any given patient is determined by an interplay of many variables including the patient's illness, which will determine a particular "trajectory" of the illness, and the patient's personal circumstances and values, including economic and social status, ethnic and religious background, and presence of family and friends.

The cases draw on the experiences of committee members, published sources, including popular biographies, presentations at meetings, and conversations with many individuals and groups. *None exactly depicts a real patient,* and each is simplified to highlight differences in patients' needs and the ways in which care may be well or poorly fitted to those needs. Some describe situations that are reasonably common but not necessarily typical. Others describe unusual situations that particularly strain care systems or underscore the inevitable limits of human arrangements in coping with every possible problem. As explored further in Chapter 4, the dying process is also affected by the health care system, including the care options available in different communities and the expertise, values, and circumstances of health care professionals.

"Joleen Wright"

This case, which draws on committee members' experiences in caring for older people with varying problems, illustrates the difficulties that clinicians face in making decisions for patients who are not fully competent mentally and who have no family surrogate to act on their behalf.

Joleen Wright, an 87-year-old woman living in a nursing home, had been pleasantly convivial and moderately demented for some time. No family or friends were known. It was very hard to discern her preferences, as she "lived in the present" and did not trouble herself about future possibilities. She had chronic hypertension and hearing and motion deficits.

Gradually over a few weeks, she started doing "poorly," walking less, eating less, and seeming more distant. Over the next two weeks, a comprehensive evaluation in her nursing home setting turned up very little. Blood tests, physical exams, and chest x-rays were all normal, but she then became short of breath and was hospitalized. By the time she arrived at the emergency room, her blood pressure had declined to dangerous levels. She had mild problems with oxygenation, probably due to pulmonary edema, and was started on monitoring and careful fluid balance. Within 24 hours, she had multiple attachments (e.g., IV, cardiac monitor, urine catheter) for monitoring and treatment and was restrained in bed to keep the connections in place. Her skin was breaking down on her shoulder blades. She was able to indicate "yes" or "no" to questions about her comfort but showed little insight or attention.

No definite reversible diagnoses surfaced despite appropriate work-up. Her condition worsened, and she faced the need for mechanical ventilation. The care team anguished over whether to continue intrusive care in the intensive care unit in order to establish a clear diagnosis or to shift toward a primarily palliative approach. Her condition continued to deteriorate, and she became minimally responsive. After a team meeting, the care team decided to institute hospice-type care and not to seek a court's involvement in getting a guardian. Joleen Wright died comfortably 36 hours later. Because no consent to autopsy could be obtained, the diagnosis remained a mystery.

"Horace Bowman"

The following case illustrates problems that patients and families can encounter with high-technology intensive care that is aimed solely at life-prolonging measures and not organized to consider the whole patient, the benefit/burden ratio of treatment, and the needs of family members for communication attentive to their concerns.

Horace Bowman was a 74-year-old man whose wife had died the year before. He had problems with angina and peripheral vascular disease but continued to smoke about a pack of cigarettes a day. He had not completed any advance directives and had been uncomfortable discussing possible future ill health.

He collapsed in the street after suffering a massive heart attack and was rushed to a major hospital center. His daughter lived across the country and flew in to be with her father. She found him unable to communicate because he was intubated, and his consciousness fluctuated. When he was alert, he clearly experienced pain and agitation.

Mr. Bowman's daughter wanted to discuss her father's chances of recovery and whether intensive care was helping. She found several physicians involved in her father's care, none of whom were willing to talk with her for more than a couple of minutes. On the fifth hospital day, the cardiac surgeon presented her with consent forms for an emergency revascularization procedure. She asked what the chances were that her father would survive and recover in any meaningful way. Rather than answer these questions, the surgeon merely noted that surgery was the "only hope." The daughter felt pressured to sign the forms.

As Mr. Bowman was being prepared for emergency surgery, he went into cardiac arrest and, despite prolonged resuscitation, died. The daughter felt that the intensive care environment deprived her of the opportunity to spend time with her father, made informed decisionmaking difficult if not impossible, and subjected her father to intrusive tests and interventions that would make her memory of his dying a continuing source of guilt and regret. She was, however, too drained of energy to complain and felt no one would respond anyway.

"Mike Pelli"

This case synthesizes the multiple phases of a child's serious chronic illness, which may at any time become life-threatening. After surgery that helped Mike gain several years, the recurrence of symptoms marked the beginning of an unpredictable trajectory toward death, a pattern also noted after palliative surgery for complex congenital heart disease and central nervous system anomalies (the two most common lethal congenital problems of infants). The case illustrates the need for ongoing evaluation and flexible care planning. It also points to a role in the process for the hospital ethics committee.

At the age of 10, Mike Pelli lapsed into a hepatic coma. He was previously diagnosed with biliary atresia (a defect of the bile ducts leading from the liver) at the age of 2 months. He was born to a single mother who was employed as a secretary and who had traditional health insurance with significant cost sharing for medications and various outpatient services (e.g., physician visits, rehabilitation).

At the age of two and a half, Mike had surgical treatment. For nearly six years, the surgery provided improved liver function; reduction in jaundice and malabsorption; and adequate growth, school performance, and development. Mike required five medications each day and multiple outpatient visits for adjustment of medications, nutritional counseling, and treatment of exacerbations of jaundice. All of this treatment placed a growing financial burden on the mother from medical expenses and loss of income when she had to take off from work to attend to Mike's medical problems. At 8 years of age, Mike began to experience repeated episodes of abdominal pain and vomiting blood. With deteriorating liver function, he required more outpatient treatment but was also admitted to the hospital several times. As a result of spending more and more time away from work, the mother lost her job and her health insurance. Mike and his mother were forced to move into a crowded apartment with relatives.

As Mike's condition deteriorated, the medical team proposed that he receive a liver transplant. This was discussed in detail with the mother and with Mike, an intelligent 10 year old. Both wanted the procedure, and Mike was placed on the transplant list. Hospital social workers noted that he qualified for government-sponsored health insurance.

Then, Mike developed severe hepatic coma and was admitted to the pediatric intensive care unit. Without a liver transplant, his prognosis was very poor. The hospital ethics committee evaluated his medical condition, the prognosis with and without transplantation, the patient's and the mother's wishes, the obligations to the patient, and the issues related to defining when treatment no longer benefits Mike. The mother insisted that everything be done to keep Mike alive.

After two weeks, a donor was identified, and Mike underwent a liver transplant. He initially responded well and regained consciousness within 48 hours of the operation. However, on the third postoperative day, he complained of a severe headache, had a seizure, and became comatose. During initial discussion, Mike's mother refused discontinuation of the ventilator. A day later after strong evidence of brain death and a visit with members of the ethics committee, Mike's mother agreed to the removal of life support. As monitors and other supports were removed by a physician and nurse known to the family, relatives comforted Mike's mother.

"Martha Nielson"

This illustrative case suggests the complexities of caring for very elderly people, in this instance, a married couple. Some complexities are related to specific disease processes, in this case, congestive heart failure; others relate to the more general frailty and pattern of physical failure associated with advanced age.

Martha Nielson, an 86-year-old woman, lived with her 92-year-old husband, George, in their son-in-law's and daughter's "in-law" apartment. She was diagnosed with congestive heart failure several years earlier and used supplementary oxygen almost constantly. For the most part, she managed reasonably well and, during a period of five years, successfully underwent a hip replacement and cataract surgery, both of which improved her quality of life and functioning. She also had three hospitalizations for congestive heart failure, each of which left her somewhat weaker.

In addition, George Nielson began failing physically and mentally in multiple ways and needed more help with personal care than the family could provide. The family arranged with a local home health agency for visits by a home health aide. The first aide proved unreliable, and the next two were not much better. Finally, arrangements with another agency worked well, although after a few weeks it was clear that home care was no longer feasible. After a number of visits to area nursing homes, the daughter arranged for Mr. Nielson to enter a nearby facility that would accept Medicaid if that became necessary.

Shortly before Easter, Martha Nielson became severely short of breath, and her daughter took her to a nearby hospital, where she had been treated before. After 36 hours, her physician of seven years reluctantly concluded—following consultations—that his patient would not survive this time. He hoped that using oxygen, diuretics, and morphine as comfort measures would provide enough time for family members out of state to arrive to say their good-byes. Most were with her when she died. Mr. Nielson was too frail to leave the nursing home and did not seem to understand fully what was happening. Five months after Martha Nielson's death, George Nielson died in his sleep.

"Eduardo Santos"

This case points to the frequent problem of inadequate pain management and the experience and role of family members. It portrays, in particular, the struggles of a daughter with her own feelings and the growth she finds in solving problems about her father's care.

Camille Santos was the 27-year-old daughter of Eduardo Santos, a 67-year-old Hispanic man sent home from the hospital to die of lung cancer. Their relationship had always been one of distant love and respect, but as the father's disease progressed, his daughter became increasingly alienated and depressed and withdrawn from her family. The father tried to protect his family from the reality of his progressing disease by maintaining a positive attitude and focusing on hope.

Upon returning home, Eduardo Santos quietly complained of severe unrelenting pain, but his physician declared there was nothing else that he could do. The family felt it was disrespectful to bother the doctor, although the father finally was moaning and begging for relief. The family was immobilized and clearly unable to act. There was no durable power of attorney document, although such a document would probably not, by itself, have helped this family.

Camille Santos turned to a local hospice where a social worker provided information about feasible and effective pain management, helped her through role playing to prepare for discussions with her family and her father's physician, and generally gave her encouragement and emotional support. When the physician again responded negatively to requests for stronger pain medication, the daughter was ready to ask for referral to the hospice, which quickly provided effective pain relief and guidance about how the family should prepare for Mr. Santos' death. After her father died peacefully at home with his family at his side, Camille Santos reported that her ability to make a difference in his dying and death had changed her view of herself and given her confidence that she could do things on her own.

"Paul Bates"

Some people die unable to communicate and without a family member or other person who knows them to make decisions on their behalf. This case is adapted from a hypothetical teaching case used in an ethics seminar (S. Tolle, Oregon Health Sciences University, personal communication).

Paul Bates was a 57-year-old homeless man brought to the emergency room by a "friend" who dropped him off and left. In the emergency room, he provided a history of weight loss, cough, fever, and chills. He said that he had not previously received care in the community. After examination and testing, he was diagnosed with "necrotizing pneumonia." Shortly after admission, he got out of bed unobserved and was found unconscious in cardiac arrest. He was resuscitated after intubation, fluids, and 20 minutes of external cardiac massage. During the next 24 hours in the medical intensive care unit, Mr. Bates' condition deteriorated with evidence of septic shock, and he then became comatose. Calls to shelters, the police department, social service agencies, and other hospitals failed to uncover any family members or friends who could act as a surrogate. After five days, physicians decided to stop life support, and Paul Bates died shortly thereafter.

"Andrew Lindts"

This case illustrates a situation that is difficult not because physical, emotional, and spiritual caring were neglected but because the patient's personal characteristics and values were not responsive to this caring. The point is not to blame patients or caregivers but to caution against regarding what appear to be unfortunate outcomes as necessarily the result of failures in care.

Andrew Lindts was a 45-year-old business executive who suddenly noticed some weakness in his left leg and intermittent fatigue. A hard-driving personality, he ignored these symptoms. During a meeting, he abruptly developed generalized tremors and collapsed. He was diagnosed with a high-grade, malignant brain tumor with a likely prognosis of less than one year. He and his wife Laura were told about the diagnosis and prognosis and counseled about the options, which were highly unlikely to eliminate the tumor but might prolong his life—at the cost of significant unpleasant side effects.

Mr. Lindts appeared to accept his diagnosis not as a fatal illness but as a problem that he could overcome, just as he had overcome a variety of business setbacks. He had more than sufficient financial resources and personal connections to consult nationally regarded specialists. Despite cautions by these specialists, he demanded the most aggressive curative therapies. Even the term *life-prolonging* sounded too feeble for him to accept.

Initially, Mr. Lindts brushed off the physicians and friends who compassionately and sensitively tried to help him understand his medical situation and prognosis. For a while, he eagerly accepted positive thinking as a curative tool and consulted with its most optimistic adherents. As his symptoms worsened, he became increasingly depressed and wondered whether religion might help. Drawing yet again on his status and connections, he talked with several prominent religious leaders and was baptized.

Eventually confined to bed, Mr. Lindts continued to place heavy emotional pressure on family, friends, and caregivers, who coped as best they could. At the same time, he also showed signs of being ready to "let go" and told his wife and his doctor that he did not want life-sustaining interventions if he lapsed into a coma. He finally became relatively uncommunicative due both to his disease and his medications. He lost consciousness and died, with his family present, 11 months after the diagnosis. Family and friends were relieved but felt guilty about this reaction.

These cases illustrate how people approach death along many different paths. Some deaths are harder than others because of the nature of the disease, the characteristics of patients and their families, or the lack of care appropriate to these circumstances. As they seek to provide reliably excellent care for the usual kinds of patients, systems must also prepare to care well for atypical patients and problems. The remainder of the chapter considers several broad aspects of caring at the end of life:

1. determining and communicating diagnosis and prognosis;
2. establishing clinical and personal goals with patients and those close to them; and
3. fitting care strategies—physical, psychological, spiritual, and practical—to patient goals and circumstances.

DETERMINING AND COMMUNICATING DIAGNOSIS AND PROGNOSIS

Diagnosis

For life-threatening medical problems, the process of establishing a diagnosis and prognosis is more than a technical and analytical exercise for clinicians to use in developing a plan to manage patient problems. It has an important interpersonal component that includes sensitive regard for what a period of testing and investigation may involve for patients in the form of uncertainty, anxiety, dread, physical discomfort, confusion, and isolation. Sensitive regard does not necessarily imply hiding the implications or intermediate findings of the diagnostic process. That may not be possible, nor may it be wise. A testing period can provide patients a time for reflection and initial coping that may buffer somewhat the shock of a terminal diagnosis. For those spared bad news (this time, at least), the process may encourage patients and clinicians to discuss the future prospect of a life-threatening illness or injury.

Prognosis

Once a diagnosis is established, the question of prognosis often follows.[1] For patients and those close to them, estimates of survival time may guide practical decisions (e.g., financial arrangements, travel plans of distant family members) and prompt attention to the spiritual and other ramifications of dying, including the prospect of reconciliation with family or friends. As noted elsewhere in this report, predicting length of survival is not a precise science. Prognostic uncertainty complicates referral to hospice under the Medicare benefit, which requires that patients be certified as having six months or less to live. Government auditors have investigated hospice care for patients who have lived longer than six months and have issued financial penalties (see Chapter 6). These investigations may further discourage timely referral to hospice, which is a long standing problem that may be less a funtion of prognostic uncertainty than of reluctance to acknowledge the approach of death (Christakis, 1994, 1995; Christakis and Escarce, 1996).

Life expectancy is the most prominent feature of prognosis, but prognoses may also include qualitative assessments of the likely physical and mental course of the person's illness to death. Just as planning will be affected by estimates of how long a patient has, it will also be affected by the prospects for physical disability, mental dysfunction, and dependency. Prognosis is usually not a one-time assessment but rather involves periodic reassessment of a patient's prospects.

Several clinical predictive models have been developed and have demonstrated their value in helping clinical investigators, intensive care directors, clinicians, and researchers understand patient risk factors as an ele-

---

[1]This discussion draws on Berger et al., 1992; Pollack et al., 1994; Thibault, 1994; Zimmerman et al., 1994; Knaus et al., 1995; and Lynn et al., 1996.

ment in making decisions and evaluating outcomes (see, e.g., Knaus et al., 1986, 1991, 1995; Pollack et al., 1987; Tores et al., 1987; Chang, 1989; Chang et al., 1989; Diamond, 1989; Selker, 1993; Zimmerman et al., 1994; Hamel et al., 1995; Lynn et al., 1995, 1996). Notwithstanding the value of these models, establishing prognosis is not and probably can never be an exact science. The limits of prognosis involve a mix of methodological and statistical issues as well as problems related to the applicability of the models in actual clinical practice. For example, it takes a very large database to provide the information necessary for precise estimates of survival for different kinds of patients. Given the relatively small numbers of deaths among children, this poses a particular problem for those working with pediatric prognostic models (Pollack et al., 1994). In addition, the complexity of these models may limit their acceptance by physicians and families. A background paper (Appendix D) prepared by a member of this committee lays out these issues.

Communication

Physician and patient narratives reveal that the communication of grave diagnoses and prognoses is a source of profound apprehension and uncertainty (see, e.g., Nuland, 1994; ABIM, 1996b; see also more generally, Katz, 1984; Seravalli, 1988; Buckman, 1993; Gerteis et al., 1993; Strickland and DeSpelder, 1995). Poor communication can traumatize patients and families, interfere with the ability to participate in decisionmaking, and generally undermine their capacity to cope with life-threatening illness. It may likewise haunt physicians and prompt them to avoid patients in a time of particular vulnerability and need. Not surprisingly, a prominent component of initiatives to improve medical education in end-of-life care includes role playing and other exercises involving the communication of bad news to patients and families (see Chapter 8).

Clinicians, counselors, ethicists, researchers, and lawyers have contributed to guidance on how to initiate communications with patients and families about life-threatening medical problems (see, e.g., Katz, 1984; Buckman, 1993; Gerteis et al., 1993; Campbell, 1994; Minnesota Hospice Organization, 1995; Quill, 1995; ABIM, 1996b; Moldow and Carlsen, 1996; Ptacek and Eberhardt, 1996). Effective communication is a skill that, ideally, is informed by such humanistic qualities as compassion, empathy, and sensitivity. Some general principles of patient-clinician communication as well as more specific suggestions for communicating difficult news are summarized in Box 3.1 and illustrated with examples in Box 3.2. A recent review of the literature on this topic suggested that patients and physicians tended to agree on these principles but that little empirical research has been done to test differences in approaches (Ptacek and Eberhardt, 1996).

More generally, patients and family should be able to get as much information as they want; for some, that will be a great deal, for others, much less. The basic view of those caring and advocating for people who are dying is that patients and those close to them should always be able to have their questions answered fully, and they should be able to get information when they need it, day or night. These needs may not be well under-

---

BOX 3.1
Communicating a Bad Prognosis to Patients and Families

Preparing
- Accept that communication with patients and families is an obligation and an honor.
- Be prepared to listen, wait, and check understanding throughout.
- Anticipate that patients' expectations, reactions, and understanding will vary.
- Plan and rehearse the delivery of bad news, including the words, the place, and others who should be involved.
- Have someone trained to handle emotional needs ready to stay with patients and families.
- Find a private, quiet place where everyone can be seated, and try to tell the patient and family together.
- Choose a time when interruptions and patient fatigue are less likely to interfere with communication.

Communicating
- Adapt communication to what is known—and sensed—about patients' medical, emotional, educational, cultural, and other characteristics and circumstances.
- Seek guidance from patients and families about the amount and specificity of information they want, and let them control the flow of information insofar as possible.
- Use the everyday language of patients rather than the everyday language of clinicians.
- Avoid deceits that undermine trust and prevent important preparations for death.
- Allow people time to absorb and process information.
- Check people's understanding of what they have heard and consider what may need to be repeated or reinforced later.
- Assess whether discussion of options, goals, and plans should be initiated or postponed to a defined later time.
- Honor people's need for hope and reassurance.

Following
- Continue to check what people understand of previous information and what new information they are ready to hear.
- Understand that communication skills can be learned and improved, although some people will be better than others.

BOX 3.2
Examples of Communicating a Bad Prognosis

Starting	"Mr. Smith, I have some laboratory reports to discuss with you. Is this a good time to talk? Is there someone else you would like to include?
Continuing	"The reports are not encouraging. This is not easy to say, but your cancer has spread to your liver."
Listening	"You've asked me about your blood tests. I'll answer that question, but I wonder if you have a worry that lies behind the question."
Checking	"Some people are reluctant to ask questions. Is there anything you do not understand or want to talk about? We will need your help in figuring out and planning where we go from here. Can we discuss some options and plans now?"
Reassuring	"I will be here for you and so will others who we will introduce you to shortly. You will certainly have many more questions and concerns. You can always call us. We can do many things together to help you."

stood by many clinicians. Some studies have suggested that many people do not understand terms used by their physicians, and physicians tend to underestimate patients' desires for information (McCormick and Conley, 1995). Moreover, clinicians who see patients on very tight schedules that are arranged to meet productivity or profit objectives may not provide patients and families with the opportunity to raise their most troubling questions.

Although recent decades have seen a generally beneficial emphasis on patient autonomy and more open communication about death, the committee cautions that it may be neither humane nor absolutely necessary to impose explicit communication on those people who regard talking about death as unwise, unlucky, or a violation of their spiritual beliefs. Moreover, those who have experienced discrimination and deprivation may distrust a judgment that their prognosis is terminal and the suggestion that aggressive attempts to prolong life will be ineffectual and even hurtful. Thus, sensitivity to the social and cultural values and experiences of patients and those close to them is important in guiding communications about care at the end of life.

Some patients, including infants and mentally incapacitated people, are not directly involved in discussions of diagnosis or prognosis or in decisions about care. Parents, adult children, and others play the central role. Communicating with older children and adults with greater but still limited mental capacity presents special challenges both in communicating information and considering treatment preferences. (See Chapter 7 for a discussion of legal issues.)

Parental grief, variations in children's emotional and intellectual development or maturity, and uncertainty about what a particular child can cope with make deciding when and what to tell children a particular challenge (see, e.g., Bluebond-Langer, 1978; Wass and Corr, 1984; Smith et al., 1993; Stevens, 1993; Kliegman, 1994; Buckingham, 1996). Children may draw conclusions about their condition from adult behavior without being explicitly informed; to assume that they are unaware can lead to neglect of their fears and anxieties. If secrecy or pretense was the primary stance 30 years ago, today the dominant view endorses open communication matched to the child's conceptual and emotional maturity and desire to talk.

Table 3.1 presents a framework for caregivers' communication with dying children. In addition to diagnosis and prognosis, communication about fears, wishes, pain or other symptoms, and preferences or feelings about treatment also presents especially sensitive issues for children at different levels of development and for their parents.

ESTABLISHING GOALS AND PLANS

Sensitivity to patients and family values is also important in communication to establish goals and plans for end-of-life care. One fundamental principle of patient-centered care is "to ask, not assume: to ask patients what they want to know, to suggest questions that patients might have" and to develop culturally sensitive interview protocols to elicit patient perceptions, expectations, and preferences and goals (Gerteis et al., 1993, pp. 39–40). A related principle is to understand that preferences and goals may change as an illness progresses so that some concerns recede in importance as others become more dominant.

Sometimes, a patient's preference may be to defer as much as possible to the physician, the hospice team, or family and to avoid direct discussion of options, risks, and benefits (Medica Foundation, 1994; Koenig and Gates-Williams, 1995). Thus, physicians, nurses, social workers, and others caring for dying patients cannot assume that patients will wish to discuss death explicitly or will want to be actively involved in planning their care. Physicians, likewise, cannot assume that patients will initiate a discussion of preferences and expectations, although some patients and families certainly will. Whether patients, families, or physicians initiate a discussion, many of the communication strategies presented in Box 3.1 will apply.

Some goals, such as those related to symptoms, life-sustaining interventions, and other clinical matters, may be explored with physicians, nurses,

TABLE 3.1 General Suggestions for Age-Appropriate Communication for Dying Children

Ages	Main concept of death	Communication approach
0-2	None	Provide maximum physical relief and comfort
2-7	Death is reversible, a temporary restriction, departure, or sleep	Minimize child's separation from parents. If parents unavailable, provide reliable and consistent substitute. Correct misperceptions of illness as punishment for bad thoughts or actions. Evaluate for feelings of guilt, resentment.
7-11/12	Death is irreversible but capricious	Evaluate for fears of abandonment, destruction, or body mutilation. Be truthful and open. Provide details about treatment. Reassure that treatments are not punishments. Maintain access to peers. Foster child's sense of control, mastery.
12+	Death is irreversible, universal, personal, but distant	Reinforce comfortable body image, self-esteem. Allow ventilation of anger. Provide privacy. Support reasonable measures for independence. Be clear, honest, and direct. Maintain access to peers. Consider mutual support groups.

SOURCE: Adapted from Wass, 1984. Used with permission.

and other clinicians as well as family. Discussion of goals related to existential or spiritual issues may involve trained chaplains and social workers. Social workers may also be very much involved in discussions of finances, the availability of services, and coping mechanisms. One challenge for those involved with dying patients and those close to them is to establish effective communication among members of the health care team and relevant administrative personnel. The goals of care need to be clear and accepted by all.

For some people, it may be feasible and valuable for communication about end-of-life care to begin well before a diagnosis of incurable illness. For example, a physician with an established relationship with a patient may, during a routine medical visit, initiate a brief discussion about preferences in the event of a catastrophic illness or injury or about the identification of a surrogate decisionmaker. The advantages of early discussion may include encouraging at least basic preparations for the unexpected (e.g., signing a durable power of attorney); reinforcing the relationship between clinician and patient; and laying the foundation for later, more specific discussions (Teno and Lynn, 1996). This kind of communication may be less likely to occur when patients lack a continuing relationship with a personal physician.

Elements of Advance Care Planning

The details of advance care planning may be highly specific to patients and families, but certain general elements can be identified. These elements are not so much a matter of specific documents—although such documents can be very useful—as they are parts of an ongoing process that includes discussions with patients and those close to them about what the future may hold; what the patient and family want to achieve as life ends; what options are available—and what their potential benefits and burdens are; what preferences should guide decisions; what practical issues should be anticipated; and, depending on the circumstances, what immediate steps should be taken. In this broad sense, advance care planning provides an important basis for a cooperative effort, first, to understand people's physical, emotional, practical, and spiritual concerns; second, to prevent distressing and unwanted interventions; and, finally, to secure what the patient, family, and care team will regard as a good death.

In addition to raising a variety of practical issues and actions, those offering support may suggest that patients and families go through a values exercise to clarify what they hope for and fear. One approach to such an exercise is included in Box 3.3.

Advance care planning often includes written directives. The directives and their legal context are discussed in Chapter 7. Table 3.2 suggests the kinds of issues to be raised with patients depending on their health status, cultural backgrounds, and preferences. In general, the guidelines for communication identified earlier in Box 3.1 will apply to advance care planning discussions.

The stability of patient preferences about treatment at the end of life is an important concern but one not investigated in depth. What might seem desirable when death is a distant, abstract possibility may be frightening when one is actually diagnosed with an eventually fatal disease. Once people

BOX 3.3
Values Questionnaire Adapted from the
Vermont Ethics Network

The following questions can help you think about your values as they relate to medical care decisions. You may use the questions to discuss your views with your health care agent and health care team. (If you fill out this worksheet and want it to be part of your Durable Power of Attorney/Health Care, sign it in the presence of witnesses and attach it to your DPA/HC form.)

1. What do you value most about your life (e.g., living a long life, living an active life, enjoying the company of family and friends)?
2. How do you feel about death and dying? (Do you fear death and dying? Have you experienced the loss of a loved one? Did that person's illness or medical treatment influence your thinking about death and dying?)
3. Do you believe that life should be preserved as long as possible?
4. If not, what kinds of mental or physical conditions would make you think that life-prolonging treatment should no longer be used?
—Being unaware of my life and surroundings
—Being unable to appreciate and continue the important relationships in my life
—Being unable to think well enough to make everyday decisions in severe pain
—Discomfort
—Other (describe)
5. Could you imagine reasons for temporarily accepting medical treatment for the conditions you have described? What might they be?
6. How much pain and risk would you be willing to accept if your chances of recovery from illness were good (e.g., 50/50 or better)?
7. What if your chances of recovery were poor (e.g., less than 1 in 10)?
8. Would your approach to accepting or rejecting care depend on how old you were at the time of treatment? Why?
9. Do you hold any religious or moral views about medicine or particular treatment? What are they?
10. Should financial considerations influence decisions about your medical care? Explain.
11. What other beliefs or values do you hold that should be considered by those making medical decisions for you if you become unable to speak for yourself?
12. Most people have heard of difficult end-of-life situations involving family members or people in the news. Have you any reaction to these situations? If so, describe.

SOURCE: Adapted from Vermont Ethics Network, 1996. Used with permission.

have become quite ill, they—and those close to them—may still change their perceptions of the benefits and burdens of continuing or foregoing treatment. A large study of seriously ill hospitalized patients found that most patients desired cardiopulmonary resuscitation during their initial interview and 70 percent expressed that preference two months later. Of those preferring resuscitation initially, 85 percent maintained that view whereas of those preferring no resuscitation, 69 percent sustained that view (Rosenfeld, Wenger, et al., 1996). Dialysis patients in another study varied greatly in their desires that previously prepared advance directives be followed as compared with allowing surrogates to exercise discretion (Sehgal, 1992). Given these considerations, communication about goals, options, and preferences should not be envisioned as a single event but as a process that occurs as a patient moves toward death.

Issues in Advance Care Planning

Overall, experience with advance care planning indicates that continued investigation is needed to determine the value and limits of such planning and the factors that make it more or less likely to occur and to be helpful to patients and clinicians. The general literature on decisionmaking and decision implementation and the research on advance care planning specifically suggest that effective advance care planning depends on several factors (see, e.g., Lo et al., 1986; Brunetti et al., 1991; Emanuel, 1991; Sachs et al., 1992; Emanuel, 1994; Emanuel and Emanuel, 1994; Morrison et al., 1994; Virmani et al., 1994; Emanuel et al., 1995; Lo, 1995; SUPPORT Principal Investigators, 1995). These factors include:

- *patient and family knowledge.* As indicated earlier, some patients and families may want to defer to physician judgments and choices. Patient knowledge is also a consideration in advance care planning. Research suggests that a significant proportion of patients are not familiar with such instruments as living wills or durable powers of attorney, that patients may not understand the language used in these instruments, and that patients may be more optimistic about their prospects and options than is warranted (Murphy et al., 1989; Joos et al., 1993; Teno, Lynn, Wenger, et al., 1997). Interventions to inform patients and provide them the opportunity to complete advance directives have generally shown increases—often substantial—in the proportion of patients with advance directives (Reilly et al., 1994; Baines, Barnhart, et al., 1996; Hammes and Rooney, 1996; Teno, Lynn, Wenger, et al., 1997). In contrast, one study of interest in advance directives found that the 5 percent of patients who were not at all interested in advance directives were more likely than the other 95 percent to have spent time in an intensive care unit (Gilligan and Jensen, 1995).

TABLE 3.2 Adapting Advance Care Planning to Patient
Circumstances: Possible Issues and Actions

Health status	Issues for discussion	Actions	Persons to lead action
Healthy	Surrogate decisionmaker	Suggest completion of durable power of attorney	C
	Health concerns	Discuss possibilities in a medical emergency	C, P
	Preferences or beliefs	Discuss values and preferences with surrogate	P
		Document strong preferences in patient record	C
Diagnosis of serious illness	Surrogate decisionmaker	Complete durable power of attorney	P
	Prognosis and options	Discuss possible and likely outcome states in relation to care options	C, P, F
	Preferences or beliefs	Discuss values and preferences in the event of an emergency	P
		Document preferences in patient record	C
Diagnosis of life-threatening illness	Surrogate decisionmaker	Determine status and location of durable power of attorney documents	C, P, F
	Preferences	Discuss and document preferences for end-of-life care and make arrangements as appropriate	C, P, F
	Goals	Discuss hopes and expectations for the last stage of life	C, P
	Contingency plans	Make specific plans for likely complications and urgent situations	C, P, F

TABLE 3.2 Continued

Health status	Issues for discussion	Actions	Persons to lead action
Advanced age	Surrogate decisionmaker	Determine status and location of durable power of attorney documents	C, P, F
	Preferences	Discuss and document preferences for end-of-life care and make arrangements as appropriate	C, P, F
	Goals	Discuss hopes and expectations for the last stage of life	C, P
	Contingency plans	Make specific plans for likely complications and urgent situations	C, F

NOTE: C, caregiver, P, patient; F, family. SOURCE: Adapted from Teno and Lynn, 1966.

• *patient and family socioeconomic characteristics.* Some research suggests that those most likely to have an advance directive are white, elderly, educated, and tend to plan for the future. For example, one study found that 34 percent of people with estate wills also had advance directives, while only 7 percent of those without estate wills had such directives (Sachs, 1994). Another report indicated that African Americans and Hispanic Americans were less willing than others studied to complete advance directives (Caralis et al., 1993).[2]

• *clinician characteristics and clinician-patient relationship.* Little specific appears to be documented about clinician characteristics associated with greater or lesser discussion and acceptance of patient goals and preferences for end-of-life care. For example, the SUPPORT study found that only about 60 percent of the physicians who had received information on patient prognosis actually reported that they had the information and only about a third recalled receiving information on patient preferences, but the investigators did not report data on physician characteristics linked to these

---

[2]In some cultures, the value clash may be acute. For example, a small study of Navajos found that 86 percent believed that talking about advance directives is a "dangerous violation of traditional Navajo values and ways of thinking" (Advance Care Planning Conflicts with Navajo Values, in *Advances/A Bridge*, Issue 1, page 6, 1996).

results (SUPPORT Principal Investigators, 1995). Elsewhere, the study investigators have reported that some physician behaviors were associated with specialty status (e.g., cardiologists being less likely to write DNRs than pulmonologists or intensive care specialists) (Hakim et al., 1996). More generally, many believe that the dominant medical culture makes it difficult for physicians to accept patient wishes to forego treatment, at least when clinicians see some chance for successful treatment (see, e.g., Katz, 1984; Schneiderman et al., 1993; Nuland, 1994; Annas, 1995; and Chapter 8 of this report).

• *characteristics of educational and decisionmaking processes*. Inadequate processes for patient and family advance care planning and lack of clinical information about patient prognosis and preferences have been identified as problems. Efforts to improve information, decisionmaking, and outcomes have sometimes proved disappointing. Most notably, one stimulus to the consideration of new strategies is the disappointing results of a major intervention to improve discussions and knowledge of hospital patients' preferences through information and counseling (SUPPORT Principal Investigators, 1995). The patients assigned to the intervention (or their surrogates) were not more likely to report a discussion with a physician about resuscitation or prognosis, to have their preferences known to their physician, to have DNR orders documented, to have them documented earlier, to spend fewer days in the intensive care unit, or to have different levels of resource use. Almost half the DNR orders were documented during the last two days before death, and barely half of patients who preferred not to be resuscitated had DNRs written (Hakim et al., 1996). The percentage of patients with some kind of advance directive was essentially unchanged at about one in five, but those in the intervention group who had such directives were more likely to have them documented in the medical record (Teno, Lynn, Wenger, et al., 1997).

• *organizational structures and processes*. Increasingly, organizational systems are viewed as major determinants of practice patterns including practices related to care at the end of life (Pritchard et al., 1994; Reilly et al., 1994; Berwick, 1995; Blumenthal and Scheck, 1995; Solomon, 1995). The focus then becomes identifying and remedying faulty processes rather trying to identify, change, or punish faulty individuals. The SUPPORT investigators discovered considerable differences among the five medical centers they studied, and factors associated with these differences are still being studied. In general, it might be expected that values and practices might differ from general community hospitals to highly specialized academic medical centers. Likewise, an organization with strong computer-based patient records and information systems should be better able to document patient directives, make information readily available to clinicians, and provide data allowing outcomes to be assessed and problems identified. Individual studies suggest that it is possible to have high rates of advance directive documentation (Hammes and Rooney, 1996).[3]

•   *cultural and legal factors.* The influence of cultural values and beliefs on patient and family preferences and behaviors has been suggested above and in Chapter 2. The role of medical culture is evident throughout this report. The most obvious attempt by public officials to support patient preferences is the Patient Self-Determination Act (PSDA). The PSDA is still relatively recent. Its implementation has been complicated and its effects remain uncertain. Chapter 7 considers the PSDA and other legal considerations in end-of-life care, and Chapter 6 considers economic issues. The specific effects of financial incentives on advance care planning have yet to be adequately studied. Cultural differences also appear to play a role both in the individual use of advance directives and physician regard for such directives (Sehgal et al., 1996).

Given this multiplicity of influences on advance care planning and the limited evidence of the effectiveness of written directives, it is not surprising that a number of observers have questioned the emphasis on such documents (see, e.g., Lynn, 1991; Lo, 1995; Solomon, 1995; Emanuel, 1996). One commentator has argued for the testing of more rigorous models of structured decisionmaking that draw on studies of shared decisionmaking that focus on factors that are most amenable to change (Emanuel, 1995b). Others stress the need to change organizational processes, structures, and values. Chapter 5 focuses on such changes in the broader context of efforts to assess and improve the quality of care.

FITTING CARE TO GOALS AND CIRCUMSTANCES

Fitting care to patient goals and circumstances involves periodic appraisal by patients, families, clinicians, and others of a number of factors. Box 3.4 highlights questions that will be relevant for most patients, except those whose dying process is so rapid that palliative and other interventions are precluded.

---

[3]Following a foundation-funded program in La Crosse, Wisconsin, that involved common patient education materials that are available in virtually all of the area's health care institutions, a study found that 85 percent of adult residents who died in the community had written advance directives, 81 percent of the directives were found in the patient's record, and the most common document (77 percent) was a power of attorney for health care (Hammes and Rooney, 1996). Analysis of the experience of decedents with and without some kind of advance directive suggested that patients without directives were somewhat more likely to have resuscitation attempted and to be hospitalized during the last six months of life.

Dimensions of End-of-Life Care

Care at the end of life is particularly intense in its attention to different dimensions of the illness experience. These dimensions, each of which may vary in importance at different stages in the process of dying, include the physical, emotional, spiritual, and practical.

The Physical Dimension of Care

Physical comfort is a basic priority in care for those who are dying. Physical care emphasizes the prevention and relief of symptoms and includes attention to hygiene, nutrition, skin care, and other physical factors that affect patient well-being.

Beyond the initial evaluation of a patient and the development and acceptance of a care plan, physicians may be most active in evaluating and managing especially difficult symptoms such as intractable pain. On a day-to-day basis, high-quality physical care is, in large measure, a function of high-quality nursing care that considers individual patient circumstances (e.g., proximity of death) in responding to symptoms (e.g., suctioning secretions). Nursing care includes both professional services and care by family and others close to the patient. Physical therapists, pharmacists, nutritionists, and others play variable roles depending on specific patient needs, and the availability of family care can be a major consideration in determining whether home hospice care is feasible for a patient. (The concept of the palliative care team is discussed further in Chapter 4.)

Good end-of-life care requires solid familiarity with the incidence of specific symptoms associated with various illnesses and understanding of symptom pathophysiology and complexity, especially coexistence of multiple symptoms. Box 3.5 lists major physical and psychological symptoms that dying patients may experience, depending on the nature of their disease and other variables. Sometimes these symptoms are a result of efforts to cure illness or prolong life. As is true in caring for all patients, the first step in excellent end-of-life care is conducting a careful patient history and examination to identify medical and personal factors that may be responsible for the patient's symptoms.

In addition, family and other nonprofessionals involved with caring for someone with advanced illness may need to be prepared to recognize and cope with physical and emotional symptoms and to recognize when to seek professional help. Hospices typically assist with such preparation. The American College of Physicians (1995) has prepared a home care guide for family, friends, and hospice workers caring at home for people with advanced cancer. The guide, which offers much information and advice that would be useful for other advanced illnesses, covers a wide range of physi-

---

BOX 3.4
Assessments Needed in Devising Palliative Care Plan

Disease status and symptom assessment
- What is the diagnosis and the prognosis?
- How is the disease likely to affect the patient?
- What other current physical or emotional problems (e.g., substance abuse) are relevant?
- What symptoms are present, and what symptoms are likely to emerge?

Preferences and goals
- Have patient and family preferences, beliefs, and goals been discussed?
- Has a surrogate decisionmaker been identified if the patient becomes unable to participate in decisions?
- Have appropriate documents been completed and preferences recorded in the patient's record?

Emotional status and spiritual assessment
- How does the patient feel about his or her situation?
- What are his or her hopes and fears?
- Should assistance from a pastor or other spiritual counselor be suggested or arranged?
- Has the patient been sufficiently assured that he or she will be cared for and will not be abandoned (assuming that reassurance can be truthfully offered)?

Family assessment
- How are family and closely involved others managing?
- How have they managed difficult situations in the past?
- How well do they understand the patient's condition and prospects?

---

cal problems (e.g., tiredness, nausea, pain), emotional issues (e.g, companionship, depression, anxiety), and practical concerns (e.g., getting information from medical staff and help from community agencies).

The Psychological Dimension

The psychological dimension of end-of-life care, which encompasses both cognitive function and emotional health, calls for openness and sensitivity to the feelings and emotional needs of both the patient and the family. It includes—but is not limited to—the identification and treatment of depression, anxiety, and other common psychological problems identified in Box 3.5. Care typically combines clinical and nonclinical elements. For example, depression can often be clinically diagnosed and managed with medications and psychological interventions, but spiritual and other forms

- Do they need physical, emotional, or practical support?
- What special problems need attention (e.g., presence of young children in the home, other family illnesses, communication or cognitive problems, history of violence or substance abuse)?

Functional status
- What can the patient do for him or herself, and where is help required?
- What kind of assistance (e.g., removal of physical obstacles to bathroom access, total physical care) is needed and from what source?

Therapy review and evaluation
- What medications are being used and with what results? What potential drug interactions require monitoring?
- On the basis of patient status, should medications be continued, adjusted, or discontinued?
- What nonpharmacological therapies are being used or should be considered?
- What health care providers are involved in patient care? Is the level and mix appropriate?
- What are the benefits and burdens (for patient, family, and caregivers) of the therapies being provided, and what are the alternatives?

Resource review and evaluation
- What professional and nonprofessional personnel are available to support the patient and family?
- Are physical facilities in the home adequate (e.g., bathroom accessible)? How do transportation, economic, and other relevant resources match patient and family needs? What else can be done?
- Can resources be used more effectively or efficiently?

of caring may complement or—for some—supplant typical medical treatments for depression.

The controversy over assisted suicide has focused particular attention on the role of depression in desire for assisted suicide (see, e.g., Lee and Ganzini, 1990; Cochinov et al., 1992; 1994; Block and Billings, 1995; Ganzini and Lee, 1997; Groenewoud et al., 1997). The diagnosis and management of depression in people with advanced illness is, however, important in its own right, although conventional treatments such as slow-acting medications or psychotherapy may be of limited value for those with a limited prognosis or restricted communication capacities.

Psychological caring involves recognizing and managing emotional barriers to accepting incurable illness and preparing for death. For example, when a family insists—against completely uniform medical advice—that "heroic" life-prolonging measures be attempted for an irreversibly uncon-

BOX 3.5
Major Physical and Psychological Symptoms

Pain
Key dimensions of pain include intensity, duration, burden felt by patient. Generally, pain is categorized as somatic, visceral, or neuropathic depending on its apparent origin. Uncontrolled pain significantly interferes with all aspects of a patient's functioning. Depression and demoralization may unnecessarily result from untreated pain at the end of life. The 1993 edition of the *Oxford Textbook of Palliative Medicine* (Doyle et al., 1993) devotes 40 percent of its discussion of specific symptom management of pain.

Anorexia-Cachexia Syndrome
This syndrome involves diminished appetite (anorexia) and wasting of muscle mass (cachexia). Decreased eating means that the energy a patient takes in does not cover the energy he or she expends. Cachexia affects a majority of terminal cancer patients and is also common in patients with chronic organ system failure and those with AIDS and dementia. Malnutrition may confound attempts at specific therapy for a life-threatening disease so that patients are unable to tolerate adverse side effects or to undergo rehabilitation.

Weakness and Fatigue (asthenia)
Tiredness may be caused by both disease and treatment. It may also be the result of malnutrition and disrupted sleep patterns. Extreme tiredness may interfere with the patient's ability to move, bathe, or go to the toilet. It may cause dizziness, possibly leading to falls.

Dyspnea and Cough
Dyspnea (shortness of breath) is caused by an inability of the lungs to work in proportion to the demands of activity. It may result from a number of pulmonary, cardiac, neuromuscular, and psychological conditions. Difficulty in breathing requires either an increase in ventilation or a decrease in activity.

Nausea and Vomiting
Nausea (feeling that one may vomit) and vomiting are common symptoms for patients with terminal cancer and AIDS and also may be side effects of life-prolonging therapies such as chemotherapy and medications. Rates vary with type of cancer and gender.

Dysphagia
Dysphagia is the difficulty some dying patients have in swallowing food and liquids. Neuromuscular diseases and cancer are common causes of this problem. Swallowing is a complex process, involving 25 muscles, 5 cranial nerves, and the medulla oblongata, and interference with any of these components may case dysphagia. Inability to swallow will affect hydration, nutrition, and medication. It can sometimes be bypassed by tube feeding, although that raises problems of its own.

BOX 3.5 Continued

Bowel Problems

Constipation may be caused by certain medications, emotional stress, reduced intake of food and liquid, or decreased activity. Diarrhea is less common than constipation in cancer patients but is considerably more common in HIV-infected patients. Bowel incontinence is a major disability for dementia and stroke patients, causing serious burdens to patients and their families.

Mouth Problems

Dying patients may be troubled by various mouth problems, including dry mouth, sores, dental problems, and infections. These symptoms, which are uncomfortable or painful in themselves, tend to make eating, drinking, and taking of medication unpleasant, and they thus may lead to dehydration and malnutrition. Meticulous moistening and cleanliness can be among the most important services to prevent suffering in a patient nearing death.

Skin Problems

Skin problems that cause distress may arise from the underlying disease, treatments for the disease, or both. Problems include itching, dryness, chapping, acne, sweating, extreme sensitivity to touch, dark spots, and pressure sores. In addition to causing physical discomfort, skin problems may be perceived by patients as indignities to be hidden from others.

Lymphedema

Tissue swelling due to the failure of lymph drainage may be caused by infection or by therapies such as surgery and radiation. It is often uncomfortable, unsightly, and movement limiting.

Ascites

The accumulation of liquid in the abdomen occurs in 15 percent to 50 percent of terminal cancer patients and in virtually all patients who die of liver failure. Ascites cause a feeling of bloating, as well as discomfort from the stretching.

Confusion

Confusion is a mental state in which patients react inappropriately to their environment because they are disoriented or bewildered. Confusion may be caused by decreasing mental capacity or by medications and may render patients unable to care for themselves. They may mistake their own abilities and overexert themselves or lose their balance. Confusion also complicates communication between patient and family or caregivers.

Dementia

A common cognitive complication in the older elderly and in younger patients with such diseases as AIDS and stroke, dementia may begin with subtle symptoms, such as apathy, social withdrawal, and difficulty in concentrating. If progressive, dementia moves through deterioration in verbal and motor responses to a complete inability of patients to move about or care for themselves.

continued on next page

BOX 3.5 Continued

Anxiety
Anxiety is a biological and emotional reaction to stressful situations, including diagnosis of an incurable illness and the approach of death. If the sense of dread, danger, or tension is severe, it may interfere with the ability to eat or sleep and may be associated with shortness of breath, nausea, diarrhea, or increased heart rate.

Depression
Although emotions such as sadness are common with the approach of death, clinical depression is a more serious condition. At its most severe, depression is syndrome of sad mood and overwhelming despair that saps the psychic and physical energy that is necessary for coping with illness. It may interfere with appetite, sleeping, personal hygiene, and social interactions, including communication with family and caregivers. In some cases, depressive symptoms may be caused by a chemical imbalance created by medications or disease.

Source: Doyle et al., 1993; *Stedman's Medical Dictionary*, 1994; ACP, 1995.

---

scious patient, the specific response may depend on the extent to which the family is understood to be expressing grief, guilt, religious teachings (or, possibly, misunderstanding of these teachings), or inadequate knowledge of the patient's condition. The appropriate response might be to arrange conversations with a social worker, psychologist, chaplain, or clinician skilled in explaining medical problems to laypeople. A hospital ethics committee may also be invoved.

One issue that many cancer, AIDS, and other patients are confronting is prolonged survival following the diagnosis of life-threatening illness that involves a high likelihood of death and intensive medical interventions (NCI, 1990; Nessim and Ellis, 1991; Zampini and Ostroff, 1993; Loscalzo and Zabora, 1996; Sullivan, 1996). Another problem for cancer and AIDS patients is that these illnesses still tend to be stigmatizing even for those whose physical problems are still minimal.

Emotional care extends beyond a patient's death to concern for grieving families and friends (IOM, 1984; Zimmerman, 1986; Buckingham, 1996). In cases of sudden death, bereavement care may be all that can be offered. Such care may range from providing a time and a place for survivors to be alone with the body to extensive grief counseling.

The Spiritual Dimension

For many, the approach of death inspires a search for meaning, peace, or transcendence that can replace fear and despair with hope and serenity (see, generally, Hoy, 1983; Reed, 1986, 1987; Sodestrom and Martinson, 1987; Hay, 1989; Kaczorowski, 1989; Speck, 1993; Byock, 1996, 1997a). Hope for a cure may persist in those with incurable illnesses, but other kinds of hope can also be a bulwark in the face of death. One can have hope of comfort, personal growth, love, reconciliation, courage, renewed happiness for one's family, or illumination about the mystery that is death.

The search for meaning or spiritual comfort in the face of death is often guided by religious and philosophical beliefs. Even for patients and families without a religious or philosophical belief system, counseling or discussions with chaplains, carefully selected hospice volunteers, or others with special empathy and insight may prove comforting. The needs of "nonreligious" people sometimes, however, create "a measure of confusion" for those who are not accustomed to this perspective (Speck, 1993, p. 517).

The role of spiritual caring is, in principle, widely recognized in hospital provisions for chaplains and religious services and inclusion of chaplains or other religious advisers in hospice and hospital palliative care teams. How well trained and prepared these individuals are to provide spiritual support dying patients and their families needs more systematic study as does the nature and variability of support provided to patients and families by the religious congregations with which they are personally affiliated.

Because nurses spend considerable time with patients, they are often well placed to identify those who could benefit from discussion of spiritual issues. Some clinicians and patients will find prayer or other shared spiritual experience comfortable and comforting. Marked religious differences between patient and caregiver can, however, sometimes create problems.

The clinician's role is, at a minimum, to avoid obstructing spiritual explorations. Such obstruction is unlikely to be willful but instead to reflect the clinician's own discomfort with death as an existential phenomenon rather than a technical problem to be analyzed and solved. In any case, "to ask people to assess where someone has reached in the personal search for existential meaning is quite daunting" (Speck, 1993, p. 517).

Spiritual—like emotional—caring embraces those close to the patient and extends beyond the patient's death. Sensitive end-of-life care has traditionally made provision for religious rituals, such as the "last rites" of the Catholic Church, the Islamic rituals around the time of death, or the after-death and burial practices of the Jewish faith.

The Practical Dimension

Individuals and organizations helping those with advanced illness, especially illness expected to end in death, can do much to alleviate the practical burdens that typically accompany such illness. They can advise and assist patients and families in arranging home health services, in making changes in physical features of the home, in shopping for groceries and doing other routine errands, in coping with visitors, and in juggling work schedules.

The willingness of those in the community to be of help can make an important difference in the experience of patients and families. Beyond providing pastoral care and friendly visitors, churches can deliver very concrete help in the form of meals, home repairs, transportation, and shopping. Neighbors who rally round those in distress not only provide practical help but symbolize community values. Employers can be flexible about working hours, vacation time, and reemployment opportunities for caregivers. Groceries and pharmacies can deliver to homes. In dozens of ways, communities can be supportive—or can leave very sick people and their families to fend for themselves. Clearly, the latter course makes caring well for those approaching death a much more emotionally, practically, and financially burdensome task.

Box 3.6 suggests just some of the practical issues that dying patients and those close to them may have to face. Some are not applicable to those who die suddenly or very quickly, and some are more relevant to those whose dying is managed in the home rather than in an institution.

The practical often overlaps with the physical, emotional, and spiritual dimensions of caring, and these three latter dimensions also mix with each other. For example, helping someone maintain a positive self-image—so important in emotional well-being—may require assistance with the most mundane matters, such as bathing, shaving, or shampooing hair. On a more profound level, in achieving a sense of meaning or peace or transcendence, a person may find that physical discomfort or disfigurement shifts from being an overwhelming problem to a peripheral concern. Conversely, delusions and other mental side effects of disease or medications can impede a person's spiritual journey. The basic point is that caring that attends to one need may serve other needs as well.

Variations in Emphases and Models of Care

Care for a dying patient may include preventive, life-prolonging, rehabilitative, and palliative care in varying proportions depending on the patient's medical problems and preferences. For example, for a patient for whom death is thought to be weeks, months, or even years distant, preventive services such as influenza immunizations may help extend meaningful life. For a patient who will be confined to bed for an extended period, meticulous skin care can prevent distressing pressure ulcers.

Rehabilitative care may be appropriate for patients who can be restored to a higher level of functioning that provides them with more control

BOX 3.6
Practical Dimensions of Care for Patients and Families

Knowledge and Communication

• What to do for pain and other symptoms: quick, clear reference guides for relieving symptoms and getting additional help; clarification of treatments and symptoms, for example, that dehydration may cause fewer problems for those near death than trying to treat it.

• How to make decisions: discussion and accessible documentation of preferences and surrogate decisionmaker.

• Who to call: phone numbers for health care coordinator (e.g., hospice nurse) and other team members; pharmacy, medical equipment company, and others whose services are not arranged by health care coordinator; family and friends to be notified of death or imminent death.

• What to do after death: provision for religious and other rituals (e.g., funeral, memorial service, wake); consideration of organ donation; disposition of the body by burial or cremation; arrangements for small children, pets.

Physical Environment and Personal Care

• What to provide for immediate comfort and control: suitability of bed, chairs, coverings, bed- or chairside resources (e.g., telephone, commode), natural and artificial light.

• How to manage personal care: bathing; shaving; hairdressing; dressing.

• How to permit privacy or companionship when wanted.

• How to provide physical access and safety: floor coverings, bathroom, hallways, refrigerator, outdoors, car or other transportation.

Family and Others Close to Patient

• What to do for primary companion and caregiver: employment issues; housekeeping or caregiving help; respite from caregiving; grief.

• What to do for children and other dependents: babysitting; homework; visiting with patient; planning for death; funeral; bereavement.

• Who to be on call in emergencies.

Financial and Other Practical Issues

• How to handle short-term finances: bill paying; record keeping; access to money, checks; health insurance information.

• What to do about longer-term finances: records of assets and liabilities; access to safety deposit box; estate planning, completion of will.

• How to manage household: food preparation; cleaning; laundry; shopping; property maintenance.

and reduces burdens on caregivers. Although there may be no prospect of cure or long-term survival, some therapeutic interventions may allow a patient to live meaningfully for a somewhat longer time. This time may be just a few weeks or months, but such extra time can be precious, for example, to those anticipating a family wedding or birth.

As curative trials fail or symptoms intensify, the emphasis on comfort care becomes more important. At this stage, use of antibiotics and other care intended to prolong meaningful life may continue, or they may be foregone in favor of care that comforts but does not seek to prolong dying. Concern about a patient's quality of life while dying is central and not to be lost in preoccupation with technical assessments and tasks.

Good patient management is generally aided by clarity about the goals of care. If the goal is life extension, then symptom treatment may be subordinated to survival, and substantially burdensome interventions may be appropriate, because they are consistent with the patient's wishes. If the goal is a good death, then symptom management is pursued vigorously even if that pursuit has the unintended, though foreseeable, consequence of compromising survival; burdensome diagnostic and therapeutic interventions aimed at the illness are rarely appropriate in this context.

Table 3.3 shows one way of envisioning shifting emphases of care as they might relate to patient and family goals, disease stage, attitudes, preferences, interventions, effects, and other elements. Time in the different categories may vary enormously. In particular, many medical problems are not curable, and those who experience them may spend much of their life supported by life-prolonging or symptomatic care or both. Some of these people will, in fact, die of other problems; and, if death is not sudden, the care for those problems may be superimposed on the longer-standing condition.

For situations in which the categorizations in Table 3.3 fit well, many clinicians find them helpful because concepts and terms help organize and regularize care plans. The labels serve as a shorthand for communicating a coherent plan of care.

Nevertheless, Table 3.3's clear-cut categorization of strategies may not work well for a broad range of complicated situations. In particular, it is reasonable to think that people, even when very ill, may want to pursue multiple goals: maintaining a positive self-image, continuing a social role (e.g., as a virtuous family member), limiting impoverishment, avoiding physical suffering, prolonging life, and retaining control. Also, for many patients, various overall courses of care are possible. The potential effects of each possible plan of care on achieving each goal are different and uncertain. In such situations, which might be quite common, shorthand labels for plans and goals (e.g., a goal of life extension versus a good death) would poorly reflect reality. Instead, trade-offs among goals are central and

TABLE 3.3 Primary Emphases of Care for Those with Different Goals Related to Life-Threatening Illness or Injury

Aspects of Care	Primary Care Goal		
	Curative	Life-prolonging, palliative	Symptomatic, palliative
Impact on disease	Eradicate	Arrest progression	Avoid complications
Acceptable side effects	Major	Major-moderate	Minor-none
Psychological attitude	"Win"	"Fight"	"Accept"
Preference for CPR	Yes	Probably	Probably not
Hospice candidate	No	No	Probably
Symptom prevention/ relief	Secondary	Balanced	Primary
Support for family	Yes	Yes	Yes
Advance care planning	Yes	Yes	Yes
Bereavement support	Not usually	Sometimes	Usually

SOURCE: Adapted from Baines, Gendron, et al., 1996.

reflect a gradual evolution of understanding about what can actually be achieved in light of responses to time and treatments.

New Models of Care at the End of Life: Mixed Management

Although health care and public language have been comfortable with a "transition from cure to care" concept, the committee concluded that this traditional conceptualization does not capture or support the reality of simultaneously pursuing a broad array of desired ends. Figure 3.1(A) represents this traditional view of patient management in a typical trajectory of cancer death. It shows that early in the course, curative efforts and life-prolonging therapies are offered, and then at some point, the futility of these therapies is recognized. The objectives of care switch to palliation of symptoms during the remaining months of life.

Although Figure 3.1(A) seems a rational model, it may limit the acceptance of new ideas about the benefits of various therapies for those who are dying. Further, it is not enough to emphasize control of symptoms once they are well established. If identified and impeccably managed earlier in the trajectory of illness, many of the symptom problems that afflict dying patients could be either eliminated or more readily managed.

For example, the body does not usually accommodate physiologically to chronic pain (Meyer et al., 1994; Woolf and Doubell, 1994). Indeed, unrelieved painful stimuli may alter the neurotransmission of pain in the central nervous system, with consequent hypersensitization and the development of an enhanced pain state, now more difficult to manage (Coderre et al., 1993). Recent studies show that early intervention may actually prevent pain from occurring in certain forms of advanced cancer (Hortobagyi et al., 1996; Paterson et al., 1996). The use of prophylactic bisphosphonate to prevent adverse skeletal events in patients with multiple myeloma and breast cancer provides a tangible example of the concept of prevention as part of palliative care. Psychosocial problems, confusional states, and, possibly, the cachexia-anorexia-asthenia syndrome are other problems that can be more successfully managed if a preventive model of care is adopted.

One way of graphically reflecting the adoption of this principle is shown in Figure 3.1(B). Although an improvement upon Figure 3.1(A), this model continues to clearly separate palliative from curative or life-prolonging therapies. It suggests that the two are mutually exclusive and that there are no therapies that can sometimes prolong life, sometimes palliate, and sometimes do both. Adoption of this model would continue to result in the neglect of therapies that are normally viewed as curative or life-prolonging but that also may be used to prevent or relieve symptoms.

Consider, for example, the current realistic aims of therapy for metastatic non-small-cell carcinoma of the lung and carcinoma of the pancreas with chemotherapy. Recent clinical trials show only modest or very modest evidence that such therapy prolongs life (Non-small Lung Cancer Collaborative Group, 1995; Chlebowski et al., 1996; Moore et al., 1996). These trials, however, do document major benefits to patients in terms of relief of pain, easing of shortness of breath, improvements in nutrition, and the maintenance of better functional status. In this case, the use of chemotherapy should be regarded as effective palliative therapy.

As in other areas of medical care, early recognition and treatment of a problem and use of preventive measures when problems may reasonably be predicted can limit the ultimate severity of pain and other symptoms. This implies the need to clearly identify and reassess the goals of treatment throughout a course of illness.

For many patients at the end of life, mixed management is the appropriate conceptual model of care. It allows ongoing efforts to extend life while still preparing for death and comforting the patient and family. For example, a patient with severe chronic obstructive pulmonary disease might

A. Traditional Model for Cancer Care

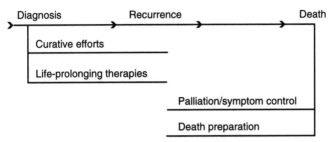

B. Revised Model for Cancer Care

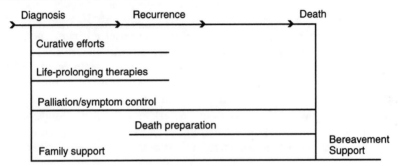

C. Mixed Management of Various Eventually Fatal Illnesses

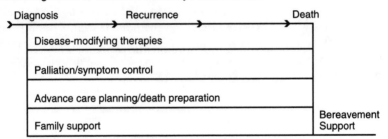

FIGURE 3.1   Alternative models of end-of-life care.

reasonably want a trial on a ventilator and also the opportunity to say farewell in case the trial failed and the ventilator was to be withdrawn.

Figure 3.1(C) reflects the reality and ideal of end-of-life care in which therapies are not rigidly divided into preventive, curative, rehabilitative, palliative, and other categories but are creatively considered for their potential benefit (or burden) regardless of a patient's prognosis. This is consistent with Table 3.3, which distinguished curative, palliative, and other primary goals of care rather than categorizing therapeutic approaches that may, in fact, serve different goals for different patients. It is also consistent with Chapter 1's definition of palliative care as involving the prevention and relief of suffering through early identification and impeccable assessment and treatment of symptoms, both physical and psychological.

Mixed management near death may be commonplace in the care of the frail elderly but does not seem to be as frequently articulated or practiced with those facing the end of life with chronic organ system failure or cancer. It seems likely that attending to "ongoing negotiation" rather than one dominant goal of care might well merit development for these patients.

This need is underscored by the fact that prognosis for many courses to death are ambiguous, even very near to death. In one study of severe congestive heart failure, half of patients who died were—on the day before they died—assigned prognoses of a greater than 50-50 chance to live two months (Lynn et al., 1996). Rather than counsel patients about a likely imminent downward trajectory, the team should ensure that the patient understands the limits of what medicine can do to prolong life and that all attempts will be made to palliate and prevent suffering. Clinicians need to engage patients and families in realistic discussions about the risks of death and provide them full opportunity to ask questions and make plans. Because people will vary in what they want to know and decide, clinicians need to be especially sensitive to patient cues about their desires.

CONCLUSION

Care at the end of life has both a specific focus on those approaching death and a very expansive interest in the patient's family and friends; the health care team; and, ideally, the larger, caring community that tends to its members in both health and sickness. This caring community most immediately includes neighbors, co-workers, employers, and members of religious and voluntary service organizations, but it also extends to those in government and communications whose policies or images may nourish the caring spirit or subvert it.

Major objectives of end-of-life care are to prevent and relieve pain and other distressing symptoms while respecting patient preferences and dignity and offering concern and reassurance to patients and those close to them. Care at the end of life attends to physical, emotional, spiritual, and practical dimensions of the experience of life-threatening illness. It involves a continuing process of assessing and reassessing needs and the therapies and other assistance intended to help patients live well while dying.

The experience of dying is significantly determined by systems of care. They can powerfully support care along all its dimensions or they can put formidable obstacles in the way of good care at the end of life. The next chapter explores the structures of health care that shape how people die.

4

The Health Care System and the Dying Patient

*Why are you afraid? I am the one who is dying! . . . But please
believe me, if you care, you can't go wrong. . . . Death may get
to be routine to you, but it is new to me.*
                    Anonymous, *American Journal of Nursing,* 1970

With help and support from family, friends, and others in the community, many people can live their lives, while dying, with some or considerable independence from the health care system. Many, if not most, however, draw heavily on that system for care—and caring—in the form of
clinical services, counseling, and practical assistance with both medical and
nonmedical needs. Thus, while the role of family and community resources
should be acknowledged and strengthened, it is also essential to understand
how care systems serve patients well and poorly and to identify the system
characteristics that contribute to poor care. Such understandings, which
will depend on better data and research than now exist, will help provide
the basis for steps to remove the impediments to good care and to fortify
the foundations for reliably excellent care.

In general, care systems—both as discrete organizations and as un-
evenly connected arrays of community institutions and services—require
people (supported by facilities and processes) who are prepared to determine what care is appropriate, to arrange its provision, and to monitor
performance for consistency with organizational and external norms.
Broadly, this means having the capacity to provide or arrange for

- symptom prevention and relief;
- attention to emotional and spiritual needs and goals;
- care for the patient and family as a unit;
- sensitive communication, goal setting, and advance planning;
- interdisciplinary care; and
- services appropriate to the various settings and ways in which
people die.

These process of care elements are, in a sense, statements of expectations for the care system. Most of these elements were discussed in Chapter 3, which emphasized the importance of sympathetic but clear consideration of prognosis and goals and fitting care strategies to circumstances. This chapter considers the major settings of care in which people die and identifies questions about the ways care is structured, provided, and coordinated. It concludes by considering aspirations for an ideal care system and what this implies for the mix of organizations, programs, settings, personnel, procedures, and policies that make up care systems.

Unlike new mothers or women undergoing mastectomies, who have recently been the subject of highly publicized criticisms of early discharge, dying patients are not themselves a potent lobbying group and their survivors are often exhausted, grieving, and expected to put their lives back together and move on. Thus, health care professionals, managers, and others have a particular responsibility to press for care systems that people can trust to serve them well as they die.

CHARACTERIZING CARE SYSTEMS

Trying to present a coherent picture of health care systems as they serve—or fail to serve—those who are dying is not easy. First, the two million people who die each year have both variable and common characteristics and needs. Second, the organizations and personnel that may be involved in end-of-life care are likewise numerous and variable. Nationally, there are roughly 6,000 hospitals, 16,000 nursing homes, 11,000 to 15,000 home health care and hospice agencies, 650,000 generalist and specialist physicians, 2 million nurses, tens of thousands of social workers involved in health care,[1] and numerous other categories of health personnel and facilities including several hundred health maintenance organizations (HMOs) and other managed care and health insurance arrangements. Third, data about care at the end of life are very limited.

Even the term *health care system* has no fixed meaning. It can be used in at least four different ways—not because people are being careless in their language but because the term is intrinsically general and capable of applying to several situations. First, the term health care system may be used to describe and analyze a community's or region's array of health care

---

[1]According the U.S. Bureau of Labor Statistics, there were 666,000 "degreed Human Services Workers" in 1995 (Gibelman, 1997), which is the category that includes social workers. The National Association of Social Workers has 160,000 members. The committee did not locate a specific count or estimate of those employed by health-related organizations or otherwise involved in health care rather than other human services.

organizations and services, whatever their relationships. This is consistent with one dictionary definition of a "system" as a set of objects grouped together for classification or analysis (*The American Heritage Dictionary*, 3d ed.). In this usage, the health care system in New York City could be characterized as an aggregation of loosely interacting (sometimes cooperating, sometimes competing, sometimes self-absorbed) components within a large, socially and economically complex geographic area. Fragmentation has been cited as the key characteristic of such systems in the United States (Shortell et al., 1996). Although they may be viewed as rather disorderly systems, they are—analytically—still systems rather than nonsystems.[2] The deficiencies of community health care systems, in the past, prompted a variety of voluntary and regulatory efforts to plan and control the development of health resources (especially facilities and advanced technologies). In part as a result of their weaknesses and in part as a result of shifting political tides at the community and national level, these sorts of health-planning mechanisms have largely been abandoned in favor of more market-based strategies.

In a second and broader sense, the term health care system may also encompass the norms, public policies, and social values that shape the delivery of health care in a community or a society. This is consistent with another dictionary definition of a "system" as the prevailing social order (*The American Heritage Dictionary*, 3rd ed.) Thus, a reference to the Canadian health care system or the American health care system may signify not just a collection of institutions and personnel but also a culture.

A third and much narrower use of the term applies to a particular entity that integrates a comprehensive range of health care services and the facilities and personnel to provide those services (Coddington et al., 1996; Shortell et al., 1996). The integration is formal and institutionalized through explicit controls related to personnel, budgets, and other matters. Systems in this sense may be more or less geographically concentrated, as is the Henry Ford Health System in Michigan, or geographically dispersed, as is the U.S. military health care system, which is not only national but international.[3] Finally, an even narrower use of the term is as a rough synonym for

---

[2]The term *nonsystem* is, however, useful in directing attention to serious faults in the mechanisms that structure routine or expected transactions among system components or that govern the distribution of resources relative to demand or need.

[3]Integration is not an "either/or" characteristic but a continuum. That continuum is clearly evident in the nation's managed care organizations, which range from fairly strongly integrated systems such as Henry Ford to weakly linked entities based on limited and often unstable contractual relationships. A hospice organization is a specialized care system that emphasizes palliative care for terminally ill people and their families and that may—like managed care organizations—be more or less strongly integrated. Medicare hospice regulations favor at least moderate levels of integration.

a provider organization such as a hospital, nursing home, or hospice program.

In this chapter, the discussion tends to focus on community health care systems, but it will be clear that such systems are embedded in a national health care system and include organizational systems as components. The committee uses the term *care system* to highlight the special role in care for terminally ill patients—and frail individuals more generally—of nonmedical services such as spiritual and bereavement counseling, respite care, and housekeeping assistance. In addition to formal or organized health care systems, informal care systems can also be distinguished; they include the family, religious communities, and folk culture (Kleinman, 1978; Kleinman et al., 1978). These systems play a central role for many if not most patients and families, but they were not the focus of this study.

ILLUSTRATIVE CASE HISTORIES

To illustrate the variability of care for those who are dying, this section presents several more cases. As in Chapter 3, these cases do *not* exactly describe a single patient or institution or represent statistically typical patients. The cases synthesize committee experiences, cases in the medical literature, research findings, and specific problems reported to the committee. Several describe situations that particularly strain care systems.

"Ellen Arthur"

This case, synthesized from the hospice literature and committee experiences, illustrates a patient and family for whom a limited range of hospice services work well and whose personal circumstances support living well while dying.

Ellen Arthur, a 78-year-old retired teacher diagnosed with kidney cancer, underwent surgery and a trial of experimental chemoimmunotherapy. Tests then showed that the cancer had spread to her lungs and bone. She was incurably ill but not imminently dying and could reasonably be expected to live for another year, perhaps two. She felt fairly well except for mild fatigue. She and her husband were financially comfortable, well educated, and surrounded by supportive family and friends. They reviewed the durable power of attorney and related documents that they had prepared many years ago.

After several months of fairly normal activity, pain and weakness began to require an increasing amount of medication. Ellen Arthur's physician concluded that she could very well die within the next six months— probably less—and certified this so that she qualified for the Medicare hospice benefit. Her physician coordinated care with the hospice medical director who, in turn, worked with the patient, her family, and an interdisciplinary team to implement the care plan as initially designed and later adjusted as the illness progressed. A hospice nurse was the center of the care team, which focused on two primary problems—fluctuating pain and fatigue. Protocols allowed the nurse to adjust pain medications within defined boundaries, and she advised ways to prevent or soothe other symptoms. For example, she suggested ice chips and glycerin swabs to ease dry mouth and advised balancing rest and activity to reduce the burden of fatigue. The family needed little other direct service from the hospice. Physical therapy and other medical services were not indicated, and the family found emotional and spiritual comfort in their friends and their faith and in reviewing their life together. Friends also pitched in to provide occasional practical help with meals, errands, cleaning the house, and respite time.

John Arthur was informed about how to recognize changes in his wife's condition, especially signs that death was imminent. He knew that if something happened that he could not handle—seizures, for example—he could call the hospice any time, day or night, and help would be sent. The Arthurs were informed that if they called 911 in such an emergency, the protocol for paramedics in their jurisdiction required attempts at resuscitation and other interventions and transport to the hospital. Ellen Arthur died at home with her husband at her side.

"Solomon Katz"

This example, adapted from a case analyzed in The New England Journal of Medicine *(Morrison et al., 1996) illustrates aggressive medical culture, nonbeneficial and even inhumane technical interventions, and disregard for patient and family concerns and preferences. It is marked by fragmented services and failure to provide appropriate referrals to hospital and community resources. No one had overall responsibility for this patient's care and well-being.*

Solomon Katz, a 75-year-old retired postal worker, experienced progressive weakness in his left leg for over a year, but he sought care in the emergency department only after he fell and could not get up by himself. After an array of tests, he was diagnosed with lung cancer metastatic to the brain. He accepted medication but refused a lung biopsy. Hospital staff described him as "in denial," but a psychiatric consultant assessed him as reacting appropriately and capable of making his own decisions. He revealed that his wife died of cancer two years earlier; he did not want to go through the treatments she had. After continued pressure from the oncology team, he agreed to a biopsy, which confirmed the previous diagnosis. They offered options for life-prolonging but invasive treatment; he declined. He was discharged home with home care and follow-up appointments at two clinics. The medical staff did not refer him to the hospital's social work staff, and no one sat down with Solomon Katz and his family to talk with them about the prognosis, palliative care options, or their concerns and preferences. He did not keep his follow-up appointments, but no one checked to see why.

Three months later, Mr. Katz was again brought to the emergency department following grand mal seizures. He was lethargic and could not talk; a CT scan showed progression of the brain tumor, including partial brain stem herniation. He was started on intravenous medications and fluids, and then oxygen and nasogastric tube feedings. The neurology team wanted to resect the brain tumor. His son, a grocery store clerk, refused surgery and asked for a do-not-resuscitate order on the basis of his father's previously expressed wishes. During the next three weeks, Mr. Katz was minimally responsive but repeatedly removed the nasogastric tube despite restraints. After pressure from the hospital staff, the son agreed to insertion of a percutaneous gastrotomy tube. On the following day, Solomon Katz died of a cardiac arrest with no family present. The son was upset by the entire experience, particularly when he later learned that his father's dying could have been a less brutal experience and that his care could have been managed differently with an emphasis on understanding his goals as his life ended and providing physical and emotional comfort. The case attracted the attention of the hospital ethics committee, which concluded such clearly inappropriate care indicated serious system problems. It began to mobilize an institution-wide effort at self-examination, staff education, process changes, and quality measurement and improvement.

"Dorothy Chang"

The next case presents a middle-age woman who died in an intensive care unit following a cascade of complications related to a bone marrow transplant and other medical problems. When it was time for life support to be ended, a protocol was followed that emphasized patient comfort and attention to the family.

Dorothy Chang was a 54-year-old woman with aplastic anemia who received a bone marrow transplant in August. She tolerated the procedure well, but her discharge from the hospital was delayed due to recurrent bacterial infections. Her infections resulted from a narrowed esophagus. An attempted corrective procedure was complicated by rupture of the esophagus and a life-threatening infection that required placement of a drainage tube in the chest and intravenous antibiotics in the ICU. She remained intubated with recurring pneumonia.

The pneumonia slowly improved, but a trial with removal of the ventilator failed. Significant muscular weakness developed, exacerbated by chronic steroid use. A tracheostomy was performed, and a feeding tube was placed with some difficulty. In early November, a head CT scan revealed a lesion consistent with a fungal brain abscess. Despite treatment, another CT revealed advancing disease, and a brain biopsy suggested *Aspergillus* infection, which occurs mainly in immune-compromised people and is very resistant to treatment.

Ms. Chang's condition declined further. She became minimally responsive, and her husband agreed with her physicians that further life-supporting treatment would only prolong death. With support from the hospital's comfort care team, Ms. Chang was moved to a more private area where her family could be with her when the ventilator was removed by an experienced physician known to the family. After all monitors and other supports were removed except an intravenous morphine drip, she was given intravenous morphine and midazolam to ensure that she would not experience distress. After the ventilator was disconnected, her breathing became irregular and stopped, and then her heartbeats began to pause before ceasing. Her family remained quietly with her for a period after death was declared. Following this patient's death after more than four months in the ICU, the ICU director decided that this case needed a careful review to identify any flaws in the unit's performance and areas for improvement. The initial assessment was that both the intensive treatment and its eventual withdrawal were appropriate for the patient's particular combination of problems but that the decision for esophageal dilation should be reviewed with gastroenterologists.

"Millie Morrisey"

The problems of appropriate end-of-life care for nursing home patients are increasingly being recognized. This case illustrates both inadequate expertise in palliative care and faulty organizational procedures for assuring that patient and family wishes are respected.

Millie Morrisey, an 86-year-old retired clerical worker, suffered from Alzheimer's disease and congestive heart failure. Before her illness became so severe, she and her niece had discussed her future, and she prepared a living will that expressed her wishes, including that resuscitation, mechanical ventilation, and other life-prolonging measures not be attempted in a medical crisis. She did not want to burden her niece, and she accepted that nursing home care would be the best option when she could no longer safely be left by herself, which happened about a year later.

After two years of nursing home care, Millie Morrisey developed pneumonia and respiratory distress. As had been its custom, the nursing home staff called an ambulance. Documentation of preferences—which included foregoing antibiotics, mechanical ventilation, and tube feeding—were neither sought nor readily accessible in her chart. The hospital quickly admitted her to the ICU, initiated antibiotics and mechanical ventilation, and used physical restraints so that she would not dislodge the tubes and lines to which she was connected. She mostly did not seem to understand what was happening and was agitated and tearful. After three days during which her niece informed the ICU team of her aunt's wishes, Millie Morrisey was successfully withdrawn from the ventilator and died a few days later, receiving comfort care only. The niece was still upset, and the nursing home staff concluded they needed to avoid similar problems in the future. The nursing director learned that she could participate in a new statewide working group comprised of many health care, social service, and religious organizations that were attempting to devise clinical and administrative guidelines to understand and honor patient and family goals and to assure excellent end-of-life care.

"Darrell Henson"

This case demonstrates the involvement of nontraditional family. It also underscores the role that poor quality care can play in turning a patient's attention to suicide.

Darrell Henson, a 67-year-old owner of a small business, was diagnosed with prostate cancer. He had surgery and remained in remission for two years. Around Thanksgiving, the cancer reappeared in bone metastases, and Mr. Henson began to suffer terribly from pain and nausea. The medications prescribed by his physician did little to help, but the physician feared being accused of overprescribing narcotics and was reluctant to do more. Mr. Henson begged his companion, Charles Jones, to help him die because life seemed unendurable with such pain. Mr. Jones, distressed by his companion's suicidal thoughts, called another physician, one who had cared for his mother. This doctor visited Mr. Henson at home, did a careful assessment of his pain and other symptoms, and developed a care plan that emphasized effective pain relief and supportive home services. Although not a conventionally religious man, Mr. Henson was relieved not to violate the prohibitions against suicide taught to him in childhood. He was able to remain home, celebrate Christmas with his companion and their friends, and—despite weakness—say his goodbyes before dying in January.

"George Lincoln"

This case illustrates the disruptions that may be caused by health care restructuring and consolidation.

George Lincoln was an 84-year-old retired engineer whose health gradually deteriorated as multiple organ systems began to fail. Through his former employer's health plan, he had long been enrolled in a large HMO. He had been pleased with the HMO, which arranged much appreciated hospice care when his wife died of breast cancer several years earlier. Then, however, the HMO was sold to a corporation with out-of-state headquarters, his personal physician was not on the new provider list, many of his numerous medications were switched to lower-cost drugs, and referral to a cardiologist experienced with very old patients proved difficult. Mostly confined to his home (and often to his bed) and experiencing considerable physical distress but still mentally alert, Mr. Lincoln concluded—with considerable equanimity—that "my time is coming." He raised the issue of hospice care with his new primary care physician. He discovered that the HMO's long-standing relationship with a community hospice had been terminated in favor of referrals to a fairly new organization. Mr. Lincoln was not told that as a Medicare beneficiary he was not limited to this hospice, and he found the new hospice provided a much-reduced level of care—and caring. He was, in any case, too fatigued and depressed to complain.

The cases above and in Chapter 3 highlight some of the positive and negative features of the care systems available to dying patients and those close to them. They vary in the degree to which care systems help the process of dying be, as described in Chapter 1, free from avoidable distress and suffering for patients, families, and caregivers; in general accord with patients' and families' wishes; and reasonably consistent with clinical, cultural, and ethical standards. Some examples were constructed to show patients who suffered reasonably avoidable distress; some involved disregard for patient and family wishes and perhaps violated clinical or ethical standards; several showed people and institutions attempting to cope with changing expectations or to correct problems. The sections below consider different settings of care from a more general analytical perspective.

SETTINGS FOR END-OF-LIFE CARE

As described in Chapter 2, people die in many settings—mainly hospitals, nursing homes, and homes. Each setting is appropriate and feasible under some circumstances and not under others. Not only are home, hospital, and nursing home settings quite different from each other, each category encompasses great variability. This discussion starts with the hospital because it is still the most frequent site for end-of-life care, despite increased pressure from various sources to shift care to other settings. Later sections consider nursing homes, home care as part of a hospice program, home care without hospice, and coordination of care within and across settings. Transitions from one setting to another create many problems as the weak or even nonexistent links among health system components are exposed. Consistent with other chapters, one problem in drafting this chapter was the relative lack of descriptive and evaluative data on the experience of dying patients and the effects of different settings and processes of care.

Hospitals

Although the situation is changing, more deaths occur in hospitals than in other settings, and most people receive some hospital care—brief or extended—after being diagnosed with serious progressive illness. Nonetheless, curing disease and prolonging life are the central missions of these institutions. Hospital culture often regards death as a failure, in part because modern medicine has been so successful in rescuing, stabilizing, or curing people with serious medical problems and in part because a significant minority of acutely ill and injured patients who die often do so before the end of a normal life span.

A major challenge in hospital care is identifying better ways to maintain vigorous efforts to cure illness and prolong life while, at a minimum, avoiding needless physical and emotional harm to patients who die. Every hospital's goal should be to provide as good a death for the patient and family as a patient's illness and circumstances permit.

Shortcomings in hospital care have been documented in a number of areas. A large study that attempted both to understand hospital care of patients with advanced illnesses and to improve that care identified opportunities for improvements in patient-physician communication, understanding and honoring of patient preferences, and symptom management (SUPPORT Principal Investigators, 1995). It also found considerable amounts of intensive interventions in the days before death, a finding that the investigators found troubling but that some critics argued might be appropriate and consistent with patient's wishes (Emanuel, 1995b; Lo, 1995). The study also found that the strategies designed to improve care did not appear to have modified behavior or outcomes

Other studies, cited in Chapters 3 and 5, have found problems related to unrelieved symptoms in hospitalized patients, poor documentation of patient preferences for care, early discharge of dying patients, and underuse of home care. As discussed further in Chapter 6, the financial incentives for hospitals to discharge patients early warrant reexamination in the context of end-of-life care.

The growth of hospice combined with pressures to minimize hospital use is shifting more care to other settings, often the home, sometimes a nursing home. This shift can be expected to continue as physicians, nurses, social workers and others working with hospitals, hospices, nursing homes, and professional and community education programs help dying patients and their caregivers understand how to cope with the period of dying and the moment of death without reflexively turning to hospitalization.

The committee identified a number of basic issues and questions that will be generally relevant for hospitals caring for gravely ill and dying patients. They are offered in part as a guide for hospitals concerned about understanding and improving care and in part as a guide to the formulation of a research agenda. For the most part, the issues and questions outlined below translate into matters of staffing and procedures involving personnel with appropriate attitudes, skills, and knowledge; in some cases, they involve physical design of facilities.

• How well are patients and families informed about who is responsible for care, what they can expect, and who they can look to for information and assistance? How specifically are the preferences and circumstances of patients and families determined, assessed, recorded, and accommodated? Are processes focused narrowly on written orders or more broadly on advance care planning? What provisions are made for children, non-English speakers, cultural minorities, and others who may not fit routine administrative and clinical procedures?

• What internal or external expertise is available to help clinicians, patients, and families with clinical evaluation, symptom prevention and management, advance care planning, and decisions about foregoing or withdrawing treatments, bereavement support, and other matters? How is this expertise organized and shared? Are other staff routinely educated about the availability of this expertise and expected to use it when appropriate?

• Have hospital personnel been trained in methods of communicating bad news, discerning patient and family wishes and concerns, and respecting dignity through their language and other behavior?

• What structures and processes—for example, ethics committees—are in place to prevent, moderate, or mediate conflicts among clinicians, families, payers, and others?

• What care options are available for dying patients within the hospital, for example, a designated area of palliative care beds governed by different rules regarding visiting hours and other matters for dying patients? Do explicit criteria and processes guide decisions about the use of these options, and are relevant staff throughout the hospital aware of them? Can hospital procedures and the physical environment be modified in other ways (e.g., in the ICU) to reduce stress and discomfort for patients and families?

• Are ICU staff, specialty services, and other personnel trained to recognize patients (and families) for whom the goals of curative or life-prolonging care should be reconsidered with particular attention to the goals of physical and emotional comfort and symptom relief? Are procedures in place for arranging appropriate care and consultations? Are the important roles of nurses, social workers, and others recognized and supported?

•   What structures and processes are in place to help patients and families with transitions to or from the hospital and other care settings? What relationships exist with nursing homes, home care agencies, hospices, and other organizations that care for or assist dying patients? What effort has been made to identify community resources, such as bereavement support groups, and to deliver information on these resources to patients and families?

•   What clinical practice guidelines, symptom assessment protocols, and other tools are in place to guide clinical evaluation and care for different kinds of patients who have a high probability of dying (e.g., the very frail elderly with acute illness, victims of catastrophic accidents)? Have practices for foregoing or withdrawing life-supporting technologies (e.g., mechanical ventilators) been reviewed to determine whether they can be modified to reduce distress for patients, families, and staff?

•   Are clinical information systems in place that reliably document and update advance planning decisions, symptom assessments, care processes, patient responses, and similar matters? Do they provide clinical decision support in the form of easy access to guidelines, prescribing protocols, and other information relevant to symptom prevention and relief?

•   What structures and processes are in place to evaluate and improve the quality of care provided to dying patients? How is accountability for such care managed? Is information about quality of end-of-life care available to the public?

The committee assumes that every hospital will find areas in which its practices can be improved, but differences among hospitals make it unlikely that any single model of end-of-life care can be sensibly recommended or imposed. Hospitals that routinely care for dying patients may be large or small, financially secure or precarious, well or ineptly managed. Depending on their location in suburban, urban, or rural areas, they may experience difficulties in recruiting well-trained medical, nursing, and other personnel. Some hospitals are highly specialized and relatively impersonal, whereas others provide routine acute medical care with a more personal character. The latter may or may not have academic connections, including residency and research programs and consultation links. All face financial constraints or pressures in the form of Medicare reimbursement practices, managed care contracting and payment mechanisms, state and local budget cutbacks, shareholder expectations for for-profit organizations, and increasing numbers of uninsured Americans. (Chapter 6 looks at financing issues in more detail.)

Notwithstanding this variability, the message of this report is that each hospital should be held accountable for identifying its shortcomings and devising strategies to improve the quality and consistency of care at the end of life. The same holds for other organizations and settings of care.

Nursing Homes

The care of dying patients will be an increasingly important issue for nursing homes in future years as the number of older people most at risk for nursing home admission grows and as hospitals and managed care plans continue to minimize hospital stays. Home care agencies, however, are caring for some patients who might previously have been admitted to nursing homes, although the extent to which home care substitutes for inpatient care is debated and the growing cost of home care is creating increasing concern (see the discussion later in this chapter).

Between 1985 and 1995, the number of nursing home residents grew almost 4 percent to about 1.5 million people, but the number of residents per 1,000 people age 65 and over dropped (Strahan, 1997). The number of nursing facilities declined by over 12 percent. The total number of beds increased by about 9 percent but the number of beds per 1,000 population dropped. About two-thirds of nursing homes are for-profit organizations, many of them part of national or regional chains. About two-thirds of nursing homes are certified by both Medicare and Medicaid, and only 4 percent are not certified by either. The large number of facilities (around 16,000 in 1995) and, to some degree, their relative isolation from both the rest of the health care system and the community present some particular difficulties for quality monitoring and improvement.

During the 1970s and 1980s, an increasing amount of attention was directed to the quality of care in nursing homes and the integrity of nursing home management (IOM, 1986; Kane and Caplan, 1990). One result was the 1987 Nursing Home Reform Act, which set forth a variety of regulatory requirements and directions for improvement in nursing home care and management. Care for nursing home residents approaching death was not a major issue during this period. Rather, the focus was primarily on eliminating neglect and mistreatment, preventing physical and mental deterioration and restoring function to the degree possible, and respecting patient dignity and autonomy. As nursing homes attempt to market specialized services or units for care of Alzheimer's, postsurgery, and other patients, the mix of objectives and services will change from the more traditional emphasis of many facilities on generalized long-term care. How these changes might encourage or complicate improvements in end-of-life care is unclear.

Nursing home residents are, altogether, a heterogeneous group. For some patients admitted to nursing homes, death is expected within a relatively short period. Others spend years in a nursing home before their final decline. Many residents are more robust than suggested by common images of frail, bed-bound human beings who are practically at death's door (Caplan, 1990). The committee believes, however, that it is essential to direct more explicit and open attention to the manner of dying in nursing homes and the ways in which care can be improved for dying patients (McCullough and Wilson, 1995; Parkin, 1996; Tolle, 1996b).

One might expect that nursing homes would be well prepared to care for dying patients. Their residents are virtually always functionally impaired. Most require attentive personal nursing care involving oral hygiene, skin care, bowel and bladder care, and nutrition. Some may be anxious, depressed, or fearful. Most who enter a nursing home and stay for more than a few months will die there or after transfer to a hospital. They will not again live at home.

Nursing homes differ from hospitals in many respects, including the low level of physician involvement, relatively low ratios of registered nurses to patients/residents, and the amount of care that is provided by nursing assistants or aides (IOM, 1996c). Staff may not be trained in caring for dying patients and may not provide adequate palliative care, sometimes because physician medication and other orders are not flexible enough. As a matter of routine or as an accommodation to a home's limited resources, residents may be transferred to hospitals, and thus, their dying hours or days are spent in an unfamiliar place with unfamiliar people.

Although nursing homes have been criticized as too often "neither homelike nor known for their quality of nursing care" (Aroskar, 1990), the experience of nursing home patients who die is not well documented. As has been found for other patients, those in nursing homes often suffer from inadequate pain management (Ferrell et al., 1990; Sengstaken and King, 1993; Morley et al., 1995; Wagner et al., 1996).

One analysis by the Washington Home and Hospice found that for the 108 patients who died in its long-term care section, the average length of stay before death was 3.4 years but the range was from 4 days to 30 years (Cobbs and Barry, 1996). The most frequent cause of death was pneumonia. Cancer caused 17 percent of the deaths among the nursing home patients compared to 50 percent in the hospice and home care groups. Only five of the nursing home deaths were considered unexpected. About 60 percent of patients who died required pain medication (usually morphine), and about 12 percent were transferred to the hospital around the time of death. All the patients had documented advance directives.

More descriptive analyses of the experiences of nursing home patients who die would be useful in better understanding care in this setting and identifying its strengths and limitations for different categories of patients/

residents. Questions to be asked about end-of-life care in nursing homes parallel in some respects those for hospitals. They include:

• How well are patients/residents and families informed about who is responsible for care, what they can expect, and who they can look to for information and assistance? What structures and processes are in place to prevent, moderate, or mediate conflicts between clinicians and families?

• How specifically are the preferences and circumstances of residents and families determined, assessed, recorded, and accommodated? Do formal protocols exist for advance care planning, developing physician orders related to life-sustaining treatments, and assuring this information is available when needed? How is this information shared with paramedics and hospital staff if transfers become necessary?

• What practice guidelines, symptom assessment protocols, and other tools are used to guide patient assessment and care? Do they cover the basics of supportive care, including appropriate hydration; nutrition; skin and mouth care; and care for pain, shortness of breath, anxiety, depression, and other symptoms?

• What structures and processes are in place to evaluate and improve the quality of care provided to dying patients? Have practices for patient transfer, communication about changes in patient status or withdrawal of life-supporting technologies, and other decisionmaking been reviewed to determine whether they contribute to avoidable distress for patients, families, and staff?

• How adequate is physician and nursing support for patient care? What education and training related to end-of-life care are available to nursing home staff including all who have contact with patients and families?

• What internal palliative care expertise is available to guide physical, psychological, spiritual, and practical caring for dying patients and those close to them? Are staff routinely educated about the availability of this expertise and expected to use it as appropriate? What relationships exist with external sources of consultation and assistance?

• Are those patients perceived to be dying segregated from other patients? If so, why and with what consequences?

Testimony presented to the committee indicated that nursing home and other long-term care organizations are "deeply challenged" by end-of-life care and decisions and that even "natural death" can be an occasion for sorrow and anxiety (Parkin, 1996). Staff may be uncertain about what the law requires or permits, what religious practices need to considered (especially if the facility is sponsored by a single religious group), what clinical and nonclinical caring is needed and appropriate, the extent to which a resident is competent to participate in decisions, and how to handle disagreements. The spiritual dimensions of caring may be neglected.

These issues are more systems rather than individual issues, and they need attention at the systems level. Moreover, "an informed corporate conscience" is needed (Parkin, 1996). Ethics committees are helpful, but more than ethical problems are involved.

Home Care

Home Care with Hospice

In the United States, hospice care is usually intended to help people die comfortably at home, although inpatient care and inpatient hospice programs have a role (see generally, Zimmerman, 1986; Mor, 1987; Buckingham, 1996). Hospice-like services and palliative care may be provided by a wide variety of organizations—hospitals, nursing homes, physician groups, HMOs—that are not officially certified. Some do not designate themselves as hospices. Most care for adults, especially cancer patients. A few programs, often associated with inpatient pediatric services, focus on specialized care for dying children, a small but clinically and psychosocially complex group (Martinson, 1978; Howell, 1993; Wass and Neimeyer, 1995; Buckingham, 1996).

In 1996, the National Center for Health Statistics (NCHS) estimated that there were about 1,100 hospices (Singh et al., 1996). For 1994, the Health Care Financing Association reported 1,682 Medicare-certified U.S. hospices. The National Hospice Organization (NHO, 1996a) reports that it "has knowledge of" 2,800 operational or planned hospices (2,200 are members of the NHO). The higher numbers include hospice units that are part of hospitals, nursing homes, and home health agencies. Hospices may be independent organizations (about 30 percent according to NHO, 1996a) or may be organizationally affiliated with home care agencies (22 percent), hospitals (28 percent), or larger integrated health systems. Ninety percent of hospices are owned by not-for-profit organizations, but ownership by for-profit organizations is growing (from about 3 percent in 1992 to 7 percent in 1996) (Singh et al., 1996).

Hospices—as organizations concerned exclusively with dying patients and those close to them—are intended to provide workable and reliable structures and procedures for turning palliative care principles into practice. For example, hospices should back up their commitment to "be there" for patients by

- being accessible to patients and families 24 hours a day, 7 days a week, in a sense reproducing on an outpatient basis one of the potential advantages of inpatient care;

• constructing interdisciplinary teams that, taken together, have the necessary knowledge and skills needed to provide comprehensive and continuous care; and

• developing organizational procedures, interpersonal strategies, and care protocols to guide the provision of services in response to common physical, emotional, spiritual, and practical problems faced by patients and their families.

Because hospice programs are designed specifically for dying patients and those close to them, some of the questions relevant to hospitals and nursing homes are not directly relevant. Nonetheless, questions can be asked about how hospice care is organized and managed to fulfill the commitments outlined above. These questions include

• How well are patients and families informed about who is responsible for care, what they can expect, and who they can look to for information and assistance? How are the preferences of patients and families assessed, recorded, and accommodated?

• What practice guidelines, symptom assessment protocols, and other tools are used to guide patient assessment and care? What structures and processes are in place to evaluate and improve the quality of care? What are the criteria for admitting patients?

• What internal and external resources and expertise are available to provide 24-hour coverage, physical and emotional care, spiritual support and counseling, practical assistance, and other aid for patients and families associated with hospice care? What education and training related to end-of-life care are available to hospice personnel?

• If home hospice care proves insufficient for a patient's needs, what are the arrangements for hospital or nursing home care?

• How is physician support for patient care organized? Are patients' personal physicians encouraged to continue with patients after enrollment in hospice?

• What structures and processes are in place to prevent, moderate, or mediate conflicts involving families, patients, or staff?

In their 1987 book, Mor and Masterson-Allen concluded from their survey of the literature that the typical hospice patient: had cancer; was white, about 65 years old, seriously functionally impaired, and close to death; and had very strong informal support. The committee found no evidence that the typical hospice patient is strikingly different today, although pediatric and noncancer patients are becoming somewhat more common. Data from the 1993 National Home Care and Hospice Survey found that 71 percent of hospice patients were aged 65 or over, 78 percent were white, over half were married, and the first diagnosis was cancer for 70 percent of patients (Singh et al., 1996).

These data are in part a reflection of the emphasis by early hospice advocates and providers on cancer patients. In part, they are a function of the Medicare benefit, in particular, its provision that death be expected within six months. This provision, which is more applicable to cancer patients than to those with many other diagnoses, is one manifestation of a more general objective of limiting total spending on intensive palliative services for those with terminal illnesses (see Chapter 6).

As noted earlier in this report, the designation of someone as terminally ill and likely to benefit from primarily symptom-oriented rather than life-prolonging care is more difficult for some diseases than others. NHO has attempted to provide guidance for hospices regarding when patients with noncancer diagnoses might be identified as likely to have six months or less to live (NHO, 1996a; see Appendix F). Beyond its particular prognostic focus, this exercise may also encourage more consideration of how patients with noncancer diagnoses can benefit from better palliative and supportive care over the course of their less predictable and often more extended incurable illnesses. Even more broadly, this kind of work may contribute to improved care for those with serious chronic illness who are not considered to be dying.

Early studies comparing hospice and nonhospice care did not find as much difference in symptom control as advocates might have expected, although the difficulty of conducting research and the variability of research settings and designs have complicated comparisons. In their review of the literature, Morand (1987) concluded that "available data show that hospice clearly does not result in patients experiencing increased pain . . . [and] some comparisons report that hospice may achieve small but significant differences in pain control" (p. 140). They reach similar cautious conclusions about the mixed findings of research on hospice effects on other symptoms, psychosocial variables, and bereavement. Mor concluded that "hospice appears to deliver the kind of service that patients and their families want . . . [so] they appear to be satisfied with it and have fewer regrets about the orientation of the care received than do nonhospice patients" (p. 156). An analysis undertaken after the authors' literature review suggested that traditional measures were not sensitive enough to reveal any special effects of hospice care so a "quality of dying" measure was devised to assess what patients wanted during their last three days of life (as reported by the principal caregiver) (Wallston et al., 1988). The researchers concluded that patients receiving hospice care were more likely than conventional care patients to die in a way consistent with their desires (in particular, being free from pain and being able to stay at home as long as desired).

Perhaps because hospice programs are now generally accepted as a desirable option for patients and families who desire it, comparisons of hospice and other care do not appear to be a research priority. It is reasonable, nonetheless, both to encourage a better understanding of the strengths and limitations of hospice care and to support further research on particular processes of care—in any setting—that contribute to patient and family well-being. Relatedly, because fewer than 20 percent of those who die each year are enrolled in hospice programs, more needs to be learned about the needs and circumstances of those not enrolled.

Home Care without Hospice

Home care through alternative arrangements is important for people who do not qualify either for inpatient care or for hospice programs. This latter group includes many people with serious chronic illness (e.g, congestive heart failure, chronic obstructive pulmonary disease) who may not be perceived as dying, although they are recognized as having an illness that will likely end in death. Many eventually will die in hospitals or nursing homes rather than at home.

Overall, home care involves a mix of people receiving short-term care (e.g., after surgery) and long-term care.[4] About two-thirds of those characterized as consumers of home-and-community-based long-term care are cared for entirely by informal caregivers who are primarily female (Hing and Bloom, 1990; Pepper Commission, 1990). (Family care has been described as a "euphemism for wives and daughters" [Holstein and Cole, 1995, p. 17]). About 14 percent of home care patients are cared for solely by formal caregivers, and the rest receive a mix of formal and informal care. For Medicare beneficiaries, use of formal home care has been growing rapidly (Bishop and Skwara, 1993). The number of home care visits grew from 37.7 million in 1988 to 208.6 million in 1994 while the number of persons served per 1,000 enrollees grew from 49 in 1988 to 93 in 1994 (HCFA, 1996b).

In 1996, the NCHS estimated that there were 9,800 home health care agencies, about 80 percent of which were certified by Medicare or Medicaid, usually by both (Singh et al., 1996). Another estimate put the number

---

[4]Long-term care has been described as a "set of health, personal care and social services delivered over a sustained period of time to persons who have lost or never acquired some degree of functional capacity" (Kane and Kane, 1987, p. 4). It has also been characterized as "the stepchild of the new ideology of curative medicine" (Holstein and Cole, 1995, p. 16).

of agencies at 14,000 (NAHC, 1993). About 4,000 home care agencies are certified by the Joint Commission on Accreditation of Healthcare Organizations (one of two national certifying organizations).

Another option for keeping people at home involves the use of day care services designed specifically for people who are able (with or without special assistance) to leave their homes for supportive care. In addition, people unable to live independently or with families may be cared for in residential board and care homes. Studies have found from 18,000 to 65,000 such homes, some of which are licensed, others not (IOM, 1996a). The involvement of these settings in care at the end of life is largely unknown.

The quality and availability of home care services can reduce the distress, dysfunction, and family stress for many whose trajectory toward death is unpredictable or marked by relative stability punctuated by occasional crises, which may or may not prove fatal (Thorpe, 1993). Patients may develop a strong attachment to home care nurses and other personnel, although frequent discontinuity of personnel is a problem. More generally, the quality and cost-effectiveness of home health care are continuing concerns (see, e.g., Perrin et al., 1993; Kane et al., 1994; Shortell, Gillies, et al., 1994; IOM, 1996a). Quality concerns focus on such issues as

- the training, skills, oversight, and even honesty of paraprofessional personnel;
- the adequacy of attention to symptom relief, psychological problems, and family circumstances;
- the high levels of personnel turnover;
- the management capacities and integrity of agencies including those that provide contract personnel;
- liability for negligence;
- needs assessment and referral to higher levels of care; and
- effective regulation and accreditation strategies.

The committee noted these quality issues with concern. Although it did not locate analyses focused specifically on patients approaching death at home without benefit of formal hospice care, it expects that their experience is quite variable. Some may receive good palliative care, whereas others may receive care that is inattentive to their symptoms and emotional needs. The debate about the cost-effectiveness of home care in averting nursing home or hospital use is reviewed in Chapter 6. For end-of-life care at home without hospice, questions generally should raise the issues noted in earlier sections for both home hospice care and nursing home care.

COORDINATING CARE WITHIN AND ACROSS SETTINGS

Seriously ill patients often move among many different health care settings where they are cared for by many different physicians, nurses, and other personnel. Coordinating care among various personnel and units within a single setting can be difficult enough. Coordinating care during transitions from one setting to another presents even greater challenges, especially when different organizations and funding sources are involved.

Procedures to Smooth Transitions

Because coordination and continuity of care are well-recognized trouble spots for health care organizations, hospitals, nursing homes, and other institutions, a variety of structures and processes have been created to smooth the transition of patients into and out of their organizations. Such structures and processes usually figure prominently in the requirements of accrediting organizations. They include the development of defined procedures for patient transfers (e.g., defining why, when, where, how), follow-up mechanisms, and standardized interorganizational relationships among hospitals, home care agencies, nursing homes, hospices, and other organizations that are or should be involved. Formally integrated health care systems, as described earlier, attempt to provide even stronger mechanisms for coordination, including designated primary care providers and integrated patient information systems. The various structures and processes for coordinating care may or may not be organized with particular attention to the needs of dying patients and their families, and this committee was not able to assess their strengths and limitations in this area.

Broader and more intensive community education may help patients, families, and providers become more aware of the range of health care and other resources available to patients approaching death, including those for whom hospital care is not appropriate but who do not qualify for hospice care. These resources may not be narrowly focused on such patients but nonetheless may be valuable, especially if their potential is more explicitly understood and the ways of integrating them into the care processes and transitions are identified. Thus, community groups might develop inventories of resources available to dying patients not only from health care institutions but also from churches, other charitable organizations, support groups, and agencies serving special populations, such as older individuals, children, or people with disabilities.

For example, a statewide task force in Oregon has developed a booklet listing for every county those resources that may be helpful to dying patients and their families (see Appendix C). This initiative has also included intensive efforts to make advance care planning in nursing homes more effective so that patients are not hospitalized contrary to their preferences and so that information about patient wishes or surrogate decisionmakers goes with patients when hospitalization is appropriate (Tolle, 1996b). The most visible element of the strategy is a bright pink form that is designed to provide such information clearly but without the expectation that such a form can cover all circumstances. (The form is reproduced—not in color— in an addendum to this chapter.) Accompanying the use of the form is an intensive educational effort intended to reach into every nursing home, hospital, paramedic unit, and similar organization and into homes as well, where the form might be clipped on the refrigerator to be easily located. Although those involved did not feel that their circumstances or resources made a clinical trial possible, they are attempting to collect longitudinal information and data about actual institutional practices that will allow them to assess the effects of the initiative.

Interdisciplinary Palliative Care as a Coordinating Strategy

Interdisciplinary palliative care teams are another way of providing and coordinating different kinds of care. Care teams may play various roles for patients and those close to them, and they may be differently composed and organized in different settings. Patients and families and others involved in caring for patients are considered members of the care team as well as the focal point of the caring process. For some patients, especially hospitalized patients, "formal" members of the care team may be a major presence. For others, particularly those dying at home, the care team may be a helpful but relatively minor and intermittent presence. The care team exists, in any case, to support the patient and family, not to intrude upon their efforts to deal with the personal, social, emotional, philosophical, or spiritual experience of dying.

Home Hospice Teams

A core element of palliative home care is the interdisciplinary care team (Mor, 1987; Hull et al., 1989; Ajemian, 1993; Buckingham, 1996). In addition to health professionals and others, most home hospices stress the need for a family member or someone else who can serve as a primary caregiver for a patient who wants to die at home. Some will not accept patients without a person who can be so designated (NHO, 1996a). Finding a person or persons to serve in that role is difficult but possible for some patients and not possible for others. Hospital-based hospices are more likely to serve patients who live alone or have employed caregivers (Mor, 1987). Some community hospices operate inpatient units that also serve such patients, and others have arrangements with nursing homes or hospitals.

For hospice organizations, the interdisciplinary team is directly responsible for patient care in the home. The team may also support staff in institutions, such as hospitals and nursing homes, that can provide most or all such care using their own personnel. To be eligible for Medicare payment, a hospice must have an interdisciplinary team that includes at least a physician, registered nurse, social worker, and counselor and must designate a nurse to coordinate care for every patient (HCFA, 1996a). Core nursing, physician, and counseling services must be provided by employees or volunteers. Additional requirements also apply to records, training, and other matters.

Central to the care team are a nurse and a social worker. The other members of a typical team are depicted in Figure 4.1.

The nurse typically provides services—either directly or by calling on other professionals as needed—to help the patient cope with progressive illness. She or he also acts as case manager, often in tandem with a social worker. The nurse is usually responsible for ongoing assessment of the patient's physical and emotional status, developing a plan of care, working with physicians to adjust medications and other treatments for physical and psychological problems, educating family members about how to avoid problems (e.g., odor) and what to do if a problem (e.g., a seizure) occurs, monitoring family status, arranging additional help as needed, and generally being available to answer questions. The specific nursing care and consultation needed for a dying patient varies depending on the nature and stage of his or her illness.

The social worker typically shares case management responsibilities and helps the patient and family with personal and social problems by providing psychological assessment and counseling, advocating for them with health care providers and others, offering information and help with interpreting information, and assisting with practical matters (Loscalzo and Zabora, 1996). In one report on hospice cancer patients in the United States, about 75 percent of formal supportive counseling was provided by social workers (Coluzzi et al., 1997).

Most hospices employ physicians, nurses, and social workers (and administrative personnel). Less intensively involved personnel may work part-time or on a contract basis. Hospices as a matter of philosophy and tradition (as well as Medicare certification requirements) stress volunteerism.[5]

---

[5]Medicare requires that volunteer staff be sufficient to provide administrative or direct patient care equal to at least 5 percent of total paid patient care hours (42 CFR Section 418.70[e]).

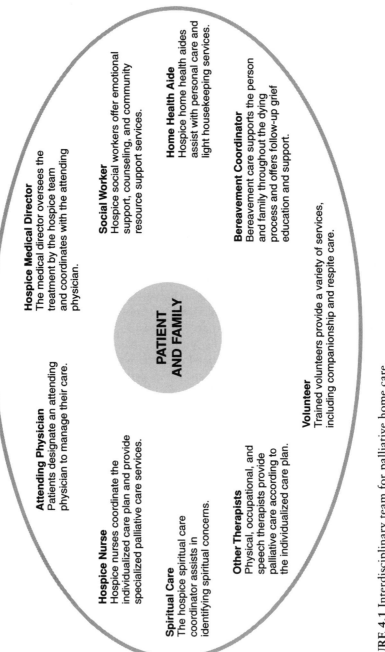

Hospice Medical Director
The medical director oversees the treatment by the hospice team and coordinates with the attending physician.

Social Worker
Hospice social workers offer emotional support, counseling, and community resource support services.

Home Health Aide
Hospice home health aides assist with personal care and light housekeeping services.

Attending Physician
Patients designate an attending physician to manage their care.

Bereavement Coordinator
Bereavement care supports the person and family throughout the dying process and offers follow-up grief education and support.

Hospice Nurse
Hospice nurses coordinate the individualized care plan and provide specialized palliative care services.

Spiritual Care
The hospice spiritual care coordinator assists in identifying spiritual concerns.

Other Therapists
Physical, occupational, and speech therapists provide palliative care according to the individualized care plan.

Volunteer
Trained volunteers provide a variety of services, including companionship and respite care.

PATIENT AND FAMILY

FIGURE 4.1 Interdisciplinary team for palliative home care.
Source: Adapted from Minnesota Hospice Organization, 1995. Used with permission.

Some hospices depend heavily on volunteers or contract personnel instead of employed staff. Volunteers serve in many capacities and are generally screened to match their talents and interests to organizational and patient needs. Some provide the key clinical services while others provide emotional and practical support to patients and families or perform administrative and informational tasks for the hospice.

A hospice patient may stay under the care of his or her personal physician, and many patients and physicians prefer such continuity. Alternatively, the hospice medical director may serve as the patient's attending physician. In the committee's experience, it is sometimes difficult for the personal physician to stay involved if house calls are required. Also, some otherwise excellent physicians may not be comfortable with an established hospice team, and others may not be fully familiar with the principles and techniques of palliative care, including appropriate use of opioids. Even if a patient is transferred to a hospice-based physician for good reasons, the personal physician can stay involved to provide support and information that may be useful for the hospice team. Many patients and families who have had a long-standing relationship with a physician undoubtedly would appreciate further communication, such as a call when death is near and a call or letter afterwards.

Effective teamwork requires active and continuing effort by all team members and by those responsible for overseeing their performance. For palliative care teams, the challenges are many (Ajemian, 1993). Team members come from very different professional backgrounds, which creates the potential for role conflict. Sorting out and maintaining clear responsibilities for decisionmaking, information provision, and other tasks is important if people are to know what is expected of them. Even so, conflict management may still be necessary. Part-time staff and volunteers, however important, can be awkward to fit with an established team, and relationships with others who have cared or are caring for the patient can become strained. For example, if hospice personnel are involved with the care of a long-term nursing home patient, staff at the nursing home may have established a close relationship with that patient and may be upset if their care for the patient is ignored. Coordination is a pervasive and continuing challenge that requires a balance between the time required for coordinating activities and the time devoted to the activities themselves (e.g., caregiving, documentation).

Inpatient Palliative Care Teams

Clearly identifiable inpatient palliative care teams have not been routine for nursing homes or hospitals. Medicare-certified hospices must have an interdisciplinary palliative care team (HCFA, 1996a). The Joint Commission on Accreditation of Healthcare Organization's standards for nursing homes call for an interdisciplinary team whose responsibilities include care planning and, by implication, palliative care for those needing pain management and similar care (JCAHO, 1996a). For hospitals, Joint Commission standards refer generally to teamwork and interdisciplinary collaboration but do not explicitly call for an interdisciplinary team in care for dying patients (JCAHO, 1996b).

It is the committee's experience that many hospitals and nursing homes have no personnel with clearly designated palliative care expertise. Hospital ethics committees may help resolve conflicts among patients, families, and clinicians about care goals for gravely ill patients, but this is not equivalent to expertise in symptom prevention and relief or in other aspects of palliative care.

Depending on an institution's objectives and characteristics, the options for developing palliative care expertise include interdisciplinary care and consulting teams or designated individuals who may be called upon to provide or assist with palliative care. The care team may be the option best suited for the varied and complex needs of seriously ill, hospitalized patients, whereas designated personnel and care protocols may be reasonable for nursing homes that can call on outside experts for consultation about more difficult situations including those that might otherwise appear to call for hospitalization.

In some cases, members of a designated hospital-based palliative care team may function less as regular caregivers than as consultants, particularly if the hospital does not have an inpatient palliative care unit (Abrahm et al., 1996). Such a team would typically function in an environment in which a variety of curative, palliative, rehabilitative, and other services are provided and in which very sick patients with many different diagnoses and problems are treated. The members of the team would help physicians and nurses care for patients with refractory pain or other especially difficult problems in symptom prevention and management. In an academic medical center, this kind of palliative care team might consist of one or more physicians, specialist nurses, social workers, pharmacists, and chaplains.

In some environments, other approaches may make sense. For example, one academic health center that served mainly as an emergency and trauma facility for a disadvantaged inner-city population established a supportive care team for hopelessly ill patients (Carlson et al., 1988; Campbell and Frank, 1997). In this case, the team consisted of a clinical nurse specialist and a small, rotating group of physicians.

The availability of a palliative care team should not imply that those routinely caring for dying patients can do without the clinical and interpersonal skills and attitudes needed to prevent and relieve common causes of distress for dying patients and those close to them. Nurses are central in this regard.

Given the current medical culture, the organization of a palliative care team may reinforce the role of ethics committees and others in helping hospital staff recognize when aggressive diagnostic or life-prolonging interventions are inappropriate and how to communicate sensitively with patients and families to help them focus on what can be done. Members of such a team may also play an important part in undergraduate and graduate medical education and in research to build a stronger knowledge base for end-of-life care. They may provide consulting services to hospice care teams, nursing home staff, and others faced with particularly difficult clinical problems. Educational and research roles of palliative care specialists are discussed further in Chapter 8.

Managed Care as a Coordinating Strategy

As indicated earlier, this report uses the term *managed care* broadly to refer to organizations that direct patients to a limited panel of health care providers, pay providers in ways that encourage economical use of services, and/or employ administrative and educational mechanisms to control access to expensive services. Although not usually counted among such organizations, hospice is a form of managed care applied to certain terminally ill patients.

Conventional HMOs and managed care arrangements have not yet enrolled a large proportion of the Medicare population overall.[6] Nationwide, only 10 percent of Medicare beneficiaries are enrolled in HMOs. However, in California, Oregon, Arizona, and Hawaii, the figure is over 30 percent, and in some Oregon counties, it is over 40 percent (Zarabozo et al., 1996). Although Medicare enrollment in HMOs underrepresents those most likely to die (e.g., the oldest old and functionally impaired), an increasing number of older people can be expected to be enrolled in managed care when they die (Zarabozo et al., 1996). A portion of these individuals will, however, be cared for and die in nursing homes, and much of this care will be paid for by private funds or Medicaid. Although state Medicaid programs may be considering managed care for poor, functionally impaired recipients, its feasibility and benefits for most nursing home patients is not clear.

The pros and cons of using conventional managed care to cover people with serious chronic illness have been debated, although little attention has

---

[6]The situation for younger adults and children who are eligible for Medicaid is quite different. States are increasingly shifting these beneficiaries to some form of managed care.

focused on those considered terminally ill (Schlesinger and Mechanic, 1993; Miles et al., 1995; Jones, 1996a,b; Miles, 1996; Paris, 1996; Post, 1996; Spielman, 1996; Virnig et al., 1996). The federal government has funded a number of social health maintenance organization (SHMO) and other demonstration projects specially designed to improve coordination of care and quality of life for frail elderly people (Vladeck et al., 1993). Research suggests that such plans are more likely to use case managers to monitor patient needs than conventional managed care plans, and they tend to provide somewhat different patterns of care for patients compared with fee-for-service settings (Harrington and Newcomer, 1991). Regardless of the pros and cons of SHMOs, they are not now available to most Medicare beneficiaries with serious chronic illnesses, including terminal illnesses.

Several HMOs, for example, several Kaiser plans, have long operated their own hospices, but most are thought to contract with hospices, as is likely the case for other organizations such as risk-bearing medical groups or integrated health systems. Some managed care organizations have established arrangements for managing the care of seriously ill individuals that closely parallel hospice programs in some respects but that may be more flexible (e.g., not explicitly limited to patients expected to live six months or less) (Blackman, 1995b; Baines, Gendron, et al., 1996; Della Penna, 1996; Emma, 1996). These arrangements may be viewed by organizations as sufficiently valuable on the bases of cost, quality, and patient satisfaction that they are included in their standard benefit package rather than priced separately as an additional benefit.

In comparison to traditional fee-for-service medicine, several positive features have been attributed to managed care (most often cohesive, integrated health plans such as well-established staff- or group-model HMOs). These features—which, if implemented effectively, parallel the model of palliative care—include[7]

- more attention to preventing medical problems,
- greater continuity of care,
- reduced levels of inappropriate treatment,
- better use of health care teams coordinated by primary care clinicians, and
- coverage of services not included in traditional health insurance.

The usual criticisms of managed care—particularly for people with chronic, progressive, or advanced illnesses—are that

---

[7]For further discussion of potential advantages and disadvantages of managed care, see, for example, Brown, 1983; IOM, 1993a, 1996b, 1997; Miles et al., 1995; Jones, 1996b.

• managed care plans have been designed primarily to serve relatively healthy and younger populations;

• they tend to attract or keep healthier individuals, while those who are less healthy stay with or move back to programs such as traditional Medicare;

• the composition of physician panels and use of other practitioners reflect the composition of the enrolled population and the plan design and thus may not match the needs of chronically ill patients;

• current capitated payment methodologies and a competitive marketplace make it very much in the financial interest of health plans to avoid enrolling patients with serious chronic illness; and

• these same financial incentives encourage underservice.

The information available to the committee primarily involves HMOs and not other forms of managed care, and very little is known specifically about care for those who are dying. Evidence of underservice or poorer outcomes is mostly speculative or anecdotal.

A few studies do, however, reinforce concerns about the effect of some managed care arrangements on people with serious chronic illness (see, e.g., Shaughnessy et al., 1994; Ware et al., 1996a, b; but also Brown et al., 1993). A recent study of a sample of frail elderly Medicare patients in a single integrated health system with both HMO and fee-for-service (FFS) patients concluded that the "HMO studied here served frail enrollees in ways that increased rather than reduced total and preventable hospital readmissions" compared to FFS beneficiaries (Experton, Li, et al., 1996, p. 1). The same researchers also found, in a related analysis, that about the same proportion of HMO and FFS patients used some home health services but that the HMO members who used home health care services received significantly fewer services than FFS members (Experton et al., 1997). The researchers suggested that the HMO should investigate premature hospital discharges and access to post-acute care" (Experton, Ozminkowski, et al., 1996). The study found no difference in total hospital days, emergency room use, or use of skilled nursing or rehabilitation services. Again, these findings are consistent with other research, which suggests possible problems in the treatment of people with serious chronic illness who need further attention from managed care plans, policymakers, and researchers.

In Minnesota, Miles and colleagues indicate that health plans ration the use of hospice care, visiting nurse care, respite care, and spiritual and psychological counseling for end-of-life care (Miles et al., 1995). He notes that such practices are "not unique to end-of-life care" but that their application to those approaching death "promises to be a hot spot" (Miles et al., 1995, p. 304).

More generally, the committee heard some concerns from hospice organizations about the practices (actual or feared) of managed care organizations. One concern expressed to the committee involved the "micromanagement" by some HMOs of care for nonMedicare patients enrolled in hospice (Murphy, 1996; Tehan, 1996). Practices mentioned included denial of certification for appropriately intensive home care or for appropriate hospitalization for palliative care. Such practices have quality as well as financial implications. They may reflect that newer managed care organizations serving mainly younger patients are unfamiliar with hospice. Thus, just as those in fee-for-service medicine may need education about palliative care and hospice programs, so may those in managed care.

REVISITING THE CARE SYSTEM AT THE COMMUNITY AND NATIONAL LEVELS

The concerns raised earlier in this chapter and the promise of initiatives such as those described in this report led the committee to consider characteristics of community care systems that would more effectively and reliably serve dying patients and their families. Such systems would offer comprehensive community health care and other resources that would permit greater integration of care across settings and more flexibility for patients, families, and clinicians. As depicted in Box 4.1, "whole-community" approaches to end-of-life care would draw on the medical and nonmedical approaches to care described in Chapter 3. They would also accommodate patients with unusual conditions and circumstances as well as those with more typical situations. The aspirations of whole-community approaches to care at the end of life include:

• making palliative care available wherever and whenever the dying patient is cared for;
• promoting timely referral to hospice for patients whose medical problems and personal circumstances make hospice care feasible and desirable;
• allowing more flexible arrangements for patients whose prognosis is less predictable but for whom palliative services would be valuable in preventing and relieving symptoms and discouraging unwanted or inappropriate life-prolonging interventions;
• encouraging, when possible, the continued involvement of personal physicians after patients' referral to hospice;
• promoting fuller and more sensitive discussion of diagnosis, prognosis, and care objectives; and, by taking these steps,
• helping dying patients and their families to plan ahead and prepare for dying and death.

BOX 4.1
A Whole-Community Model for Care at the End of Life

Programs and settings of care suited to the needs and circumstances of different kinds of dying patients

- Home hospice programs
- Other palliative care arrangements for patients who do not fit the home care model
  —Day programs in hospitals and nursing homes, similar to those developed by geriatricians
  —"Step-down" arrangements including nursing homes that permit a less intensive and less expensive level of inpatient care when appropriate
  —Specialized inpatient palliative care beds for those with severe symptoms that cannot be well managed elsewhere
  —Respite programs to relieve families of patients with a long dying trajectory (e.g., those with Alzheimer's disease) that imposes major physical and emotional burdens on families

Personnel, protocols, and other mechanisms that support high-quality, efficient, timely, and coordinated care

- Practical and valid assessment instruments and practice guidelines for patient evaluation and management that can be applied at both the individual and organizational level
- Protocols for evaluating patient's need for referral or transfer to other individual or organizational caregivers
- Procedures for implementing patient transitions in ways that encourage continuity of care, respect patient and family preferences and comfort, and assure the transfer of necessary patient information
- Consulting and crisis teams that extend and intensify efforts to allow patients to remain home despite difficult medical problems or crises
- Ongoing professional education programs fitted to the varying needs of all clinicians who care for dying patients
- Performance monitoring and improvement programs intended to identify and correct problems and to improve the average quality of care

Public and private policies, practices, and attitudes that help organizations and individuals

- Provider payment, coverage, and oversight policies that, at a minimum, do not restrict access to appropriate, timely palliative care and, as a goal, promote it
- Support systems provided through workplaces, religious congregations, and other institutions to ease the emotional, financial, and practical burdens experienced by dying patients and their families
- Public education programs that aim to improve general awareness, to encourage advance care planning, and to provide specific information at the time of need about resources for physical, emotional, spiritual, and practical caring at the end of life

The component resources of an ideal system to serve these objectives would include a mix of organizations, programs, settings, personnel, procedures, and policies. A system with these components would reflect the understanding that there is not just one way to care for dying patients. The people, tools, and other resources would need to be available in many settings and be flexible enough to respond to patients who do not comfortably fit the routines and standards that serve most patients well.

Clearly, the elements of such a whole community system represent an aspiration. The difficulties faced by those seeking to improve care at the end of life will vary from community to community, and some elements may be easier to achieve than others. Overall, however, this model implies effort on multiple levels—within individual health care and other organizations and government agencies and through cooperative community, regional, and national initiatives.

CONCLUSION

Desirable and obtainable care for those approaching death is determined by both individual and system characteristics and their interactions. The individual's disease, clinical status, emotional state, and preferences determine much about what clinical care is appropriate. Personal values, financial circumstances, family structure, and other patient or family characteristics set limits on what is possible or, at least, what is more or less difficult to accomplish.

Over these individual conditions, clinicians and health care organizations typically superimpose a template or protocol that guides but need not rigidly dictate care. The nature of this template or protocol may, in turn, be partly determined by such factors as medical culture, locale (e.g., urban or rural), supply of health care resources (e.g., hospital beds, physicians, organized hospices), delivery system integration, organizational mission and leadership, community norms, statutory requirements, research linking processes of care with outcomes, and internal and external mechanisms for monitoring and improving the quality and outcomes of care. The committee believes that many problems with care at the end of life reflect disincentives for good care and that strategies to improve care will need to focus on change at the system rather than the individual level.

As noted in Chapter 3, in reaction against medical and technological overreaching, efforts to improve care systems for the dying share certain emphases with more general efforts to make health care more patient-centered and more concerned about patients' quality of life, not just their physiology. Although it is very much concerned with systems of care, the patient-centered care perspective tends to emphasize what is desirable and appropriate for the individual patient. Quality improvement strategies tend to be more population-oriented in their emphasis on institutional goals, priority setting, and statistical analyses. Both have emerged in an environment even more strikingly characterized by efforts to cut the cost of health care under the rubric of managed care.

Overall, patient-centered, quality-improving, and cost-driven strategies for care of those with advanced or terminal illnesses may complement each other; they also may conflict. Chapter 5 considers ways of identifying how well care systems serve patients and those close to them. Chapters 6 and 7 consider some of the economic and legal factors that may support or impede good outcomes.

ADDENDUM

Physicians' Orders for Life-Sustaining Treatment
(Used with permission of the Center for Ethics in Health Care, Oregon Health Sciences University)

Note: The form as actually used is bright pink for visibility and tamper resistance.

Physician Orders
for Life-Sustaining Treatment

Last Name of Patient/Resident
First Name/Middle Initial of Patient/Resident
Patient/Resident Date of Birth

This is a physician order sheet based on patient/resident wishes and medical indications for life-sustaining treatment. If in the clinical record, this should be first page. In other settings, locate in a prominent place. When need occurs, first follow these orders, then contact physician. Any section not completed indicates full treatment.

Section A
Check One Box Only

Resuscitation. Patient/resident has no pulse and is not breathing. For all other medical circumstances, refer to "Section B, Emergency Medical Services (EMS)" listed below.

☐ Resuscitate   ☐ Do Not Resuscitate (DNR)

Section B
Check One Box Only

Emergency Medical Services (EMS)

☐ **Comfort Measures Only:** Oral and body hygiene, reasonable efforts to offer food and fluids orally. Medication, positioning, warmth, appropriate lighting and other measures to relieve pain and suffering. Privacy and respect for the dignity and humanity of the patient/resident. Transfer only if comfort measures fail.

Call 9-1-1/code only if EMS is desired:

☐ **Limited Interventions:** All care above and consider oxygen, suction, treatment of airway obstruction (manual only), wound care.

☐ **Advanced Interventions:** All care above and consider oral/nasal airway, bag-mask/demand valve, monitor cardiac rhythm, medication, IV fluids.

☐ **Full Treatment:** All care above plus CPR, intubation and defibrillation.

Other Instructions: _____

Section C
Check One Box Only

Antibiotics

☐ No antibiotics except if needed for comfort
☐ No invasive (IM/IV) antibiotics
☐ Full Treatment

Other Instructions: _____

Section D
Check One Box Only

Artificially Administered Fluids and Nutrition (oral fluids and nutrition must be offered if medically feasible)

☐ No feeding tube/IV fluids (provide other measures to assure comfort)
☐ No long term feeding tube/IV fluids (provide other measures to assure comfort)
☐ Full Treatment

Other Instructions: _____

Section E

Discussed with: ☐ Patient/Resident ☐ Health Care Representative ☐ Court-appointed Guardian
☐ Other (specify): _____

THE BASIS FOR THESE ORDERS IS:

Signature of Physician (mandatory)	Physician Name (type or print)	Time and Date Signed

© CENTER FOR ETHICS IN HEALTH CARE, Oregon Health Sciences University, 3181 SW Sam Jackson Park Rd, L101, Portland OR 97201-3098   (503) 494-4466

How to Change "Physician Orders for Life-Sustaining Treatment"

This form, "Physician Orders for Life-Sustaining Treatment," should be reviewed if:

(1) The patient/resident is transferred from one care setting to another, or
(2) There is substantial permanent change in patient/resident health status, or
(3) The patient/resident treatment preferences change.

First, review "Patient/Resident Preferences as a Guide for Physician Orders for Life-Sustaining Treatment" (Section F). Second, record the review in "Review of Physician Orders for Life-Sustaining Treatment" (Section G).

Finally, if this form is to be voided, draw a line through the "Physician Orders" and/or write the word "VOID" in large letters, then sign or initial the form. After voiding the form, a new form may be completed. *If no new form is completed, full treatment may be provided.*

Section F — **Patient/Resident Preferences as a Guide for Physician Orders for Life-Sustaining Treatment**

I have given significant thought to life-sustaining treatment. The following have further information regarding my preferences:

Advance Directive	☐ NO	☐ YES - Attach copy
Court-appointed Guardian	☐ NO	☐ YES - Attach copy of documentation

I expressed my preferences to my physician and/or health care provider(s) and agree with the treatment orders on this document. Please review these orders if there is a substantial permanent change in my health status such as:

Close to death	Advanced progressive illness
Permanently unconscious	Extraordinary suffering

Signature of Patient/Resident or Guardian/Health Care Representative (optional)

Signature of Person Preparing Form (optional)	Preparer Name (type or print)	Time and Date Prepared

---

Section G — **Review of Physician Orders for Life-Sustaining Treatment**

Date of Review	Reviewer	Location of Review	Outcome of Review
			☐ No change ☐ Changed, FORM VOIDED, new form completed ☐ Changed, FORM VOIDED, *no* new form
			☐ No change ☐ Changed, FORM VOIDED, new form completed ☐ Changed, FORM VOIDED, *no* new form
			☐ No change ☐ Changed, FORM VOIDED, new form completed ☐ Changed, FORM VOIDED, *no* new form

5

Accountability and Quality in End-of-Life Care

The days when medical care was a small private matter between patient and general practitioner are long gone and will never return.

Rashi Fein, *Medical Care, Medical Costs*, 1986

The relationship between patient and practitioner—this once small, private matter—is now enmeshed in a very large and complex system that delivers the benefits of medical progress to the people of the United States. That system depends on an often bewildering array of organizational, financial, and monitoring arrangements that link medicine, government, business, and other institutions. By fragmenting the patient-physician relationship and often putting personal physicians at a distance from their dying patients, these arrangements may diminish the knowledge and intimacy that contributes to a professional's feeling of individual responsibility. The unintentional result may be to leave no one participant clearly responsible for a patient's overall experience.

Thus, at the individual, organizational, and community level, cultivating responsibility and establishing accountability for the quality of care for patients approaching death are especially important tasks. This chapter begins by examining basic concepts of accountability and quality. It then presents evidence of quality problems in end-of-life care and reviews basic concepts of quality assessment and improvement. The discussion particularly emphasizes the importance of broadening the understanding of outcomes relevant to dying patients and those close to them. The last two sections consider instruments for measuring quality and guidelines for improving clinical practice. This discussion should be read in the context of other chapters of this report that discuss additional avenues for protecting and improving the quality of care.

This chapter—consistent with the rest of this report—emphasizes that a comprehensive strategy for improving care at the end of life must focus not only on the structures, processes, and outcomes of care but also on the environmental factors—such as laws, financing mechanisms, and educational programs—that shape the delivery of care. Unless environmental causes of poor quality care are understood and addressed, efforts to improve organizational and individual behavior may prove disappointing. In this context, quality measurement and improvement strategies should

- allow clinicians and others directly responsible for end-of-life care to evaluate and improve what they are doing on a continuing basis;
- help policymakers, patients, families, and the public to hold organizations and individuals accountable for how reliably and effectively they care for dying patients; and
- support systematic research on the effects of different clinical, organizational, and financing options for end-of-life care and on the effectiveness of alternative strategies for improving care and outcomes for patients and those close to them.

Overall, the committee concluded that more effort is warranted to assess patient experiences at the end of life; to evaluate the benefits and burdens of common end-of-life interventions (e.g., mechanical ventilation), including how they are experienced and valued by patients and families; to understand how perceptions, values, and preferences may change during the course of dying; and to improve physician understanding of patient and family preferences. As emphasized throughout this report, the knowledge base about the dying process and the effectiveness of different care strategies is limited. This, in turn, limits efforts to establish and refine standards or benchmarks against which care processes and outcomes can be assessed and improved.

CONCEPTS OF ACCOUNTABILITY AND QUALITY

Accountability

Under the banner of accountability, a variety of public and private policymakers, purchasers, health care organizations, researchers, and others have joined together to develop new methods to monitor and influence patient care in hospitals, managed care plans, and other settings. Dictionary definitions of accountability emphasize the state of being answerable or being obliged to report, explain, or justify (see, e.g., *The Amercian Heritage Dictionary*, 1993). The concept immediately raises the question—"accountability *for what?*" This report argues that health care personnel and organizations have, in general, not been held responsible for the quality of care for dying patients. In the absence of systems that can measure outcomes and identify problems across care settings, even those who identify themselves as responsible for supportive end-of-life care—palliative specialists, hospice personnel, ethics consultants, chaplains, and others—may not always know whether they are fulfilling their responsibilities.

The concept of accountability also raises the question—"accountability *to whom?*" The health professions have traditionally defined their accountability with reference to those they serve (e.g., patients, students) and to their fellow professionals and the standards of performance they have collectively created. For more than a century, however, state and federal governments in the United States have been developing regulatory mechanisms to supplement or, in some instances, replace professional accountability. A recent IOM report defined public accountability for those serving Medicare beneficiaries as involving not only beneficiaries but also "the larger public as interested parties and taxpayers" (IOM, 1996b, p. 31). In addition, private organizations, including hospitals, health plans, and other organizations, have established mechanisms of accountability. As a result, any one clinician or health care organization may be accountable to multiple parties whose expectations may not be fully compatible.

A third question—"*how* are professionals and organizations to be held accountable?"— requires a complex answer that involves a mix of social norms, regulations, economic incentives, measurement tools, and information reporting mechanisms. The notion of accountability to one's own conscience and a recognized set of ethical standards (e.g., the Hippocratic Oath or one of its successors) is appealing because it implies an internalized, ever-vigilant control mechanism. It is also part of what defines and dignifies a profession. It likewise provides a basis for trust that patients' vulnerability will not be exploited by physicians and other health professionals for "power, profit, prestige, or pleasure" (Pellegrino, 1991, p. 80). External regulations, reporting requirements, and accreditation standards have a role to play, but the imposition of external rules and monitoring does not make up for a lack of trust or trustworthiness.

The "invisible hand of the market" is yet another mechanism of accountability that relies on decisions by millions of informed consumers (and their agents) that, in theory, reward good performers and penalize poor performers. In health care, making quality a meaningful factor in such decisions is, today, an embryonic undertaking in which the quality of end-of-life care is largely invisible. Price is a more easily understood and comparable variable and the extent to which purchasers actually consider quality in their decisions is controversial.

Quality of Care

The quality of health care should contribute to the quality of living and the quality of dying but, as noted in Chapter 1, it is not synonymous with them. Another IOM committee has defined quality of care as "the degree to which health services for individuals and populations increase the likelihood of desired health outcomes and are consistent with current professional knowledge" (IOM, 1990, p. 21). This definition covers both individuals and populations, which is consistent with increasing concerns about how resources can be employed to the greatest social advantage. The definition acknowledges the relevance of professional knowledge, which includes experience and judgment as well as the important but still limited results of biomedical and clinical research. Notably, the definition deliberately omits resource constraints on the grounds that judgments of what constitutes excellent, acceptable, or unacceptable quality should be independent of constraints on resources. Decisionmakers cannot and should not, however, ignore resources in making decisions about what level of quality is desirable and affordable for a particular institution, population, or community. This means paying attention to quality and value both for those covered by public and private insurance arrangements and for those excluded from such arrangements.

Similarly, although the definition of quality of care applies generally, the specifics will differ depending on patient circumstances and goals of care. That is, the desired outcomes for a dying patient will differ in some respects from the outcomes desired when prevention of a disease is still relevant or cure is still possible. Even for patients diagnosed with incurable illnesses that are likely to prove fatal within a matter of months, the outcomes that are meaningful early in the dying trajectory (e.g., physical functioning and independence) may become less so as the progress of the disease and the imminence of death makes such outcomes less realistic and heightens the relevance of physical and emotional comfort, resolution in personal relationships, and issues of spiritual meaning or peace.

Quality Assessment and Improvement

Quality of care may be assessed in several ways (see, e.g., Donabedian, 1966; IOM, 1990; Blumenthal, 1996). Assessments may be implicit (e.g., rated by clinicians without reference to defined standards) or explicit (e.g., based on written criteria). They may be used to judge performance (e.g., rate it acceptable or unacceptable, or better or worse than for a comparable organization) or to improve performance (e.g., identify reasons for poor outcomes) or both. Assessments may be internal (e.g., clinical audits undertaken by those providing care) or external (e.g., undertaken by purchasers, government officials, or others not involved in providing care). External processes have involved such mechanisms as licensure, accreditation, information reporting, performance ratings or comparisons, inspections, and penalties for noncompliance, some of which have been evolving for over a century.

In recent years, reliance on external strategies has been criticized as costly and relatively ineffective, and strategies emphasizing internal responsibility for continuing improvement in quality have been encouraged (see, e.g., Batalden and Buchanan, 1989; Berwick, 1989; Berwick et al., 1990; IOM, 1990; Horn and Hopkins, 1994). Continuous quality improvement (CQI) models (sometimes termed Total Quality Management or TQM) are generally described in terms of a set of reinforcing principles for implementing change. These principles include targeting systemic defects (e.g., burdensome protocols for patient referral) rather than individual mistakes; encouraging close relationships among the participants in health care transactions (e.g., physicians, patients, purchasers); using planning, control, assessment, and improvement activities that are grounded in statistical and scientific precepts and techniques; feeding statistical information back to practitioners on how their practices may differ from their peers' or depart from evidence-based standards for practice; standardizing processes to reduce the opportunity for error and link specific care processes to outcomes; and striving for continuous improvement in contrast to merely meeting established goals or criteria (IOM, 1992).

Typical of quality improvement strategies reflecting these principles are the guidelines recommended by the American Pain Society for the treatment of acute pain and cancer pain (APS, 1995). The guidelines, which focus on inpatient care and address institutions rather than single individuals, are summarized in Box 5.1. They do not explicitly consider the special circumstances of dying patients but are consistent with the discussion in Chapter 3.

EVIDENCE OF QUALITY PROBLEMS IN END-OF-LIFE CARE

Conventionally, several broad types of health care quality problems have been differentiated (see, e.g., IOM, 1990). They are *overuse of care* (e.g., unwanted treatments or hospitalizations; diagnostic tests that will not inform patient care but may cause physical and emotional distress); *underuse of care* (e.g., failure to assess and treat pain; late referral for hospice care, premature hospital discharge); *poor technical performance* (e.g., errors in surgical technique); and *poor interpersonal performance* (e.g., inept communication of difficult news). In general, underuse of care is more difficult to detect than overuse. For example, in population-based analyses, it may be difficult to distinguish problems of inadequate access to care from problems of undertreatment for identified patients (IOM, 1990).

Care at the end of life is characterized by problems in each of these areas. Said differently, systems have much room to improve the extent to

---

BOX 5.1

Guidelines for Improving the Quality of Treatment for Acute Pain and Cancer Pain

- Recognize and treat pain promptly.
- Record and display patients' self report of pain at the time of their initial evaluation and after each intervention to relieve pain.
- Document processes of care and outcomes (including patient perceptions of care).
- Provide prompt feedback of process and outcomes data to the health care team.
- Make information about analgesics (e.g., potency, dosages, side effects, contraindications) easily available to all health care team members involved in writing and interpreting medication orders.
- Promise patients attentive analgesic care including verbal and written notice that pain relief is important, that patient reporting on pain is crucial, and that health care team members are accountable for responding to patient concerns (although successful pain relief cannot be absolutely promised).
- Define explicit training, competence, accountability, monitoring, and related policies for using advanced analgesic technologies (e.g., patient-controlled opioid infusion, inhaled analgesics).
- Examine the process and outcomes of pain management and seek continuous improvement through a formal, ongoing process of performance assessment and monitoring, data feedback, problem identification and process change, performance reassessment, and process revision.

SOURCE: Adapted from APS, 1995, pp. 1875–1876.

---

which they are providing the right care at the right time in the right way. Overuse and underuse of care may occur simultaneously, for example, when futile efforts to cure are continued at the expense of efforts to relieve physical and psychological symptoms and help patients and families prepare emotionally, spiritually, and practically for death. The discussion below emphasizes overuse of certain interventions (including hospitalization) and undertreatment of symptoms. Untimely referral to hospice, which has already been cited as a problem, is a form of underuse as is inattention to patient and family needs for nonmedical support. Poor technical performance, for example, miscalculation of medication dosages for pain or other symptoms, has been little studied; for purposes of this discussion it is considered an aspect of undertreatment. Problems in patient-physician communication were considered in Chapter 3, and Chapters 4, 6, 7, and 8 discuss different aspects of quality of care related to settings of care, financing mechanisms, and public policies.

The Problem of Unrelieved Symptoms

Numerous studies indicate that dying patients and patients with advanced illnesses experience considerable amounts of pain and other physical and psychological symptoms (Donovan et al., 1987; Foley, 1993; AHCPR, 1994a; Cherny et al., 1994; Miaskowski et al., 1994; Seale and Cartwright, 1994; Ward and Gordon, 1994; Donnelly and Walsh, 1995a,b; Breitbart, Rosenfeld et al., 1996; Lynn, Teno et al., 1997). Pain prevalence has been the focus of many of these studies. For example, Bonica (1990) found that 75 percent of patients with advanced cancer experienced pain; over a quarter of the patients described the pain as very severe, and 40 percent to 50 percent described it as moderate to severe. Portenoy and colleagues (1994) reported that more than 60 percent of cancer patients they studied reported pain. Several studies of nursing home patients have reported that from 40 percent to over 80 percent of nursing patients have pain (Roy and Michael, 1986; Ferrell et al., 1990; Sengstaken and King, 1993; Morley et al., 1995; Wagner et al., 1996).

The prevalence of pain is better mapped for cancer than for other diagnoses. One of the few large studies to look at a range of diagnoses (nine altogether, including three cancer diagnoses) in seriously ill hospitalized patients found severe pain reported by about 40 percent of family members of conscious patients (Lynn, Teno, et al., 1997). Pain has been reported in 30 percent to 80 percent of HIV-infected individuals with the higher levels and more persistent levels of pain reported in AIDS patients (Lebovits et al., 1989; Schofferman and Brody, 1990; Breitbart, McDonald, et al., 1996; Breitbart, 1997). Studies suggest that pain is experienced in 55 to 85 percent of patients with multiple sclerosis (Moulin, 1989). Pain is a defining characteristic of coronary artery diseases, although relief of the pain may be a less immediate priority than the diagnosis and treatment of the complications of the disease (AHCPR, 1994b).

Reports on end-of-life symptoms other than pain are more limited and, like those for pain, typically involve cancer patients. In an analysis of nine studies of cancer symptoms in the last week of life, Ingham and Portenoy (1994) found reported shortness of breath in 9 percent to 52 percent of patients, nausea in 3 percent to 71 percent of patients, vomiting in 12 to 50 percent of patients, and pain in 12 percent to 99 percent of patients (over 30 percent for 7 of the 9 studies). Donnelly and Walsh (1995b) reported that pain, fatigue, and loss of appetite were the most common and severe symptoms across a range of advanced cancers. Portenoy et al. (1994) found that 40 percent to 80 percent of the patients they studied "experienced lack of energy, pain, feeling drowsy, dry mouth, insomnia, or symptoms indicative of psychological distress" (p.183). They also found that the mean number of symptoms per patient was 11 and that the number of symptoms

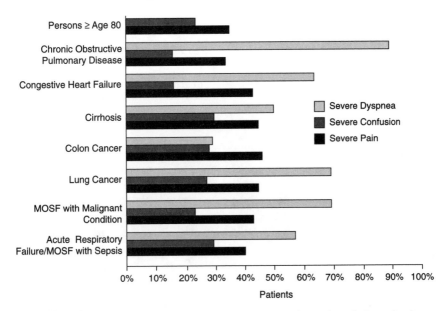

FIGURE 5.1 Rates of severe symptoms in patients three days before death, as reported by family members.

NOTE: Family members of elderly patients were not asked about dyspnea. MOSF = multiple organ system failure.
Source: Lynn, Teno et al., 1997, p. 102. Reprinted with permission from the Annals of Internal Medicine. The American College of Physicians is not responsible for the accuracy of this reprint.

was highly related to measures indicating poorer quality of life. Bruera likewise has found patients reporting multiple symptoms, with weakness, loss of appetite, and pain most common (Bruera, 1993).

The earlier cited study of hospitalized patients who were seriously ill with one of nine diagnoses reported moderate to high rates of symptoms for many patients. The results for severe pain, severe dyspnea, and severe confusion by diagnosis are presented in Figure 5.1.

A British study, which was able to compare 1987 results with an earlier 1969 study, examined symptoms for cancer and noncancer patients. The reports, presented in Table 5.1, were obtained in after-death interviews with persons identified through a sample of death certificates and determined to be knowledgeable about the decedents' care (Seale and Cartwright, 1994).

In general, prevalence and severity studies have certain limitations or characteristics that need to be recognized. For example, they are limited to

TABLE 5.1   Symptoms Reported in 1969 and 1987 for Cancer and Other Deaths in Two English Studies

	Cancer deaths (%)		Other deaths (%)		All deaths (%)	
	1969	1987	1969	1987	1969	1987
Pain	87	84	58	67[a]	66	72[a]
Trouble with breathing	47	47	44	49	45	49
Vomiting, feeling sick	54	51	21	27[a]	30	33
Sleeplessness	69	51[a]	41	36	49	40[a]
Mental confusion	36	33	36	38	36	37
Depression	45	38	31	36	36	36
Loss of appetite	76	71	37	38	48	47
Constipation	42	47	23	32[a]	28	36
Bedsores	24	28	13	14	16	18
Loss of bladder control	37	25[a]	24	55	28	23[a]
Unpleasant smell	26	19	11	13	15	14
Number of deaths (=100%)[b]	215	168	570	471	785	639

[a]Difference between 1969 and 1987 significant at the 5% level.

[b]Small numbers of deaths for whom inadequate information was available are included in the total but have been excluded from this and other tables in this book when calculating percentages.

SOURCE: Seale and Cartwright, 1994. Used with permission.

the extent that patients are unable to report symptoms because they have mental or physical problems that preclude or compromise communication.

Another limitation is that prevalence and even severity measures by themselves do not indicate the importance of a symptom to patients and families (Lynn, Teno et al., 1997). In one study of various symptoms in cancer patients, the "proportion of patients who described a symptom as relatively intense or frequent always exceeded the proportion who reported it as highly distressing" (Portenoy et al., 1994, p. 183). Thus, two patients could report the same duration, frequency, or intensity of a symptom but differ in the extent to which they found the symptom distressing or difficult to tolerate. Similarly, the same symptom may become a source of greater or lesser distress to a person as death approaches and different things become important to them.

Further, although studies reporting pain and other symptoms, particularly those involving cancer pain, are often interpreted as indicating undertreatment, some of the studies have not explicitly investigated the use, lack of use, or misuse of palliative therapies. Studies that have attempted to assess treatment directly have, however, generally found problems.

In one study that explicitly assessed pain treatment practice for cancer outpatients, Cleeland and colleagues (1994) found that 42 percent of patients were not appropriately treated. A study of ambulatory AIDS patients identified pain treatment as inadequate in 85 percent of patients; for example, strong opioids, which are recommended for patients with severe pain, were prescribed in only 8 percent of such patients (Breitbart, Rosenfeld, et al., 1996). Another study, which found pain reported by 78 percent of randomly selected patients hospitalized in an academic medical center, discovered that only 49 percent of those patients had a progress note mentioning pain in their chart (Donovan et al., 1987). Patient reports and their recording are important because caregiver recognition or estimates of pain do not necessarily match patient reports (see, e.g, Cleeland, 1989; Grossman et al., 1991; Au et al., 1994; APS, 1995).

In a study of nursing home patients, 60 percent of the patients with needs for pain management received effective pain care, whereas the rest had problems ranging from no medication to ineffective type or frequency of medication (Wagner et al., 1996). Cherny and Catane (1995) concluded that from 64 percent to 80 percent of patients admitted for palliative medicine and hospice services had inadequately relieved pain. These and other studies reporting variable pain management practices and results (Jadad and Browman, 1995; Kimball and McCormick, 1996) suggest the need for more research to understand practice patterns and their effectiveness (Wennberg, 1984, 1991).

Explicit findings of undertreatment are consistent with professional perceptions of treatment inadequacies. For example, a survey of physicians in five hospitals found that 8 of 10 physicians agreed that the most common form of narcotic abuse was undertreatment of pain (Solomon et al., 1993). In 1990, concern about unrelieved symptoms led to a statement from a National Cancer Institute workshop that "undertreatment of pain and other symptoms of cancer is a serious and neglected public health problem" (cited in AHCPR, 1994a, p. 8).

Reviews of pain research have suggested that pain can be fairly readily relieved in approximately 70 percent to 90 percent of cancer patients and that a significant proportion of the remainder can find relief short of complete sedation (see, e.g., Takeda, 1986; Walker et al., 1988; Goisis et al., 1989; Schug et al., 1990; Zech et al., 1995; Portenoy and Kanner, 1996). These and other studies also suggest that the high doses of opioids needed to relieve pain in certain patients rarely hasten death (Citron et al., 1984; Brescia et al., 1992; Wilson et al., 1992). At least one analysis of several studies of the effectiveness of the World Health Organization's pain management guidelines, however, suggested the need for more rigorous evaluation and concluded that, until then, "it would be inappropriate to judge the performance of clinicians, programs, and institutions . . ." based on whether or not they applied these specific guidelines (Jadad and Browman, 1995, p. 1872; see also WHO, 1990; Grond et al., 1991, 1993; Ventafridda et al., 1987, 1990).

Although the research base is often weaker than for pain, effective strategies also exist in many cases to relieve certain other symptoms including shortness of breath, vomiting, and depression (Cohen et al., 1991; Bruera, Miller, et al., 1992; Bruera, Schoeller, et al., 1992; Breitbart and Holland, 1993; Doyle et al., 1993; Gavrin and Chapman, 1995). Certain other problems—for example, wasting, loss of appetite, and fatigue—have proved less amenable to intervention, although Chapter 9 discusses promising directions in research for the problem of wasting and loss of appetite. Strategies to relieve these symptoms could also prolong life.

A number of comprehensive and specialized clinical guides are available to help physicians, nurses, and other health professionals provide effective palliative care for many patients.[1] These guides also suggest a number of barriers to effective palliative care beginning with inadequate clinician knowledge. Box 5.2, which is reprinted from the cancer pain guidelines of the Agency for Health Care Policy and Research (AHCPR), lists barriers to pain and the studies identifying them. It is the committee's experience that many of these barriers apply to other symptoms.

One of the major problems identified in the AHCPR pain guidelines was inadequate assessment of pain. Clinicians and researchers have developed and tested formal instruments for systematically assessing pain and thereby identifying whether change in treatment is needed. These instru-

---

[1]See Doyle et al., 1993 (and its extensive reference list); a new edition is expected in late 1997. See also Saunders and Sykes, 1993; Chernow, 1994; and Enck, 1994. See Brody et al., 1997, for an overview of comfort issues in withdrawing life-sustaining interventions.

BOX 5.2
Barriers to Cancer Pain Management

Problems related to health care professionals
- Inadequate knowledge of pain management.[1]
- Poor assessment of pain.[2]
- Concern about regulation of controlled substances.[3]
- Fear of patient addiction.[4]
- Concern about side effects of analgesics.[5]
- Concern about patients becoming tolerant to analgesics.[6]

Problems related to patients
- Reluctance to report pain.[7]
  - Concern about distracting physicians from treatment of underlying disease.
  - Fear that pain means disease is worse.
  - Concern about being a "good" patient.
- Reluctance to take pain medications.[8]
  - Fear of addiction or of being thought of as an addict.
  - Worries about unmanageable side effects.
  - Concern about becoming tolerant to pain medications.

Problems related to the health care system
- Low priority given to cancer pain treatment.[9]
- Inadequate reimbursement.[10]
- Restrictive regulation of controlled substances.[11]
- Problems of availability of treatment or access to it.[12]

---

[1] Bonica, 1985; Cleeland et al., 1986; Ferrell et al., 1992; Von Roenn et al., 1993.
[2] Grossman et al., 1991; Von Roenn et al., 1993.
[3] Weissman et al., 1991; Joranson et al., 1992; Von Roenn et al., 1993; Shapiro, 1994a, 1994b.
[4] Sacher, 1973; Bonica, 1985; Ferrell et al., 1992.
[5] Cleeland et al., 1986; Von Roenn et al., 1993.
[6] Cleeland et al., 1986; Shapiro, 1994a, 1994b.
[7] Levin et al., 1985; Dar et al., 1992; Von Roenn et al., 1993; Ward et al., 1993.
[8] Levin et al., 1985; Rimer et al., 1987; Cleeland, 1989; Hodes, 1989; Dar et al., 1992; Von Roenn et al., 1993; Ward et al., 1993; Joranson, 1994.
[9] Bonica, 1985; Max, 1990.
[10] Ferrell and Griffith, 1994; Joranson, 1994.
[11] Foley, 1985; Weissman et al., 1991; Joranson et al., 1992; Shapiro, 1994a, 1994b.
[12] Foley, 1985.

SOURCE: Adapted from AHCPR, 1994a

ments include both written or oral questions and visual or figurative elements. Some of these instruments are cited in Appendix F. In addition to their use in assessing and guiding patient care, these instruments also may be useful in monitoring provider performance and evaluating the outcomes of different types of care. As discussed in a later section of this chapter, the development of reliable and valid instruments for measuring other symptoms and determining how they affect patient well-being is a continuing need.

The Problem of Overtreatment

In the context of end-of-life care, overtreatment involves both care that is clinically inappropriate and care that is not wanted by the patient, even if some clinical benefit might be expected. Fear of unwanted treatment at the end of life is an important factor in initiatives promoting advance care planning (Emanuel, 1991; Hill and Shirley, 1992; Solomon et al., 1993). Such fear—and the loss of control it implies—may also contribute to interest in assisted suicide.

Unfortunately, documented preferences do not rule out unwanted care. For example, a study of AIDS patients reported that nearly one in two who wanted care focused on comfort were receiving aggressive curative or life prolonging treatments (Teno et al., 1991). In a large study of seriously ill hospitalized patients, about 1 patient in 10 was reported to have had care provided that was inconsistent with preferences (Lynn, Teno, et al., 1997), and doctors were often unaware of what patient preferences actually were (SUPPORT Principal Investigators, 1995). Departures from patient preferences sometimes involved more use of life-sustaining interventions than wanted and sometimes less. For the same study, investigators considered rates of medical ventilation, coma, and intensive care unit (ICU) interventions as indicators of possible inappropriate treatment in the last few days of life. In the initial phase of their study, they found that more than a third of the patients spent at least 10 days in the ICU and nearly half received mechanical ventilation during their last 3 days of life.

Another study that surveyed physicians at five hospitals on a number of issues in end-of-life care found that 55 percent of those surveyed felt that they sometimes provided "overly burdensome" treatments to patients, whereas only 12 percent said they sometimes gave up too soon on patients (Solomon et al., 1993, p. 16). Overall, when asked about the inappropriate use (but not inappropriate underuse) of several treatments, a majority expressed concern about mechanical ventilation, cardiopulmonary resuscitation, artificial nutrition and hydration, and dialysis. Each of these interventions has been the subject of considerable debate about the circumstances under which their use promises no or virtually no benefit.

Much of the recognition of overtreatment stems from countless personal experiences, some documented in print, others conveyed in conversation. In general, the committee concluded that concern about overuse of certain kinds of advanced technologies at the end of life is warranted. Given current cost containment pressures, it will, however, be important to monitor for signs of increasing underuse of such interventions. In addition, it would be useful to understand whether one factor in overtreatment is clinician uncertainty about or unfamiliarity with effective palliative care strategies, including methods of withdrawing mechanical ventilation and other life-sustaining technologies so as to cause minimum distress to patients and families (Brody et al., 1997).

DIMENSIONS OF QUALITY IN CARE AT THE END OF LIFE

The literature on quality of care has traditionally distinguished three dimensions for analysis: structure, process, and outcome (Donabedian, 1966, 1980; IOM, 1990). The emphasis in recent years has been increasingly on the outcomes of care, but quality improvement requires an understanding of how structures and processes interact with environmental and patient characteristics to produce outcomes (see, e.g., Chassin et al., 1986; IOM, 1990; Lohr, 1992; Fowler, 1995; Berwick, 1996; Blumenthal, 1996; Brook et al., 1996). Several analyses have recently focused attention on how these concepts can be useful in strategies to measure, monitor, and improve the quality of care for those approaching death (Byock, 1996; Merriman, 1996; Stewart, 1996; Teno, 1996b; AGS, 1997; Donaldson, 1997; Stewart et al., *forthcoming*).

Table 5.2 depicts the committee's general conceptualization of structure, process, and patient/family outcomes and the larger environmental context as they relate to care at the end of life (see Stewart et al., *forthcoming*, and Patrick, *forthcoming*, for alternative conceptualizations). (Economic outcomes, including expenditures for end-of-life care, are discussed in Chapter 5.)

Structures and processes of care are not neatly separable categories, but they can be generally distinguished for purposes of discussion. For analyses intended to identify contributors to good and bad outcomes, the focus is on specific variables (e.g., staffing level or pain management) and their potential for manipulation rather than on their label.

In contrast to structure and process measures, the environmental elements are essentially "givens" rather than variables that can be manipulated by those directly responsible for care at the end of life. Such elements may be particularly important for those with advanced illness. For example, a person who lives alone in a rural area where outpatient or home care resources are scarce may very well face a higher likelihood of institu-

TABLE 5.2 Dimensions of Quality in Care of Dying Patients and Related Quality Strategies

Context	Structures	Processes	Outcomes
Culture, norms, social institutions	Care settings (home, institution)	Establishing diagnosis and prognosis	Physical (symptoms, function)
Demographic	Personnel (staff, volunteers, numbers, training)	Establishing goals and plans	Psychological (emotional, cognitive)
Geography	Clinical policies (protocols, guidelines)	Providing palliative and other patient care	Spiritual
Economic system, resources	Information and decision support systems	Caring for families, bereavement care	Perceptions of care, burden of care
Political system, policies, regulations	Financial policies (free care, target profit levels)	Coordinating care including transfers among settings	Dignity, control over decisionmaking
Individual and family characteristics		Monitoring, improving care	Survival

tionalization than a city resident living with a family member. An affluent community is likely to support more health care institutions and services and attract better trained personnel, although high-technology medical centers are not necessarily better than (or as good as) community hospitals at providing supportive and appropriate care.

Structural Aspects of Quality of Care

The link between specific health care structures and outcomes is a matter of continuing dispute based on modest and sometimes conflicting research (see, for example, IOM, 1986; Mor, 1987; Relman, 1988; IOM, 1990; Lansky, 1993; SUPPORT Principal Investigators, 1995; IOM, 1996c).

Nonetheless, because structural elements are such visible and intrinsic elements of organized caregiving, the effort to identify and establish how structures affect outcomes is understandable. This effort is undergirded by a network of organizations and procedures for establishing consensus on structural standards and for accrediting or otherwise certifying that health care facilities, organizations, and personnel meet these standards.

Several organizations, including the Health Care Financing Administration, the Joint Commission on Accreditation of Healthcare Organizations, and the National Hospice Organization, have identified a variety of structural characteristics thought to increase the likelihood that dying patients will be served well. These characteristics, which generally have been emphasized hospices, have been set forth in the Medicare program's conditions of participation, materials for voluntary accreditation or certification, and documents of technical assistance. They typically involve written institutional policies related to such matters as staff credentials and composition, advance care planning, emergency response procedures, information systems, safe physical environments, and governing mechanisms that protect and respect patients.

Notwithstanding a general interest in structural elements of quality care, the mere existence of regulations and policies does not guarantee their conversion into desired processes or outcomes of care. This is another reason for the interest in continuous quality improvement strategies that focus on internal rather than external mechanisms of quality assessment and assurance.

Care Processes and Quality

Processes of care have been a major focus of public and private efforts intended to improve health outcomes (Donabedian, 1966, 1982; IOM, 1990; Wilson and Cleary, 1995; Wilson and Kaplan, 1995). The same holds true for care at the end of life (see, e.g., Doyle et al., 1993; Higginson, 1993; SUPPORT Principal Investigators, 1995; Tolle, 1996a). The broad process dimensions set forth in Table 5.2 reflect the discussion in Chapter 3 and do not identify specific variables—such as elements of pain management—that might be considered in assessing the quality of care in a particular setting. Assessments also may consider utilization statistics for various services (e.g., home nursing visits, emergency transfers, diagnostic tests, length of hospital stay) as indicators of care processes.

Sometimes, process-of-care measures (e.g., rates of influenza immunization for elderly people) are relied on as proxies for outcomes (e.g., rates of influenza and its complications) when outcomes data are unavailable or too demanding to collect with available resources. Process measures are, however, important in their own right as they help evaluators to understand how care is provided, how an intervention changes other aspects of the care process, and how processes might be improved to achieve better patient outcomes or greater efficiency. For example, the SUPPORT study, which is discussed at several points in this report, was a process intervention intended to improve decisionmaking for very seriously ill patients (SUPPORT Principal Investigators, 1995; see also the *Hastings Center Report*, Special Supplement, Vol. 25, No. 6, 1995).

Furthermore, it has been suggested that "some processes are valued more than [some] outcomes" (Teno, 1996b, p. 8). Communication with patients and families and responsiveness to their desires to be involved in decisionmaking are examples of highly valued processes. More generally, when cure or prolonged life are no longer dominant goals, the processes of caring for the body, mind, and spirit affirm the dignity and value of those approaching death and can be appreciated in and of themselves.

Broadening the Understanding of Outcomes

The limitations of mortality rates and physiological indicators (e.g., blood pressure) as measures of health outcomes or quality of care have been pointed out in other contexts (see, e.g., IOM, 1990; Patrick and Bergner, 1990; Patrick and Erickson, 1993). It is particularly obvious that other measures are necessary for examining the quality of patient and family care at the end of life. As one committee member phrased it in discussing her critical care practice, "if the quality of care in my palliative care practice were judged by mortality rates, I would look pretty bad because 85 percent of my patients die." Similarly, nursing home administrators trying to reduce inappropriate hospitalizations of dying patients have particular reason to be concerned that mortality data be used carefully in judging their performance.

Caution is particularly important when outcomes are linked to reimbursement for care. If severity of illness and other patient characteristics are inadequately considered, outcome measurements may lead to mistaken judgments about quality of care and may inappropriately reward those who achieve good scores because they avoid less healthy people (Thomas and Ashcraft, 1989, 1991; Iezzoni, 1992; IOM, 1993a; Hopkins and Carroll, 1994).

Although a focus on measures other than mortality might seem to deflect attention from death, it instead underscores that a lot more happens to most dying people than the specific event of their death. Nonetheless, the understanding of what it means to live well while dying and how to measure the quality of dying remains at an early stage.

Outcomes as experienced by patients are increasingly being recognized by clinicians and researchers. Many commonly used physiological indicators (e.g., blood pressure, cholesterol level) may not be strongly linked to outcomes as experienced by patients. Thus, outcomes related to physical and mental functioning and well-being must be identified to evaluate the impact of social, economic, medical, and other actions intended to improve individual or population health. For those approaching death, common measures of function and well-being may have only limited relevance. Conversely, measures that are particularly sensitive to the experiences of older people may not be as well suited to younger people with advanced illnesses.

In reviewing the hospice literature, Mor (1987) identified several categories of outcomes for attention. They include pain and other symptoms, performance status, satisfaction with care, psychosocial state, secondary morbidity, and site of death. A more expansive listing has been proposed by the American Geriatrics Society (AGS) as part of its efforts to focus attention on the quality of end-of-life care (AGS, 1997) (see Box 5.3). The AGS list, which has been endorsed by more than 30 organizations, includes both outcomes (e.g., satisfaction) and aspects of care processes (e.g., advance planning, aggressive care near death). To focus more narrowly on patient and family outcomes, the committee identified major categories of outcomes relevant to assessments of the quality of life for dying patients. The six categories summarized in Table 5.3 mostly parallel the dimensions of care discussed in Chapter 3 but extend them somewhat. For example, a patient's overall quality of life can be expected to reflect the patient's physical, emotional, spiritual, and practical circumstances, including those that are not specifically a function of their health status or health care. In addition, patient and family perceptions of care are increasingly recognized as important in their own right.

MEASUREMENT INSTRUMENTS AND ISSUES

It is axiomatic in the continuous quality improvement literature that "if you don't measure it, you can't improve it." To that end, a number of instruments for measuring quality of care and patient status and well-being have been developed, and work to adapt these instruments or develop others helpful in improving care for seriously ill and dying patients is proceeding on many fronts. An August 1996 workshop, convened in conjunction with the committee's August meeting, examined many instruments for measuring and assessing outcomes and quality of care in the context of quality improvement for care at the end of life. One objective was to propose a preliminary "toolkit" of instruments to measure end-of-life care (Teno, 1996b). The committee was able to read the papers drafted for the workshop, participate in the workshop, and review the workshop summary and initial recommendations. (For more information see Appendix F and www.gwu.edu/~cicd/TOOLKIT.HTM). The committee concluded that the

BOX 5.3
Quality Domains Suggested by the American Geriatric Society

Physical and emotional symptoms. Pain, shortness of breath, fatigue, depression, fear, anxiety, nausea, skin breakdown, and other physical and emotional problems often destroy the quality of life at its end. Symptom management is regularly deficient. Care systems should focus upon these needs and ensure that people can count on a comfortable and meaningful end of their lives.

Support of function and autonomy. Even with the inevitable and progressive decline with fatal illness, much can be done to maintain personal dignity and self-respect. Achieving better functional outcomes and greater autonomy should be valued.

Advance care planning. Often, the experience of patient and family can be improved just by planning ahead for likely problems, so that decisions can reflect the patient's preferences and circumstances rather than responding to crises.

Aggressive care near death—site of death, CPR, and hospitalization. Although aggressive care is often justified, most patients would prefer to have avoided it when the short-term outcome is death. High rates of medical interventions near death should prompt further examination of provider judgment and care system design.

Patient and family satisfaction. The dying patient's peace of mind and the family's perception of the patient's care and comfort are extremely important. In the long run, we can hope that the time at the end of life will be especially precious, not merely tolerable. We must measure both patient and family satisfaction with these elements: the decisionmaking process, the care given, the outcomes achieved, and the extent to which opportunities were provided to complete life in a meaningful way.

preliminary toolkit was indeed just that, preliminary and awaiting refinement. It recommended an extensive process of testing, adapting, and developing instruments that are (1) relevant to the experiences of dying patients and those close to them, (2) sensitive to the effects of changes in care, and (3) efficient and practical to use. Additional collaborative work to develop this toolkit is planned.

Instruments

Dozens, even hundreds, of instruments exist to measure health status or quality of life (McDowell and Newell, 1996). For example, one recent review reported 159 different instruments used in the 75 articles analyzed (Gill and Feinstein, 1994). Some were fairly narrow (e.g., hand grip strength,

Global quality of life. Often a patient's assessment of overall well-being illuminates successes and shortcomings in care that are not apparent in more specific measures. Quality of life can be quite good despite declining physical health, and care systems that achieve this should be valued.

Family burden. How health care is provided affects whether families have serious financial and emotional effects from the costs of care and the challenges of direct caregiving. Current and future pressures on funding health care are likely to displace more responsibility for services and payment onto families.

Survival time. With pressures upon health care resources likely to increase, there is new reason to worry that death will be too readily accepted. Purchasers and patients need to know how survival times vary across plans and provider systems. In conjunction with information about symptoms, satisfaction, and the other domains listed here, such measures will allow insights into the priorities and tradeoffs within each care system.

Provider continuity and skill. Only with enduring relationships with professional caregivers can patient and family develop trust, communicate effectively, and develop reliable plans. The providers also must have the relevant skills, including rehabilitation, symptom control, and psychological support. Care systems must demonstrate competent performance on continuity and provider skill.

Bereavement. Often health care stops with the patient's death, but the suffering of the family goes on. Survivors may benefit with relatively modest interventions.

SOURCE: AGS, 1997.

word recall) whereas others (e.g., Sickness Impact Profile) were more comprehensive. Some instruments have been tested and validated in end-of-life care; most have not. A few are designed for use with family members. Box 5.4 presents some illustrative items that were selected to indicate the kinds of questions being asked of seriously ill or dying patients and their families.

Various groups (IOM, 1990; Medical Outcomes Trust, 1995; Stewart, 1996; Lynn, 1997) have defined attributes of useful measures. Box 5.5 offers one widely cited list, which combines technical and practical methodological considerations. The main focus of the committee was more on clinical and research uses of measures than on external performance monitoring and rating.

TABLE 5.3 Categories of Patient/Family Outcome Measures for End-of-Life Care

Overall quality of life	Spiritual well-being
• Overall experience of living as perceived by patient	• Continued meaning in life • Composure despite physical distress • Readiness for death • Religious or philosophical peace
Physical well-being and functioning	Patient perceptions of care
• Specific symptoms (description or rating; "bothersomeness") • Overall comfort or distress (not just frequency or intensity of symptoms) • Functioning (given the stage of illness)	• Overall satisfaction with care • Technical and physical aspects (e.g., prevention and relief of symptoms, surroundings) • Interpersonal aspects (e.g., sensitivity of caregivers, continuity, information provided) • Consistency with patient preferences (e.g., site of care, therapies)
Psychosocial well-being and functioning	Family well-being and perceptions (before and after patient's death)
• Cognitive status • Emotional status • Social interactions • Self-image • Sense of control and dignity	• Emotional status of family members • Economic status of family • Adequacy of information and decisionmaking process • Perceptions of care provided patient • Perceptions of care provided family including bereavement support

Measurement Issues and Problems

Developing measures of patient status or quality of care that meet these requirements is a significant challenge for any arena of health care (see, e.g., Ware et al., 1988; Fowler et al., 1994), but measures appropriate to the special circumstances of dying patients and their caregivers present particular problems (Mor, 1987; Cella and Tulsky, 1990; Cohen and Mount, 1992; Byock, 1996; Ingham, 1996; Merriman, 1996; Puchalski, 1996; Roach, 1996; Stewart, 1996; Teno, 1996b; Wilkinson, 1996; Donaldson, 1997). Some problems are most relevant to ongoing quality assessment by organizations delivering care, whereas others apply mainly to researchers (see Chapter 9). Several of the problems have contributed to the reluctance of external performance monitoring or certifying organizations to include indicators important for dying patients.

Consistent with the discussion of undertreatment, pain measures have been more extensively developed and evaluated than measures for other symptoms common among people approaching death. The strategies employed in developing, testing, and refining pain assessment instruments have provided useful models and lessons for those working in other areas. Among the issues that have been identified for a variety of symptoms and circumstances are the following.

The Timing of Assessments

Timing involves two questions: when and how often to schedule assessments of patient and family experiences and perceptions. At a minimum, the committee believes that it is important to try to make assessments when death is expected within a few weeks, although this will not always be possible. Such assessments may include questions that extend back in time (e.g., to diagnosis); accuracy with respect to events may thereby suffer but the perceptions are still important. Nonetheless, because predictions of death are so imprecise, some patients may be evaluated three days before death, others three weeks before death, and others not at all. In addition, many patients will be unable to be interviewed because of cognitive impairment or some other reason. Thus, interviews with families may be important as a source of more representative information on patients' experiences—as well as on their own experience before and after their loved one's death (Addington-Hall and McCarthy, 1993).

Frequent assessments of symptoms may be integral to ongoing effective management of pain and other symptoms. Indeed, proponents of better pain management have urged that pain be regarded as a fourth vital sign (in addition to breathing, heartbeat, and blood pressure). The Edmonton Symptom Assessment System (ESAS), which was designed to chart nine symptoms for cancer inpatients, is intended for use twice a day and is designed to be quick and easy to use and interpret (Bruera and McDonald, 1993). Such charting may both guide day-to-day care and allow patterns of care (e.g., good versus poor symptom control) to be assessed from patient records.

Frequent assessment may not always be either possible or the best use of limited resources. For example, an extensive home and inpatient palliative auditing process developed in England calls for audits at the time of referral and then weekly (Higginson, 1993). Even with this system, early experience in its use found that audits were often missed for items related to financial matters, spiritual status, family anxiety, and communication between family and patient. In addition, a comprehensive assessment may be

BOX 5.4
Illustrative Examples of Items Proposed to Measure Individual Perceptions or Experiences

Overall quality of life
• Considering all parts of my life—physical, emotional, social, spiritual, and financial—my quality of life in the past two days was [very bad to excellent 10-point scale]. (McGill Quality of Life Questionnaire*)
• During the past 30 days, for about how many days did poor physical or mental health keep you from doing your usual activities, such as self-care, work, or recreation? [Space for number of days, plus options for "none," "don't know/not sure," and "refused."] (Centers for Disease Control Behavioral Risk Factor Surveillance Survey)

Symptoms
• During the past week, did you have any of the following symptoms? [List of 12 symptoms] If yes, how often did you have it? [4 points from rarely to almost constantly.] If yes, how severe was it usually? [4 points from slight to very severe.] If yes, how much did it distress or bother you? [5 points from not at all to very much.] (Memorial Symptom Assessment Score*)

Functioning
• Assistance [needed] with bathing (include getting supplies, supervising). [4 responses from none to must be bathed.] (Rapid Disability Rating Scale-2*)

Planning and preferences for care
• Have you and your doctor made a plan that makes sure you are not in pain or other discomfort while dying? [Yes/no.] (Teno)

difficult given that many patients are referred for palliative care very late in their illness, when the effort to help may take precedence over the effort to assess quality or outcomes. Assessment may also be difficult for patients whose probability of death is sufficiently unpredictable that they are not categorized as dying, referred to hospice or similar programs, or otherwise "captured" by those attempting to assess the quality of care. One result is that assessments are often made retrospectively—after a patient's death and using recorded data or surrogates—rather than during the dying process.

The Role of the Patient or a Surrogate as a Source of Patient Information

Seriously ill and dying patients may not be able to report for themselves because of the physical or mental impairments produced by their illness. Even a patient who can articulate that "it hurts" may not be able to rate current or recent pain in the ways required by an assessment instrument. In addition, as noted earlier, the timing of death is not easily predicted. The

- During the last week of (the patient's) life, did he/she prefer a course of treatment that focused on extending life as much as possible, even if it meant more pain and discomfort, or on a plan of care, that focused on relieving pain and discomfort as much as possible, even if that meant not living as long? To what extent were these wishes or preferences followed in the medical treatment he/she received during the last month of life? [5 point scale from not at all to a great deal.] (SUPPORT)

Experience of care
- Were you given confusing or contradictory information about your health or treatments? (Picker Institute CONT1.6*)
- Did you ever request pain medicine? [Yes/no.] How many minutes after you requested pain medicine did it usually take before you got it? [7 points ranging from right away to never got medicine.] (Picker Institute MS2.0*)
- As much as I wanted them to, members of the hospital staff asked how I was feeling and tried to comfort me. [Agree/disagree.] (SUPPORT)

Spirituality
- I believe that God loves me and cares about me. [6 points from strongly agree to strongly disagree.] (Spiritual Well-Being Scale)
- It is important to me to feel that my life has meaning. [5 points from agree to disagree.] (Missoula/VITAS*)

---

*Used with permission.
SOURCE: As indicated above and in more detail in Appendix F.

question thus arises whether a surrogate—someone such as a family member or a caregiver—can provide reliable and valid information on the patient's experience. Some studies suggest that surrogates tend to report more distress than do patients (Higginson et al., 1994). Note that the issue here is whether surrogates can "speak" for patients, not what they say about their own status or experience, which is important to assess in its own right.

The committee urges continued research to assess the degree to which patient and surrogates perceptions match (when both can be measured), the extent to which different surrogates provide different reports, the reasons for differences, and the bases for choosing a proxy. Such research is neither simple nor inexpensive but is a high priority for quality assessment and improvement for patients approaching death.

BOX 5.5
Desirable Attributes of Outcomes Assessment Instruments
Based on Criteria Developed by the Medical Outcomes Trust

Conceptual and measurement model: (a) "underlying rationale for and description of the concepts that the measure is intended to assess and the relationships between or among those concepts" and (b) "the instrument's scale and subscale structure and the procedures that are used to create the scale scores"

Reliability: "the degree to which an instrument is free of random error" or, less formally, the stability of results when the instrument is used by different raters or at different times

Validity: "the degree to which an instrument measures what it purports to measure"

Responsiveness: "an instrument's ability to detect change in outcomes that matter" to patients, clinicians, or relevant others

Interpretability: "the degree to which one can assign qualitative meaning—that is, clinical or commonly understood connotations—to qualitative scores"

Respondent and administrative burden: these involve "the time, energy, financial resources, personnel, or other resources required" of respondents or those administering the instruments

Alternative forms: "all the ways in which the instrument might be administered other than in the original ways" (e.g., to proxies rather than patients)

Cultural and language adaptations: the degree of "conceptual and linguistic equivalence between the original instrument and its adaptations"

———————

SOURCE: Medical Outcomes Trust, 1995 (material in quotes); Lohr et al., 1996.

The Relative Emphasis on Ratings of Satisfaction versus Reports About Care

Measures of satisfaction with care are widely used and sometimes relied on entirely or primarily as indicators of quality of care. Such measures have a variety of limitations, particularly those instruments that are developed informally without systematic validation (Ware, 1978; Ware and Hays, 1988; Ware et al., 1988; Ahorony and Strasser, 1993; Gerteis et al., 1993). One problem is that the gap between categories in typical rating scales (e.g., between excellent and very good or between points 4 and 5 on a five-point scale) may be different than suggested by the words or numbers used to describe categories (Ware and Hays, 1983; Teno, 1996a; Allen Russell, Center for Health Research, personal communication, May 1996; see more generally, discussions of interval and ordinal measurement in Blalock, 1979; Kerlinger, 1986). For example, the difference between a service rated excellent (or 5) versus very good (4) may be more important than the difference between a very good (4) versus a good (3) rating—both to caregivers and to competitors in a vigorous market. Indeed, those who rate a service as "only" very good or good may actually have serious concerns that the simple ratings do not reveal.

One response to the apparent limitations of ratings is to emphasize patients' reports about care (e.g., whether different options for care were explained) (Cleary et al., 1991; Gerteis et al., 1993; Teno, 1996a,b). Although this approach may be somewhat more demanding, it has the advantage of providing more specific perceptions that may be useful in correcting problems. At this time, it seems reasonable to suggest that both ratings and reports be tested (Teno, 1996a).

The Scope and Depth of the Instrument

This chapter has outlined many dimensions of end-of-life care and quality of life that warrant assessment. Unfortunately, the circumstances of many dying patients—including physical and mental status, location in a home rather than institutional setting, and family problems—may make it difficult to ask any questions, much less a large number of them. That is one reason for interest in identifying one or two indicators (e.g., patient's or surrogate's report of overall satisfaction or inadequately relieved pain) that are both attention getting and likely to point to broader quality problems. Depending on the purpose of an assessment (e.g., everyday patient care, research project), the selection of questions may vary.

The Relevance of Measures of Function

Measures of physical and psychological functioning are widely used to assess well-being and outcomes of care for people suffering from chronic illnesses or impairments, being treated for serious medical problems, undergoing function-impairing treatments, or even experiencing relatively good health. For people with advancing, eventually fatal medical problems, the relevance of particular functional indicators or capacities may change as their illness progresses. At an early stage of illness, for example, the ability to drive may seem paramount; later the ability to get out of bed may be a primary concern. How assessment instruments and their interpretation should reflect these kinds of changes needs further investigation.

The Meaning of Symptoms

Although some symptoms are more evident to observers than others (e.g., vomiting or incontinence versus pain or fatigue), the meaning of symptoms to patients and their impact on overall quality of life are intrinsically subjective (Ward and Gordon, 1996). Some may find pain or incontinence terribly distressing; others may be less affected. Some may find pain less distressing than any mental haziness induced by medications. As discussed in Chapter 1, suffering has dimensions beyond specific physical or psychological indicators. Some outcomes measures ask patients or others to assess symptoms by rating them on a descriptive scale (e.g., from no pain to severe pain). Others ask for an assessment of the effect of the symptom on the patient (e.g., from no pain to pain that is severe, continuous, and overwhelming in its impact on physical or cognitive functioning) (Higginson, 1993).

Sensitivity to Change or Differences in Patient Status

To be useful in guiding quality improvement, instruments should provide interpretable and meaningful information about changes in patient status that may occur as a function of disease or treatment. They should also be sensitive to the range of differences in patients whose care is being assessed. Some instruments are designed primarily for use in relatively healthy populations and may not capture some outcomes relevant to people with progressive debilitating or life-threatening conditions. This has been a problem with "report cards" that attempt to provide overall ratings for managed care plans but do not consider services and outcomes for people with serious acute and chronic medical problems.

The Need for Disease- or Condition-Specific Measures.

Not only the stage of illness but the nature of the illness itself may be relevant to the choice of quality or outcomes measures. In addition, providers of care may be more proficient in caring for some kinds of illnesses (e.g., cancer) than others (e.g., Alzheimer's disease). The importance of condition-specific measures is an empirical question that can, in principle, be answered by testing instruments for reliability and validity across different patient conditions. Only a few instruments have been subjected to such investigation. Some instruments were originally developed for particular categories of patients (e.g., the Health Assessment Questionnaire for arthritis patients) whereas others were not. In either case, the instruments may or may not have been used, tested, or adapted for different kinds of patients. Patient differences by diagnosis may diminish as death is thought to be imminent, in which case disease-specific measures may be less relevant at this stage.

Although measures of symptoms and satisfaction with care raise a variety of problems, spiritual constructs may be particularly troublesome both to define and translate into operational measures (Mor, 1987). A literature review by Puchalski (1996) identified 30 potential instruments for assessing spirituality or spiritual well-being. Several generally used quality of life measurement instruments include questions on spirituality. In the context of end-of-life issues, spiritual well-being has been defined in essentially nonreligious terms as "meaningful existence, ability to find meaning in daily experience, ability to transcend physical discomfort, readiness for death" (Stewart, 1996). Some measures of these qualities have been incorporated and tested in instruments for assessing end-of-life care (Byock, 1996; Merriman, 1996).

In addition to working with hospitals and hospices providing palliative care, researchers developing quality of life, quality of dying, and quality of care measures for dying patients should seek other ways to extend experience with different measures and populations. One strategy would be to continue to press the National Institutes of Health to require quality of life measures in a greater range of clinical trials and to analyze the experience of patients who die under both experimental and control protocols. The committee makes such a recommendation in Chapter 9.

GUIDELINES FOR CLINICAL PRACTICE

Recent years have seen considerable interest in the use of clinical practice guidelines to improve the appropriateness, effectiveness, and cost-effectiveness of care (see, e.g., Brook et al., 1986; Chassin et al., 1986; Lohr et al., 1986; PPRC, 1988, 1989; Roper et al., 1988; Audet et al., 1990; and IOM, 1990, 1992).[2] Practice guidelines have the potential to contribute to quality of care for dying patients in several ways as part of multifaceted quality improvement strategies.

First, by describing specific processes of care identified as effective, guidelines may improve the technical provision of care. Although experience, physical skill, attention to detail, and similar factors contribute to technical proficiency, good performance also depends on a solid under-

---

[2]Another IOM committee has defined clinical practice guidelines as "systematically developed statements to assist practitioner and patient decisions about appropriate care for specific clinical circumstances" (IOM, 1992, p. 2). Clinical guidelines may be focused on procedures (e.g., cardiopulmonary resuscitation), symptoms (e.g., pain), or illnesses (e.g., congestive heart failure). The IOM has recommended, in general, an emphasis on medical conditions rather than procedures.

standing of what constitutes effective care (e.g., selection of analgesic or route of administration) or correct performance of a technical task (e.g., giving an injection). To the extent that the evidence base is weak, as it is for much end-of-life care, the potential of guidelines to improve care is reduced. In any case, to inform potential users, guidelines should be accompanied by documentation of (a) the strength of the evidence and consensus associated with specific recommendations and (b) the processes and participants involved in developing the guidelines (IOM, 1992).

Second, guidelines that explicitly and clearly describe appropriate care for particular clinical problems such as management of specific symptoms provide a basis for problem identification and correction. Thus, they can help those responsible for detecting patterns of undertreatment (e.g., failure to prescribe pain medications at all or in sufficient amounts and frequencies) or overtreatment (e.g., use of artificial hydration when ice chips and glycerin swabs would be more comfortable for a patient nearing death).

Third, guidelines that include good explanations of possible outcomes (e.g., potential benefits and burdens of a third course of chemotherapy) can contribute to better communication and shared decisionmaking on the part of patients and practitioners. Guidelines that specify expected outcomes also provide a tool for comparing care in different settings and assessing the effectiveness of different or new interventions.

Unfortunately, the lack of interest in dying patients that is noted throughout this report is reflected in the scarcity of guidelines for end-of-life care and in the lack of a strong evidence base for developing such guidelines. Some guidelines for symptom management, for example, those for treating cancer pain, may be useful with patients approaching death, although they may not be sensitive to the shifting and balancing of goals of care that occurs as patients near death. Other guidelines focus on ethical and legal rather than clinical aspects of end-of-life care. For example, when the Milbank Memorial Fund sponsored a meeting of specialty societies in September 1996 to review clinical guidelines relevant to end-of-life care and to discuss areas for future work, almost all the examples it received from meeting participants dealt with ethical issues such as informed consent and surrogate decisionmaking.

The committee did not attempt a systematic review of guidelines, but it did review examples of guidelines for managing life-threatening illnesses that might be expected to discuss evaluation and management of the end stage of the illness. Many were silent. For example, guidelines for diagnosis and management of unstable angina developed by a private, government-funded panel do not cite advance care planning or end-of-life concerns in the discussion of patient counseling, the algorithms for medical management or cardiac procedures, or the index (AHCPR, 1994b). For heart failure guidelines (AHCPR, 1994c), the discussion of patient/family counseling refers to advance directives and advice for family members in the event of sudden death. The guidelines do not, however, cover care for patients for whom invasive therapy is rejected and medical management is failing.

Somewhat more cognizant of care issues involving patients near the end of life are several guidelines for nursing home care issued by the American Medical Directors Association (AMDA). These guidelines used several AHCPR guidelines as the basis for statements on depression, heart failure, pressure ulcers, and urinary incontinence (AMDA, 1996). The preface explicitly states that the guidelines usually assume that recovery or rehabilitation is the goal of care but that this is not always the case. For example, for patients for whom palliation of symptoms is the primary goal of care, the AMDA guidelines note that standard care (e.g., to undertake a comprehensive diagnostic workup for incontinence) may be foregone to minimize distress (e.g., avoid pain) based on a specific assessment of the benefits and burdens for an individual patient.

Considerable experience with practice guidelines has reinforced the observation that the availability of guidelines does not ensure their implementation (Eisenberg, 1986; Lomas, 1991; Lomas et al., 1991; Foley, 1995; Bookbinder et al., in press). Although new educational strategies such as academic detailing[3] are being tested as part of guidelines implementation strategies, additional approaches appear necessary to implement guidelines in ways that improve outcomes including relief of pain and other symptoms (IOM, 1992; AHCPR, 1994a; APS, 1995). These approaches include

- providing for clinician participation in the development of guidelines (to encourage "buy-in");
- incorporating guidelines in continuous quality improvement initiatives that include feedback of statistical information on organizational and clinician performance;
- integrating guidelines and outcomes measures into computer-based patient information and decision support systems; and
- linking acceptance of guidelines and compliance to health plan contracting requirements or financial incentives.

Such approaches would, in general, appear relevant both for organizations that care for a broad range of patients and those that focus more

---

[3]Academic detailing has been described as including several steps (Avorn and Soumerai, 1983 and Soumerai and Avorn, 1990). These include: interviews to establish baseline knowledge and motivation associated with a practice; programs focused on specific categories of physicians and their opinion leaders; clearly stated educational and behavioral objectives; sponsorship by a respected organization; use of authoritative and unbiased information and concise graphic materials; repetition of essential messages; active participation by physicians; and positive feedback on improved practices.

specifically on care at the end of life. Just like guidelines themselves, the effectiveness of implementation strategies cannot be assumed but must, instead, be evaluated. This process has begun in some areas of end-of-life care (see, e.g., Dietrick-Gallagher et al., 1994; Ward and Gordon, 1994, 1996).

CONCLUSION

This chapter has stressed the importance of cultivating responsibility and establishing accountability for the quality of care for patients approaching death. Central to both tasks is information that can be used to measure outcomes and quality of care, identify and correct problems, and improve system and individual performance. Methods of quality measurement and improvement are works in progress throughout the health care system. For care at the end of life, these methods are, by and large, at a fairly early stage of development. Taken together, however, various available methods and instruments do begin to capture some aspects of what Chapter 1 set forth as elements of a decent or good death—a death free from avoidable distress and suffering; in general accord with patient and family wishes; and reasonably consistent with clinical and ethical standards.

The committee here has emphasized that there is a role for both internal and external quality assurance and improvement mechanisms including guidelines for clinical practice. In general, it accepts the argument that efforts should focus on the identification and correction of systemic problems rather than searching narrowly for individual bad actors. It has stressed the importance of outcomes measures but also acknowledged that it is important to assess structures and processes of care and to understand the impact of legal, financial, cultural, and other variables. Such knowledge will help distinguish those factors that health care organizations and professionals may directly act to improve from other factors that are either not subject to influence by providers or require cooperation by others, such as those who determine how different health care services are financed. A high priority is research and methodology development involving the creation and refinement of measurement instruments relevant to goals for patients approaching death and the links between outcomes of care and the environmental, structural, and process-of-care factors that determine outcomes.

Other chapters of this report identify many sources of quality of care and accountability problems. For example, Chapters 3 and 4 have pointed to problems of coordination and continuity in a system that moves patients among many different health care settings and personnel. Chapter 6 points to financing incentives that encourage overtreatment of some patients and undertreatment of others and that generally discourage careful and time-consuming symptom assessments, counselling, and consultations. Chapter

7 will highlight the problem of anti-addiction drug policies that inappropriately target the medical use of opioids to control pain and other symptoms. In considering education and research, Chapters 8 and 9 reinforce the theme of inattention to the needs of dying patients, with the latter chapter also revisiting some methodological issues in assessing those needs.

6

Financial and Economic
Issues in End-of-Life Care

*To many people, reducing expenditures at the end of life seems
an easy and readily justifiable way of cutting wasteful spending
and free resources to ensure universal access to health care. . . .
We must stop deluding ourselves. . . .*

Ezekial Emanuel and Linda Emanuel,
The Economics of Dying, 1994

The United States has experienced years of mounting concern about
steep increases in health care spending and in the share of national resources devoted to health care. Between 1970 and 1994, personal health
care spending grew from $63.8 billion to $831.7 billion (from $310.9 to
$764.6 billion in 1992 dollars), and the percentage of the U.S. gross domes-
tic product devoted to health care rose from 7.1 percent to 13.7 percent
(Levit et al., 1996). Despite a recent slowdown in the rate of increase for
health care spending, the stress on controlling or reducing health care costs
remains intense.

Because spending on care at the end of life is so high and because much
of it is financed by government programs, the cost of end-of-life care has
attracted considerable attention. In the 1980s, analyses indicated that over
one-fourth of Medicare expenditures in a year were accounted for by the 5
percent to 6 percent of beneficiaries in their last year of life. These figures
prompted debate about whether such spending was excessive and whether
advance directives, hospice care, and futility guidelines could be promoted
to control costs as well as strengthen patient autonomy and improve care
(Jecker and Schneiderman, 1992; Lundberg, 1992; Singer and Lowy, 1992;
Fries et al., 1993; Murphy and Finucane, 1993). Analyses have cast doubt
on expectations that these strategies might make a major contribution to
containing health care costs (see, e.g., Emanuel and Emanuel, 1994; Teno,
Lynn, Connors et al., 1997). More forceful policies, such as explicit age-
based rationing, have also been discussed.

Financing of end-of-life care is also a concern for those who see incentives that in combination with cultural, legal, and other factors may impede excellent palliative care. As discussed in this chapter, financing mechanisms may encourage or discourage the use of beneficial services and may affect the mix of services, providers, and settings of care available to dying patients and their families.

This chapter examines four major questions asked about the cost of care for those who die. First, who pays for care at the end of life? Second, what is spent on this care? Third, do financing mechanisms create impediments to good care? Fourth, how might costs for care at the end of life be reduced?

WHO PAYS FOR CARE AT THE END OF LIFE?

No comprehensive national statistics document in detail the sources of payment for care at the end of life. Nonetheless, it seems clear that dying is, in considerable measure, publicly funded. Because over 70 percent of those who die each year are elderly and covered by Medicare and because thirteen percent of Medicare beneficiaries are also covered by Medicaid, those two programs undoubtedly cover a large proportion of expenses for end-of-life care. In addition to elderly people, others of those who die (e.g., some AIDS patients) are seriously enough disabled or impoverished that they qualify for Medicare or Medicaid or both. Veterans and defense health programs also pay for some end-of-life care. Moreover, some people who die without insurance or other available financial resources—for example, many homicide victims and homeless adults—die in public hospitals.

Notwithstanding Medicare's importance to its beneficiaries, the program does not cover all of their health care expenses. Data from the 1987 National Medical Care Expenditure Survey indicates that for those aged 65 or over who died in 1987, Medicare accounted for 48 percent of health expenditures during the last six months of life (52 percent for noninstitutionalized decedents and 39 percent for those in institutions) (calculated from Table 2 in Cohen, Carlson, et al., 1995). For all beneficiaries, in 1992, Medicare covered barely half (53 percent) of health care expenses with 14 percent, 10 percent, 20 percent, and 3 percent of expenses covered by Medicaid, private insurance, beneficiary out-of-pocket spending, and other sources respectively (Gornick et al., 1996).[1]

---

[1]Coverage percentages range from zero for outpatient prescription drugs and 6 percent for nursing home care to 87 percent for inpatient hospital care. Disabled beneficiaries have more of their expenses covered by Medicaid and "other sources" (25 percent and 11 percent) than do aged beneficiaries (12 percent and 2 percent). For those who qualify for federal-state Medicaid, the program is an important source of payment for nursing home care. It pays about 47 percent of all nursing home bills, compared to Medicare's 8 percent (Levit et al., 1996). Patients and families cover most of the rest of the cost of nursing home care (42 percent for aged beneficiaries but 14 percent for disabled beneficiaries) (Gornick et al., 1996).

For both decedents and survivors, Medicare coverage is particularly limited for long-term care, outpatient medications, and supportive services. For many, much of this care is either paid for out of pocket or provided by unpaid family members (Hing and Bloom, 1990; Pepper Commission, 1990). For example, although more than three-fourths of Medicare beneficiaries have some form of supplemental private insurance that is either self-purchased or provided by a former employer (PPRC, 1995), private insurance covers only 25 percent of prescription drug spending with almost 60 percent paid for out of pocket. Some dying patients qualify for the Medicare hospice benefit, which covers some prescription drugs and some nonmedical services (e.g., light housekeeping assistance, respite care). Community programs supported by other federal, state, local, or private sources provide some nonmedical supportive services (e.g., delivery of meals, transportation) to older people and those with disabilities.

Although over one-fourth of those who die each year are under 65, little information is available that describes how their care is financed. Some younger people who die are covered (directly or as dependents) by employer-sponsored health plans, and it seems reasonable to expect that this small group would (as in Medicare) account for a significant proportion of plan spending (IOM, 1993b). The liability of employer-sponsored plans for end-of-life care may, however, be limited when dying beneficiaries exceed maximum coverage limits or resign their jobs or when insured spouses resign or lose jobs as a result of absenteeism caused by their caregiving burdens.[2] Thirty-seven states provide Medicaid benefits for hospice care, which is used primarily by impoverished, nonelderly patients who do not qualify for Medicare under the disability provisions.

WHAT IS SPENT FOR CARE AT THE END OF LIFE?

Several points about spending on care at the end of life warrant emphasis. Because people who die generally have been very ill, many of these points should not be surprising. First, the small percentage of those who die each year accounts for a considerable percentage of total health care spend-

---

[2]Federal law provides that those who leave jobs under certain circumstances may be able to extend their coverage, at their own expense, for 18 or, less often, 36 months (IOM, 1993b). Few aggregate data are available on the cause of departures from employer health plans, but most are probably related to job changes, changes in marital status, retirement, switches to a spouse's health plan, and similar factors. Data on employer coverage or payments for those who die are virtually nonexistent. This is not surprising in part because death is a relatively rare event in the employer-covered population and in part because linking information on decedents to health plan coverage—or disenrollment—is expensive, although advances in computing power and the development of massive national health databases could make it easier in the future.

ing. A 1984 article (Lubitz and Prihoda) attracted widespread interest when it reported that the 5.9 percent of elderly Medicare beneficiaries who were in their last year of life in 1978 accounted for 27.9 percent of total Medicare spending. Other analyses suggest similar patterns through the 1980s and also dating back to 1960, before the adoption of Medicare (Lubitz and Prihoda, 1984; Scitovsky, 1984; Riley et al., 1986; Gornick et al., 1993; Lubitz and Riley, 1993). A more recent analysis looked beyond the Medicare population using data from the 1987 National Medical Care Expenditure Survey (Cohen, Carlson et al., 1995). This analysis estimated that total health care expenditures during the last six months of life for the 2.1 million people who died in 1987 (approximately 0.9 percent of the population) amounted to $44.9 billion in 1992 dollars (approximately 7.5 percent of total personal health care expenditures). For those aged 65 or over who died in 1987, this analysis found that spending during the last six months of life accounted for about 5.5 percent ($32.6 billion) of total spending.[3] In this same age population, another study (Scitovsky, 1994) reported that 23 percent of survivors had no Medicare payments in 1988 compared with 3 percent of those who died.

Second, as one extends the time analyzed from the year before death to several years before, the contrast between expenditures for survivors and decedents diminishes. In 1988 average Medicare payments for decedents ($13,300) were approximately 7 times those for survivors ($1,900) (Lubitz and Riley, 1993).[4] In 1978, the decedent-to-survivor payment ratio was 6.2 in the last year of life but dropped to 2.3 for the second-to-last year (Lubitz and Prihoda, 1984). For those who were 65 in 1974 and died in 1989, Medicare payments over this 15-year period were about twice as high for those who died as for those who survived (Gornick et al., 1993; see also Roos et al., 1987).

Third, the cause of death contributes to variations in expenditure levels and ratios for decedents and survivors both in the year of death and in the years before the final year (Riley and Lubitz, 1989; Scitovsky, 1994; Riley

---

[3]This analysis indicated that 15.9 percent of Medicare spending for elderly beneficiaries in 1987 was accounted for by care in the last six months of life for those who died (Cohen, Carlson et al., 1995). The authors of this study point out that the equivalent (six months) figure for the 1988 (last year of life) data reported by Lubitz and Riley (1993) is about 21 percent (because about three-quarters of Medicare costs in the last year of life are incurred in the last six months). After noting that sampling error for their 1987 data could put the figure as high as 19.4 percent, the authors attribute their lower figure to differences in study years and estimation methods.

[4]Very high-cost care does not appear to be common for Medicare beneficiaries who die. About 5 percent of decedents generated Medicare payments of $40,000 or more in 1988, although less than 1 percent of surviving beneficiaries generated such high payments (Scitovsky, 1994).

et al., 1995). Some conditions, such as diabetes and renal failure, show relatively long periods of higher decedent-to-survivor payment ratios. In contrast, payments for cancer decedents were notably higher than for survivors just for the year of death and the year before (Scitovsky, 1994). Among cancer patients, a recent analysis found that total Medicare payments between the time of diagnosis and the time of death were highest for those dying of bladder cancer ($57,600) and lowest for those dying of lung cancer ($29,200) (Riley et al., 1995). The difference was accounted for primarily by the shorter survival times for the latter group of patients.

Fourth, total Medicare payments per decedent drop as age at death increases; in contrast, expenditures increase with age for survivors (see Table 6.1). Some data, however, suggest that this pattern is less evident for accidents and heart attacks than for cancer, chronic obstructive pulmonary disease, and renal failure (Scitovsky, 1994). More generally, for Medicare beneficiaries who died between 1984 and 1991, higher levels of hospital charges (which cannot be equated with actual payments) were negatively associated with older age and a diagnosis of Alzheimer's disease and positively associated with being female, being on Medicaid, living in areas of higher population density, and having poor perceived health status (Culler et al., 1995).[5]

Fifth, lower Medicare spending for older decedents appears to be partly offset by higher Medicaid spending for those who are eligible for both Medicare and Medicaid (Temkin-Greener et al., 1992; see also Scitovsky, 1988). Also, a recent paper cites yet provisional, unpublished research at the U.S. Department of Health and Human Services as indicating "that nursing home costs rise with longevity, offsetting declining Medicare costs" (Scitovsky, 1996, p. 3). The reason for this pattern is suggested by data indicating that among those aged 65 to 74, about 17 percent of those who died had spent some time in a nursing home, but for those between ages 85 and 94, the figure was 60 percent (Kemper and Murtaugh, 1991).

Sixth, although data are limited, analyses suggest that chronic and terminal illnesses have serious financial consequences for families (Bloom et al, 1985; Beck-Friis et al., 1991; Covinsky et al., 1994, 1996). These finan-

---

[5]Also of interest is Scitovksy's analysis (1988) of sample data on decedents (mostly white and middle class) who received care from physicians at a large, multispecialty group practice. It indicated that total expenses (including expenses for care provided outside the group) were about 20 percent lower for those aged 80 or over compared to younger decedents. Expenses for hospital care were substantially lower, but payments for nursing home and home health were substantially higher for older decedents. For those aged 65 or over, total expenses did not vary by impairment status, but those who were totally impaired had substantially lower expenses for hospital care and higher expenses for nursing home care. High nursing home expenses were especially characteristic of those aged 80 and over who were totally impaired.

TABLE 6.1   Medicare Payments Per Person-Year, According to Survival Status and Age, 1976 and 1988[a]

	1976		1988	
Age	Decedents	Survivors	Decedents	Survivors
≥65	$3,488	$492	$13,316	$1,924
65–69	4,271	401	15,436	1,455
70–74	4,046	472	15,778	1,845
75–79	3,670	560	14,902	2,176
80–84	3,238	608	10,208	2,465
≥85	2,566	631	10,208	2,465
85–89	NA[b]	NA	11,422	2,578
≥90	NA	NA	8,888	2,258
Ratio, 65–69 to ≥85	1.66	0.64	1.51	0.59

[a]Approximate relative standard errors for all estimates are less than 0.02.
[b]NA=Not Available.

SOURCE: Lubitz and Riley, 1993.

cial consequences stem in part from out-of-pocket medical expenses but also from lower patient or family income that results from absenteeism, reduced working hours, or job loss related to illness or the demands of caring for an ill family member.

Seventh and contrary to some popular thinking, the increase in overall personal health care spending is not explained by growing costs for end-of-life care. Rather, it is accounted for by population growth, general inflation in the economy, and additional medical inflation, although the contribution of each component has fluctuated widely (Levit et al., 1996). An analysis covering data for 1976, 1980, 1985, and 1988 (excluding Medicare beneficiaries enrolled in health maintenance organizations [HMOs]) revealed that the share of Medicare spending accounted for by those who died had not grown during this period (Lubitz and Riley, 1993). The authors concluded that "the same forces that have acted to increase overall Medicare expenditures have affected care for both decedents and survivors" (Lubitz and Riley, 1993, p. 1093; see Table 6.2). Moreover, another analysis has esimated that the impact on Medicare spending of increasing life expectancy is small (Lubitz et al., 1995).

TABLE 6.2 Medicare Enrollment and Payments, According to Survival Status, in 1976, 1980, 1985, and 1988[a]

Variable	Year			
	1976	1980	1985	1988
Enrollment				
All beneficiaries (millions)	23.4	25.2	27.2	29.1
Decedents				
Number (millions)	1.22	1.35	1.45	1.49
Percent	5.2	5.4	5.3	5.1
Payments				
Total (billions of dollars)	15.2	31.0	57.2	73.0
Percentage paid for decedents				
Unadjusted	28.2	30.6	26.9	27.2
Adjusted[b]	28.2	30.8	27.4	28.6

[a]Approximate relative standard errors are less than 0.004.
[b]Adjusted to 1976 values for age, sex, and survival status.

SOURCE: Lubitz and Riley, 1993.

DO FINANCING MECHANISMS IMPEDE GOOD END-OF-LIFE CARE?

General Features of Insurance Plans That Might Affect End-of-Life Care

The committee searched for research on the effects of insurance on care at the end of life. It found very little. For example, the Health Insurance Experiment funded by the federal government and undertaken by Rand researchers excluded people over age 62 (i.e., those more likely to die) (Newhouse et al. 1993). What information exists is largely limited to traditional fee-for-service arrangements and may not apply to managed care, which covers a small but increasing proportion of Medicare beneficiaries.

Overall, considerable research indicates that the availability and type of health care insurance affect the use and provision of health care (see, e.g., Hadley, 1982; Lurie et al., 1984, 1986; Manning et al., 1987; Braveman et al., 1989; Hadley et al., 1991; IOM, 1993b; Newhouse et al., 1993). In part, these effects are intended and desired. For instance, health insurance eases the financial burden of illness and encourages people to get beneficial care that they might otherwise forego.[6] Insurance, however, may also encourage the use of services of little value, thus raising costs without comparably increasing value. As described below, insurers and policymakers have devised a number of mechanisms to counter this utilization effect of insurance.

Insurers have also devised responses to another problem—biased risk selection—that may have consequences for seriously ill people. Biased risk selection arises when insurance is voluntary or when people can choose among health plans with different features. Plans that disproportionately attract the sick will cost more than those that attract healthier people.[7] One result of this adverse selection dynamic is that insurers may refuse or restrict coverage to those with existing medical problems or may charge them more. Medicare is virtually universal for Americans aged 65 and over, which limits selection problems. Nonetheless, many beneficiaries voluntarily purchase supplemental coverage, and others voluntarily enroll in certified managed care plans; both choices may generate problems related to adverse selection. A particular concern is that competitive health plans may find it more economically attractive to compete on the basis of risk selection (i.e., attracting the well and avoiding the sick, especially the really sick) than on the basis of providing high-quality, cost-effective care.

Although insurance increases access to care, those without insurance do not necessarily go untreated, especially when they have acute or life-threatening problems (Hafner-Eaton, 1993). Emergency departments are forbidden by law from turning away critically ill people for lack of insurance or other financial resources. If an uninsured person is admitted for care and dies, the expenses incurred may be absorbed by the hospital (and, when possible, passed on indirectly to other payers) or covered by special public or charitable funds. If the person survives but is expected to remain seriously ill, efforts may be made to qualify the individual for public insurance or arrange a transfer to a public facility.

---

[6]Historically, the earliest sickness insurance arrangements were not designed to cover medical care expenses but to help offset wage losses and funeral expenses (see IOM, 1993b, Chapter 2, for a brief history of the evolution of health insurance). As medical care and hospital services became more effective and expensive, attempts began to be made to insure hospital care. Attempts to cover inpatient physician services followed.

[7]In most countries, the difficulties of private and voluntary health insurance have led to some kind of public insurance mandate. In the United States, several attempts since the early 1900s to establish national health insurance have been turned back. After World War II, a variety of factors encouraged a significant growth in the scope of private health insurance. Although perhaps half of those over age 65 had some form of insurance by the early 1960s, the difficulties faced by many older people in securing private health insurance eventually led to the adoption of Medicare.

Just as being without insurance does not necessarily preclude care, participating in an insurance plan does not guarantee that the plan will pay for the specific services wanted, needed, or received by those the plan insures. Health plans vary in the services they cover, and even for covered services, other restrictions, such as requirements for prior approval of hospitalization, may apply (IOM, 1989). In addition to limiting costs, the objectives of such requirements may be to improve quality of care by reducing departures from those clinical practices associated with better outcomes, to reduce patient care for which risks exceed probable benefits, or to limit exposure to iatrogenic (care-induced) illness.

Health plan restrictions that may particularly affect people with advanced illness come in many forms. These include

- *limiting the scope or level of benefits to restrict costs and encourage economical choices by consumers.* Some services may be excluded altogether; for example, Medicare excludes payment for most outpatient prescription medications. In addition, plans may require patients to pay part of the cost of a service (in the form of deductibles, copayments, or coinsurance), cover a limited number of visits or days of care, or set a cap on the dollar amount of payments for selected or all services during a defined time period. Some plans (including Medicare) set no upper limit on beneficiary liability for cost-sharing.

- *creating financial incentives for practitioners and providers to provide less care.* Plans may establish a fixed payment per day, per case, or per capita regardless of the amount of service rendered. Some health plans are paid by employers, governments, or others on a capitated (per member per month) basis, but they may pay practitioners and providers on a fee-for-service, per case, or other basis, or they may combine partial capitation with other payments.

- *requiring that patient services be authorized in advance.* Many health plans insist that special personnel review hospital admissions, medical procedures, and certain other services. They may also require that a designated primary care physician authorize referrals to specialists.

- *creating protocols or other tools to govern care.* Plans may adopt written statements that define what services are to be provided for particular medical problems, what medications are covered (e.g., formularies), and otherwise direct care to varying degrees.

- *establishing productivity standards or appointment schedules.* Such schedules may limit the time physicians can spend in evaluating patients, identifying problems and concerns (such as depression or persistent pain), and discussing care options.

- *covering services only if provided by designated physicians and other health care providers or applying higher cost sharing requirements if patients use physicians outside the plan network.* Patients may be covered only if they use providers that have contracts with or are employed by the health plan or if they obtain explicit authorization—and pay more—for the use of out-of-plan care.

• *limiting the number, type, and geographic distribution of designated providers of specialized services.* Depending on the characteristics of the provider network, patients may find specialist expertise unavailable for some problems, appointments hard to get, or travel requirements difficult.

The label *managed care* is often applied to health plans that employ one or more of the last six strategies listed above, although some use more restrictive definitions that focus on one strategy (e.g., financial incentives) or a specific combination of strategies. This report follows the less restrictive usage. In any case, the report's major concern is not with organizational labels but with specific incentives and actions that may particularly affect those with advanced illness. Chapter 4 has already considered some of the concerns about incentives used by managed care plans, which cover approximately 1 Medicare beneficiary in 10 (with some states having considerably higher proportions).

Financing Issues by Type of Service

Although care at the end of life is often associated with hospice services, this report has pointed out that only a small percentage of Medicare beneficiaries qualify for hospice benefits. Despite a general shift of care from hospitals to homes for both financial reasons and personal preferences, most older individuals still die in institutional settings, especially hospitals. Hospitals also play a major role in caring for incurably ill people who subsequently die elsewhere. Thus, the following discussion first considers hospitals, then nursing homes, hospice, and home care. The emphasis here is on the traditional, fee-for-service Medicare program and the possible effects of its financing provisions on care at the end of life. A later section considers Medicare managed care. To repeat a familiar theme, the effect of financing mechanisms on end-of-life care in different settings has been little examined.

Hospital Services

From the perspective of this report, major concerns about Medicare's hospital payment policies are that they may encourage premature patient discharge and discourage appropriate inpatient palliative services. Since the early 1980s, Medicare, which is administered by the Health Care Financing Administration (HCFA), has used a prospective payment scheme that pays for most hospital stays on a prospectively determined, diagnosis-related basis.[8] In general, the scheme assumes that hospitals will get a mix of patients in each diagnosis-related category or group (DRG), some of whom will cost more than the DRG rate and some less. The differences, it is assumed, will average out over all patients. If hospitals spend less than the DRG payment, they keep the difference. They are not, in general, compensated more if they spend more unless a patient reaches the defined outlier (very high cost) category. Although other factors are also at work (e.g., pressure from private payers and employers), the structuring of the prospective payment program is generally credited with reducing hospital stays without an offsetting increase in hospital admissions.

Because Medicare provides less generous coverage for much nonhospital care, shorter hospital stays may increase the financial burden on patients and families, especially for prescription drugs. Further, because dying patients are among the sickest of Medicare patients, the physical, emotional, and financial burdens of severely shortened lengths of stay may fall heavily on this group.

One particular concern has been that prospective payment might encourage hospitals to control costs by cutting quality and limiting beneficial care, including palliative services. Early analyses suggested that Medicare beneficiaries were indeed being discharged "quicker and sicker" and in more unstable condition, but no effects on 30-day or 6-month mortality could be readily identified (ProPAC, 1989; Kahn et al., 1990; Kosecoff et al., 1990; Rubenstein et al., 1990).

Although these initial findings were reassuring, mortality is not the only issue. Premature discharge may cause physical and emotional distress for patients and families, for example, if patients are discharged more quickly than appropriate home palliative care can be organized. In addition, some dying patients may be difficult to manage outside the hospital, even with intensive palliative services. For example, some patients experience pain that can only be relieved with radiation or other therapies available in hospitals. Not only may hospitals be discouraged from treating such patients, hospice coverage for inpatient care—whatever their justification—is very limited.[9]

---

[8]In addition to taking diagnosis into account, the assignment of a DRG to a particular patient may reflect other characteristics of a patient or a patient's care, such as age, operating room procedures, secondary diagnoses, or—rarely—costs so high that the case qualifies as an outlier. Hospital payments are also affected by their case mix and other factors.

[9]In addition, the American Academy of Hospice Physicians (Byock, 1996, p. 6) testified to the committee that "current diagnosis and treatment coding often leads to a charade in which tests are ordered and treatments begun to secure financial coverage for basic care to continue in the patient's preferred setting. This usually occurs in the hospital where the DRG for the

In response to concerns about limitations on palliative hospital care for dying patients, the Medicare program agreed to test a palliative care diagnostic code (ICD-9-CM V66.7) (Cassel, 1996). The test will help determine whether a new DRG code is needed to pay hospitals for palliative services to terminally ill patients and whether it is feasible. One question is whether it is possible to identify a homogeneous set of palliative resources—irrespective of diagnosis—so that they can be reimbursed and monitored for quality of care. The code is not intended to discourage the referral to hospice of patients who can be appropriately and feasibly managed with hospice's home and inpatient resources and coverage. Nonetheless, committee members are aware that some hospice organizations are concerned that the code could have negative effects on them.

In general, the committee urges that more attention be paid to Medicare payment policies and the hospitalization experiences of dying patients, including the experiences of those who die (and are expected to die) shortly after discharge. Relevant policies include those relating to inpatient palliative care. Among the process and outcome variables that warrant attention are trends in DNR orders and in systems for monitoring and comparing patient survival and other outcomes for hospitals and other sites of care.

Physician Services

Most physician services provided to Medicare patients (in the hospital, office, home, and nursing home or other institution) are reimbursed on a fee-for-service (FFS) basis. Since the early 1990s, these fees have been set using a resource-based relative value scale (PPRC, 1992). For beneficiaries enrolled in HMOs that receive a capitation (per person per month) payment from Medicare, different physician payment models may apply. Plans that themselves are paid on a capitated basis may pay physicians on a fully or partly capitated basis but they may also employ a discounted or other form of FFS payment that is not so different from traditional FFS. Under capitation, salary, or mixed models of physician payment, physicians may be able to earn more by seeing more patients, whereas FFS physicians can also earn more by doing more for patients.

Aside from anxieties about the general FFS incentives for overuse of surgical and other procedural services, the primary concern about

---

patient's diagnosis has been exceeded, but it also applies to maintenance of skilled nursing visits at home for patients who are debilitated but not in acute crisis." As was true for many other concerns, the committee did not locate empirical data to support or contradict this claim.

Medicare's physician payment scheme is that its payment categories and payment levels may not appropriately recognize the resources needed for high-quality palliative care in different settings. The committee also heard concerns that the channeling of payments to individual physicians may make it difficult to support a coordinated interdisciplinary team or an integrated, multi-site patient record system.

For physicians treating Medicare beneficiaries who are perceived to be dying, the most relevant fees are likely to be those for "evaluation and management" services rather than for procedural services such as surgery and diagnostic tests. Codes for evaluation and management visits differ depending on several patient or other factors (e.g., whether the visit is for a new versus established patient, for an initial versus subsequent visit, and for an office or other site of care). Within the broad visit categories, different codes exist for brief, limited, extended, and other classes of visits based on the effort or practice costs involved. Although the time and effort involved in a visit with a new patient would appear to warrant a payment differential, the distinction between new and established patients could be seen as discouraging continuity of care and encouraging switching among physicians.

Visit codes do not distinguish patients with special characteristics or needs (e.g., the frail elderly), as was recommended to HCFA by the Physician Payment Review Commission, which monitors and advises on Medicare physician payment (PPRC, 1991, 1992). Thus, the fee is the same whether or not a patient has, for example, physical or cognitive impairments or special needs for education and counseling. HCFA has responded that the special needs of these patients can either be accommodated by using a higher code (for a more complex visit) or by the averaging effect across all patients and visits. However, unless these patients are separately identified and analyzed, it is not possible to determine whether such accommodation happens in practice.

PPRC has also criticized the payments for nursing home visits as too low compared to hospital visits. It argued that "there is no sound basis for assuming the work and intensity involved in evaluating and managing nursing home patients should be any less than for patients seen in the hospital or office" (1992, p. 59).

Although guidance on how to translate actual patient encounters into visit codes has been developed for physicians and carriers who administer Medicare physician payment, some ambiguity inevitably remains. Such ambiguity combined with disputes about appropriate codes and payment levels may create particular problems for physicians trying to care well for the complex physical and emotional problems presented by patients with advanced illness that is expected to prove fatal. The committee heard concerns that carriers may not accept codes that reflect the kind of careful symptom assessment and emotionally supportive care that was discussed in Chapter 3. Medicare does not explicitly dictate the scheduling of patient visits, but restrictive interpretation of visit codes may influence physicians to limit the time spent with patients in much the same way as explicit policies do.

The committee did not identify any empirical analyses of the relative effort or practice costs for different kinds of palliative care in different care settings. Such data are needed to evaluate whether the physician fee schedule adequately compensates for palliative care services. The committee urges PPRC and HCFA to consider analyses and tests of palliative care codes for physician as well as hospital care.

Nursing Home Services

Most public funding (and about half of all funding) for nursing home care is provided by Medicaid, a joint federal-state program for which nursing home patients may qualify after spending down their own financial resources. The program pays some costs for nearly 7 in 10 nursing home residents (AHCA, 1995). In 1993, elderly beneficiaries accounted for about 12 percent of the Medicaid population but 33 percent of total expenditures, much of which was accounted for by nursing home use (PPRC, 1996). Given these proportions, it seems reasonable to expect that the controversy over Medicaid's burden on state budgets will eventually shift from cuts primarily affecting younger women and their children to focus on older people and those with disabilities.

In 1987, Congress repealed legislation providing that states pay nursing homes amounts "reasonable and adequate to meet the costs incurred by efficiently and economically operated nursing facilities." Payment levels and methods vary significantly across states and these variations have "a dramatic impact on nursing home expenditures and staffing" (IOM, 1996c, p. 62).

As of 1993, only 19 states adjusted payments based on nursing home case mix (Swan et al., 1994). Lack of case-mix adjusted payment is a concern because it may discourage nursing homes from accepting sicker Medicaid patients and from providing an adequate level of care. Overall, the combination of reduced hospital length of stays, more sophisticated medical technologies, and increasing resident age and disability are contributing to a nursing home population that is more severely ill and impaired and more demanding of nursing resources than in the past. A recent IOM study of nurse staffing levels concluded that the research literature generally indicated a "strong relationship among resident characteristics, nurse staffing time requirements, and nursing costs in nursing homes" (IOM, 1996c, p. 13).

Some nursing home patients receive hospice services under the Medicare hospice benefit. Although the Office of Inspector General (OIG) of the Department of Health and Human Services (DHHS) has raised questions about duplicate billing for these patients (OIG 1997 Workplan), little appears to be known about these patients, the care provided to them, or the degree to which nursing home personnel have the appropriate expertise for meeting their needs.

The availability, quality, and cost of nursing home care for dying patients are only a subset of troubling and difficult issues involving long-term care, which also includes much home care. Another IOM committee is expected to begin examining many of these issues in the latter part of 1997. A 1996 IOM report supported federal regulations and efforts by facilities and states to improve professional nurse staffing in nursing homes and reduce waivers of federal staffing requirements (IOM, 1996c). The same report also supported the need to increase professional nurse staffing on all nursing home shifts and specifically recommended that Medicare and Medicaid payment levels be adjusted to support a required 24-hour registered nurse coverage in nursing facilities by the year 2000. The benefits of these changes would accrue to most nursing home residents.

Hospice Services

The Medicare hospice benefit was designed specifically to increase beneficiaries' access to hospice, and about 60 percent of hospice patients are covered by Medicare (Vladeck, 1996). Hospice accounts for about 1 percent of Medicare spending, and about one-tenth of one percent of Medicaid spending (NHO, 1996a).[10] A study by the Minnesota Hospice Association indicated that about 77 percent of patients enrolled in hospice were covered by Medicare, 12 percent by private insurance, 4 percent by Medicaid, and 7 percent by other sources (Holst, 1996). In addition, informal care is a major resource for hospice patients. Data from the National Hospice Study suggest that about 70 percent or more of the hours of care provided for "long-stay" hospice patients was provided by informal caregivers (Mor, 1987; see also Murinen, 1986).

The Medicare hospice benefit was adopted following years of steep increases in Medicare spending. Not surprisingly, the benefit, features of

---

[10]Cancer is the most frequent diagnosis, accounting for 60 to 80 percent of all hospice patients (Christakis and Escarce, 1996; Strahan, 1996). Another 10 to 13 percent have heart-related diagnoses. The National Hospice Organization estimates that 1 out of 3 patients with AIDS or cancer is cared for in hospice, a much higher proportion than for heart disease. Some Alzheimer's patients receive hospice care, but predicting the length of the terminal period of this disease is difficult (Volicer, 1996).

which are summarized in an Addendum to this chapter, is circumscribed with an array of features intended to control program costs by:

1. limiting the number of qualifying beneficiaries
2. encouraging efficient and economical home care
3. discouraging in-patient palliative care.

Claims that hospice can reduce spending for end-of-life care are examined in a later section of this chapter.

To qualify for Medicare hospice benefits, patients must be certified as having a life expectancy of six months or less if the illness runs its natural course. This has limited the use of the hospice benefit to those, mainly cancer patients, whose dying trajectory is relatively (but, by no means, perfectly) predictable. Conversely, this provision tends to exclude many who might benefit from hospice services but who have conditions such as congestive heart failure whose course is very difficult to predict.

As discussed earlier in this report, the prognosis provision implies a degree of precision that does not exist. The committee was, thus, disturbed to learn that the DHHS Office of Inspector General was investigating long-stay hospice patients as part of its fraud and abuse initiatives.[11] The first audit report on a mainland hospice, released in September, 1996 claimed that the hospice erred in admitting 176 patients out of 364 patients who were either enrolled for more than 210 days or had been discharged alive over a 27-month period. The 364 cases represented about 2 percent of all patients enrolled in the hospice during that period, and the hospice overall had a median length of stay of 47 days in FY 1995 (letter from B.R. Howe to the Regional Inspector General for Audit Services, DHHS Region IV, April 29, 1996). Although hospices should not be immune from investigations of possible fraud or abuse, the committee urges regulators to exercise extreme caution in interpreting hospice stays that exceed six months as evidence of anything other than the consequence of prognostic uncertainty. To do otherwise would inappropriately penalize hospices and would threaten the trust that dying patients need to have in those who care for them. It might also discourage more timely admission to hospice of patients now referred only a few days before death, after important opportunities

---

[11]In 1995 the OIG began, under the name Operation Restore Trust, a series of investigations of fraud and abuse in home health agencies, nursing homes, durable medical equipment suppliers, and hospice organizations. The inclusion of hospice came after audits of two Puerto Rican hospices reported 77 percent of one hospice's patients were ineligible because they were not terminally ill (NHO Newsline, July 15, 1995).

for physical, psychological, spiritual, and practical support have already been missed.

In addition to eligibility restrictions, the Medicare hospice payment mechanisms are also designed to limit costs. Four levels of per diem payment rates apply as does an overall cap on payments that was set for FY 1997 at $13,974 multiplied by the number of hospice enrollees. Medicare sets a cap on aggregate hospital payments at 5 percent of total payments, and the per diem rate for inpatient hospice care is only $418.93. The use of volunteers, which reflects hospice philosophy but also limits Medicare's liability for some care, is required.

At the same time that they encourage efficiency, the aggregate caps on payments for in-patient care and total payments and the per diem rates could discourage appropriate care for some patients. For example, the current per diem of $94.17 for routine home care may discourage the use of certain costly pain medications, even when less expensive drugs fail; late-night nursing visits to deal with medical or emotional crises; the appropriate application of high-technology equipment (e.g., infusion pumps); and extensive counseling services for particularly distressed patients and families (Joranson, 1994; Brown, 1996). Even more significant, the financial constraints mean that hospice care may not be suitable or feasible for patients without family or others able to provide extensive assistance with medications, hygiene, nutrition, and other care.

The last several years have seen efforts to apply capitated payment schemes to an increasingly broad range of services and providers. Hospice has not been immune, although few if any capitated contracts are in place so far, and the discussions of capitation do not appear to envision their application to Medicare beneficiaries (Hospice News Service, 1996). Capitation contracts would involve paying a hospice a small amount each month for all members (well or ill) of an HMO or other health plan and then holding the hospice financially responsible for services to terminally ill health plan members. Capitation of hospice care has been characterized as a "high-risk" mechanism because of (1) lack of data on the incidence and variability of terminal illness in non-Medicare health plan populations, (2) variability across communities, (3) lack of effective tools to detect and deflect inappropriately early referrals, and (4) lack of other information necessary to set rates and manage financial risk. The committee does not encourage this kind of capitation of hospice services.

The committee heard some concern that physicians felt financially threatened by hospice. This fear is misplaced, to the extent that it rests on the false perception that Medicare requires patients electing hospice coverage to switch to a hospice physician and leave his or her personal physician. Some individual hospices, however, apparently do encourage such a switch which may or may not be in the patient's best interest. Regardless of who the attending physician is for a hospice patient, the direct patient care services (as opposed to general oversight or consulting services) are generally covered separately by Medicare Part B rather than folded into the hospice per diem (NHO, 1996a).

Medicare beneficiaries enrolled in HMOs may elect the hospice benefit. They are not limited to using a hospice that the HMO may have contracted with for its non-Medicare enrollees, although it is not clear how well beneficiaries are informed of their options. HMOs enrolling Medicare beneficiaries are not required to provide hospice benefits themselves (although they may), and they cannot deny access to a HCFA-certified hospice for patients who wish it. When Medicare beneficiaries enrolled in HMOs elect the hospice benefit, the usual capitation payment to the HMO is reduced to a minimal level for certain covered services not required of or provided by the hospice. For HMOs paid on a reasonable cost basis, costs are covered for services not related to the terminal condition and for attending physician services provided to a hospice patient by an HMO physician.

A few HMOs operate their own Medicare-certified hospices (Della Penna, 1996), but most do not. Some HMOs and capitated physician groups have organized internal hospice-type programs to cover younger enrollees because they believe that it is good for patients and to the plan's financial advantage to do so (Baines, Gendron et al., 1996; Emma, 1996).

Although comprehensive and detailed data are scarce, hospice coverage for those not eligible for Medicare or Medicaid appears to vary enormously in terms of what services and providers are covered and with what limitations (e.g., exclusions for preexisting conditions). Hospice coverage is said to be offered by 80 percent of large- and medium-size employers (Snow, 1997).

Home Care Services

Because the Medicare hospice benefit is limited to those with a prognosis of six months or less, it is not applicable to many patients with serious illnesses but an uncertain prognosis. For these individuals, coverage for home health services can help them secure important supportive services such as medical social services and home health aide services. A major limitation of the home health benefit is that beneficiaries must be homebound and need part-time or intermittent skilled nursing care or physical or speech therapy. Some dying patients would be able to benefit signficantly from home palliative care before they become completely homebound.

As mentioned in Chapter 4, the use of Medicare-covered home care has grown rapidly in recent years. It is one of the fastest growing segments of total program spending. Between 1988 and 1994, program payments grew more than 500 percent—from $1.9 billion to $12.7 billion—and the number of certified home health agencies has grown from approximately 5,700 to 7,800 (HCFA, 1996b). The reasons for the growth in expenditures include changes in Medicare home care policies and their judicial interpretation, an aging population, a growing supply of providers, earlier discharge of patients from hospitals, and the increased feasibility of providing advanced technologies in the home.

The increase in expenditures has prompted a comprehensive assessment of the home health benefit that is examining, among other issues, quality of care, payment methods, fiscal integrity, and effective program management (Clauser, 1994; Vladeck and Miller, 1994). One part of the initiative is demonstration projects to test a prospective per-episode payment system to encourage efficiency and cost control. Preliminary results suggest difficulties in establishing episode lengths given the skewing of episodes.

In general, Medicare coverage for home care services has provoked both support and skepticism as well as some evidence of fraud and abuse (Kane et al., 1991; IOM, 1994b; GAO, 1995a). The skepticism has largely to do with claims that home care can reduce total health care costs by substituting for hospital or nursing home care (Benjamin, 1993). One of the largest studies of home health care concluded that "home care was used mostly by those not at risk for entering a nursing home, costs increased,. . . and benefits . . . are few and fleeting" (Weissert, 1991, p. 68). Another study suggested a "complementarity" in home health and nursing home use. Home health services "tended to be used by persons with serious health problems whose disability appeared to be more a consequence of illness and whose chronicity may have been tied to the duration of the health problem . . . [whereas skilled nursing facility] use seemed to be concentrated among those with serious functional disability of potentially longer standing" (Manton et al., 1994).

Some have questioned whether any savings that do exist from averted hospital or nursing care are offset by a shift to paid home care away from unpaid care by family members (Pepper Commission, 1990). Analyses indicate that Medicare home care users are more likely than nonusers to be disabled, living alone, poor, and receiving Medicaid (Clauser, 1994). The Medicare benefit does not require a deductible, copayment, or previous hospitalization, although this may change given the concern about recent spending increases. In contrast to hospices, about half of home health agencies are for-profit, and these agencies tend to have more aide visits, fewer therapy services, longer episodes of care, and more visits per episode than other categories of agencies (ProPAC, 1996).

Medications

One of the long recognized limitations of the Medicare benefit is that it does not cover most outpatient prescription medications. The major exception is if a patient is enrolled in hospice and is prescribed drugs for symptom management. Some (usually expensive) supplemental policies cover outpatient prescription drugs. Medicaid programs generally cover outpatient medications, but a number limit the availability of medications by placing limits on the number of refills, the number of prescriptions covered in a month, or the quantity of medication (Soumerai et al., 1987; Joranson, 1994). These restrictions can interfere with effective, continuous management of pain and other problems.

Medicare's disparity in inpatient and outpatient coverage for medications may encourage the use of more expensive interventions. For example, pain relief through oral medications or transdermal patches is not covered for outpatients, but use of an infusion pump to provide pain relief at home can be covered under some circumstances (Joranson, 1994). The latter is not only more expensive but is somewhat more likely to produce certain kinds of complications. A patient without the resources to cover oral morphine and without assistance from family members might even be admitted to a hospital for intravenous or subcutaneous medications, which are covered in that setting. Ferrell (1993) points out that having morphine so administered might cost $4,000 compared with $100 for an oral morphine solution.

One study of elderly patients treated for selected chronic illnesses suggested that "limiting reimbursement for effective drugs puts frail, low-income, elderly patients at increased risk of institutionalization in nursing homes and may increase Medicaid costs" (Soumerai et al., 1991, p. 1,072). No studies appear to have specifically examined the effects of limited outpatient prescription drug policies on patients at the end of life, but it seems reasonable to expect that these policies also put this group in jeopardy as well.

WHAT ABOUT PROPOSALS TO REDUCE THE COST OF END-OF-LIFE CARE?

The discussion to this point has focused primarily on patient concerns as they are affected by efforts to limit Medicare costs. The concern with Medicare's precarious financial position is likely to make the cost of care for the dying one issue—among many—for those attempting to protect the solvency of the program.

As noted in the introduction to this chapter, various strategies for reducing the cost of end-of-life care have been put forth. Five are briefly considered below: broader use of hospice care; expanded use of advance directives; consumer choice strategies; futility guidelines; and explicit rationing of care. A suggestion not discussed below is that a closer physician-patient relationship would reduce costs associated with fragmented care, inattention to patient circumstances and concerns, litigation arising from mistrust, and similar problems (Scitovsky, 1996). The committee did not make formal recommendations on any of these options, but it does encourage continued investigation and testing of innovative strategies to discourage the use of nonbeneficial or marginally beneficial care without jeopardizing people's health and well-being.

Hospice Care

In addition to its benefits for patients and families, hospice has been proposed as a way to reduce costs, particularly for Medicare. The basic argument is that hospice saves money by decreasing the amount of expensive hospital care provided to terminally ill patients. After reviewing the literature, the committee concluded that the impact of hospice on overall health care costs remains uncertain.

Proponents of the cost savings position cite two studies—one published in 1985, which showed that expenditures for hospice patients in the last month of life are almost two-thirds lower than patients not in hospice (Mor and Kidder, 1985), and the second published in 1995, which reported that hospice saved Medicare $1.52 in Part A and B expenditures for every dollar spent (NHO, 1995). The more skeptical (see, e.g., Kidder, 1992; Scitovsky, 1994; Emanuel, 1996) point to the one randomized trial of hospice (Kane et al., 1984) showing no cost savings. Skeptics also criticize the nonrandomized studies for probable selection bias (e.g., patients who choose hospice may be more willing than others to forego aggressive life-prolonging interventions), measurement problems (e.g., reliance on charges rather than costs, exclusion of costs to families), and time period evaluated (e.g., in some studies, only one month prior to death).

One recent review of the literature suggests that for those patients for whom hospice care is applicable, cost savings of 25 percent to 40 percent may be generated in the last month of life (Emanuel, 1996). Savings in the last six months of life may drop to 10 percent to 17 percent and 0 percent to 10 percent in the last year. Because not all terminally ill patients are candidates for hospice care for the reasons described in earlier chapters, such savings cannot be readily extrapolated to all patients.

This committee believes that hospice programs should be promoted primarily on noneconomic grounds related to their emphasis on medical and nonmedical care goals, attention to families and others close to their patient, provision for nonmedical supportive services (e.g., respite care, bereavement counseling), and similar features. Nonetheless, given the accelerating financial pressures on Medicare, it is reasonable to consider continued research to identify the circumstances under which hospice care can reduce the cost of end-of-life care. One area for such research involves the application of the new guidelines for qualifying patients with selected noncancer diagnoses, which were discussed in Chapter 4.

Advance Directives

Advance directives specifically and advance care planning more generally are not health care financing mechanisms per se, and the arguments in their favor have primarily to do with patient and family control over end-of-life decisionmaking and with thoughtful consideration of peoples' goals at the end of life (see Chapters 3 and 7). Nonetheless, the potential of advance directives to reduce costs has also attracted attention. The idea is that written directives would eliminate the uncertainty or the dedication to rescue that drives clinicians treating comatose or otherwise mentally incompetent patients to provide ineffectual life-prolonging interventions. In addition, advance care planning might help some people to prepare for decisions that they may face while conscious and mentally competent (e.g., when to elect hospice care, when to accept or refuse another round of chemotherapy) and to be less susceptible to pressure from clinicians or family to agree to unwanted interventions when a crisis arises.

Some research suggests that patients who sign advance directives generate lower costs for their final hospitalizations than patients without such directives (Weeks et al., 1994). Other research, however, indicates the patient and family preferences are often not effectively communicated to or understood by clinicians (SUPPORT Principal Investigators, 1995; see also Chapter 3).

A sense of the outer limits of cost savings comes from an estimate that if every patient who died in 1988 "executed an advance directive, chose hospice care, and refused aggressive, in-hospital interventions at the end of life . . . the total savings in health care expenditures would have been $18.1 billion . . . or about 3.3 percent of all health care spending" (Emanuel and Emanuel, 1994, p. 542). The savings to the Medicare program would have amounted to about 6 percent of program spending in 1988. Clearly, it is unreasonable to contemplate universal acceptance and implementation of these measures. It is reasonable, however, to expect that some unwanted care and avoidable costs are incurred when care is provided contrary to the oral or written directive of a patient or family. Even if savings were only 10 percent of the high estimate cited above, the amounts, while small in the context of overall spending and spending increases, would not be meaningless.

The savings estimates for advance directives are, in general, vulnerable to the same criticisms that have been raised about research on hospice cost savings (e.g., that those willing to sign directives are not representative of the larger population) (Emanuel, 1996). In particular, skepticism about projections of significant cost savings rests on doubts about (1) the willingness of people to sign such directives, (2) their readiness to forego life-extending care when death is a real, not an abstract, prospect, and (3) the ability of health care systems to implement directives (Schneiderman et al., 1992; Teno et al., 1993; GAO, 1995b; SUPPORT Principal Investigators, 1995; Levinsky, 1996; Scitovsky, 1996; Lynn, Harrell et al., 1997; see also Chapters 3 and 7).

Although there is no evidence to suggest that significant cost savings would soon result, some steps could be taken to increase the potential for advance care planning to avoid some services—and expenditures—that most would agree are unwanted, ineffective, and even damaging to patient well-being. For patients who have completed advance directives (or taken similar steps), better procedures are needed to assure that information on patient wishes is readily available and considered at critical decision points, for example, the transfer of a seriously debilitated, very elderly patient from a nursing home to a hospital. The Oregon initiative described in Chapter 3 provides examples of such procedures.

Some have argued that managed care organizations are particularly well suited to encourage use of advance directives (Fade and Kaplan, 1995). A number of managed care organizations have undertaken systematic efforts to encourage greater use of advance directives (Baines, Barnhart et al., 1996; Christensen, 1996; Hammes and Rooney, 1996). Some caution is, however, warranted about promoting advance directives as a cost-containment measure in this context, and managed care organizations have particular reason to be hesitant about appearing too intent on encouraging people to sign directives limiting certain forms of care. For example, Sulmasy (1995), in discussing concerns about conflict of interest, suggested that advance directives (particularly if assisted suicide were to become legal) could be a "chillingly effective way to control the cost of managed care" (p. 245). He also notes that some have suggested lower insurance premiums for those who have advance directives (see *Washington Post*, May 2, 1993, C3).

Overall, continued efforts to encourage various forms of advance care planning and goal setting make sense at the margin, notwithstanding the social and cultural obstacles. One caveat: should people suspect that they were being pressured to sign advance directives and that such directives might be used inappropriately to limit care, then the result might be both higher costs and more use of advanced technologies that patients or families would forego in an environment of greater trust. Also, patients might try to "game" or manipulate a system that conditioned coverage on signing advance directives by later revoking the directives (assuming that such directives would continue to be revocable). As Callahan has pointed out, "advance directives were designed to assure the private good, not the public . . . to give patients a safeguard against being overpowered by overzealous physicians or institutions" (Callahan, 1996).

Consumer Choice Strategies

A market-oriented strategy to reduce health care spending proposes that those who wish aggressive but marginally beneficial treatments (or, in some versions, aggressive beneficial care) should be allowed that option but only if they absorb some of the additional costs that such a choice might entail (Eddy, 1991a; Havighurst, 1992, 1995). People could contract for a different "intensity" or "quality" or "extensiveness" of coverage as provided in different health plan options. The differences might be set forth in alternative clinical protocols for specific health care problems. Thus, one person might choose a health benefits package that covered only palliative services for persons with prostate cancer of a certain stage and prognosis, whereas another person might choose (and pay more for) a package that also would pay for curative or life-extending care under the same circumstances.

It may be unrealistic to expect people—particularly those not immediately concerned about life-threatening illness—to analyze and understand how health plans differ in their protocols for caring for myriad different illnesses and combinations of medical problems (IOM, 1993b). Nonetheless, with the support of clinicians and others, people might be helped to understand a choice—similar to that involved in electing hospice care—between an option that allowed for aggressive, curative or life-extending care for conditions with a poor prognosis and an option that provided for palliative services appropriate to the person's disease stage and prognosis.

Medicare Managed Care

Managed care strategies have the potential to reduce costs for end-of-life care in much the same way that they appear to reduce costs for healthier populations, in particular, by reducing the use of inpatient hospital services. For example, patients admitted to the hospital but determined to be likely to die within a few days may be discharged to die elsewhere if they do not meet the criteria for acute inpatient care. The overall impact of such strategies on the cost and quality of care would vary depending on the regard given to the wishes of patients approaching death and the alternative care available (e.g., hospice, nursing home, home health care). Alternative care will offset some of the savings from avoided hospitalization unless it also prevents rehospitalization or is provided on an unpaid basis.

As discussed in Chapter 4, the proportion of Medicare beneficiaries enrolled in HMOs is small, although much higher in a few states and growing nationwide. Although research examining patients who die is very limited, the results are consistent with other research that raises concerns about hospital discharge and home care policies and practices as they affect the frail elderly, the chronically ill, and other vulnerable groups.

The point is not that managed care organizations cannot provide good care for terminally ill patients but that financial incentives may tempt some to avoid enrolling the ill people or to behave in ways that compromise the quality of care for those with life-threatening illnesses. Speaking generally of the chronically ill, Jones has argued that market dynamics argue "for investing less, at the margin, in improvements or plan features that increase value to the chronically ill" (Jones, 1996b, p. 4). He identifies strategies that plans might use to discourage enrollment by the chronically ill. These range from using advertising images that suggest that the plan is for healthy not ill people to "keeping the numbers and availability of specific types of health professionals, clinic facilities, and other resources that attract the chronically ill to a minimum, thus ensuring long waiting times" (Jones, 1996b, p. 4). Governments, accrediting bodies, and other standard-setting organizations can attempt to devise standards that minimize these strategies. Unless, however, the financial incentives for capitated plans to avoid the chronically ill are changed, avoidance strategies can be expected to continue.

What can be done to change incentives? One approach is to devise a scheme for paying health plans that adjusts capitation payments to compensate them properly for the risk they assume in enrolling sicker people but that also avoids overpaying for healthy enrollees. Despite some success in improving methods for risk-adjusting payments, no method yet appears equal to the challenge (Newhouse et al., 1989; IOM, 1993b; Newhouse, 1994; Ellis et al., 1996; Gruenberg et al., 1996; Jones, 1996b). As far as the committee is aware, no special attention has been paid to the question of adjustments for those who die, and methods usually either use full-year participants only or annualize adjustments. Any explicit adjustment in rates to account for deaths could raise policy and political questions if it appeared to pay plans more if their members died. Current proposals to cut the Medicare capitation payment to HMOs across-the-board rather than to risk-adjust payments would, if anything, intensify the incentives to avoid people with serious health problems.

Another approach relies on performance measurement and reporting schemes that would identify, publicize, and discourage poor performance and that also would identify apparently good performance that was mainly a function of having a relatively healthy group of enrollees. Issues in measuring the quality of care have been discussed in Chapter 5. Given the difficulties that existing schemes are having in devising feasible and informative measures for a modest array of relatively common health problems, collecting sufficiently sensitive process and outcomes measures for the most vulnerable patients appears to be a distant although desirable prospect. Moreover, the strategy would not be successful unless the negative effects of being identified as a poor performer were strong enough to overcome financial disincentives to being identified as a good plan for chronically ill people (and thereby disproportionately attracting them).

A third approach to encourage health plan interest in sicker people is to devise special payment strategies for people with serious chronic illnesses or for patients with life-threatening illnesses who do not fit the hospice model (Jones, 1996b; Lynn, 1996b). Jones has discussed how Medicare, Medicaid, and very large employers might develop competitive care arrangements for people with specific chronic illnesses that would balance cost, quality, and access objectives in relation to the special needs of these patients (Jones, 1996b). He argues that Medicare could take the lead in experimenting with such options. For terminally or seriously ill Medicare patients who do not fit the current hospice model, Lynn has suggested the creation of coverage that would favor lower-technology supportive care provided by multidisciplinary teams (Lynn, 1996b). The thrust of this proposal is, however, not to save money but to make supportive care more available without increasing costs. Nonetheless, a test of such an option (or two or three variants that might be expected to have different cost effects) might indicate the extent to which such a strategy might affect overall costs and the extent to which it was accepted by patients, families, and practitioners. The generalizability of findings from such a test would need careful attention.

Of some interest in this regard, Medicare is considering tests of special capitation payment arrangements for patients with end-stage renal disease (Farley et al., 1996). Researchers assessing strategies for establishing such payments conclude that more work remains to be done on several design and technical issues before such arrangements are feasible. They also note that enrollee protection policies (e.g., quality assurance programs, grievance and appeal procedures) are particularly important for chronically ill Medicare beneficiaries who "may be especially vulnerable to reductions in access or quality resulting from cost cutting actions by plans" (Farley et al., 1996, p. 141).

Futility Guidelines

Futility has been defined in a number of ways (Veatch and Spicer, 1992; Halevy and Brody, 1996). Miles, for example, has suggested that it be viewed as "a medical conclusion that a therapy is of no value to a patient and should not be prescribed" (Miles, 1992, p. 310). Such conclusions might best be applied through professionally developed guidelines that focused on therapies that "a vast majority of people would not accept for themselves" (Miles, 1992, p. 313). Another view, which also argues for professional guidelines and for qualitative definitions of futility, suggests that futility might be viewed in probabilistic terms as a point on a continuum where the probability of benefit is very low, perhaps 1 in 100 (Schneiderman, 1994). Others have suggested community-based guidelines, such as those developed in Denver and Sacramento (Murphy and Barbour, 1994; see also Appendix C).

Expectations that "futility" guidelines would produce large cost savings should be restrained. Based on their analyses of data on a large group of seriously ill hospitalized patients, Teno and colleagues found that guidelines limiting treatment for patients with only a 1 percent or less chance of surviving 2 months would have saved about 13 percent of hospital charges for these patients (Teno, Murphy et al., 1994). They emphasized, however, that most of these savings came from 12 patients, 6 of whom were under age 51 and probably would not be very likely targets for aggressive care-limiting guidelines. They also found that 90 percent of all patients with this poor prognosis died within a week and that about a third died after life-sustaining treatments were withdrawn. The authors interpreted this as indicating that "some limits on aggressive treatment are already in place" (p. 1206). In a smaller study of pediatric intensive care unit (PICU) patients and a definition of futility that was deliberately broad for analytical purposes, Sachdeva et al. (1996) found a very small number of futile care days in the PICU and thus a small potential for savings based on limiting care.

Rationing

Rationing is another term with varied meanings (see, e.g., Aaron and Schwartz, 1984; Mechanic, 1985; Brook and Lohr, 1986; Reagan, 1988; Grumet, 1989; Morreim, 1989; Englehardt, 1991; Hadorn and Brook, 1991; Wiener, 1991; Hall, 1994). One traditional view sees rationing as the fair allocation of a specific limited resource (e.g., food during famine, organs for transplant). A more expansive definition includes limiting consumption of a potentially beneficial good or service by various explicit or implicit means (e.g., ability to pay, inconvenience, queuing, limits on technological innovation). Both these concepts of rationing exclude strategies for eliminating clearly inappropriate or harmful care and, instead, focus on care that may have some but not "enough" benefit to warrant coverage.

Determinations about what constitutes enough benefit or what constitutes essential—not just beneficial—care are partly subjective and partly scientific questions (Brook and Lohr, 1986; Eddy, 1996). One problem is that the evidence base for such determinations is very limited. Although it will continue to expand, evidence will still be unlikely to provide a firm foundation for treatment decisions about many specific combinations of patient circumstances (e.g., an 80-year-old man with mild dementia and congestive heart failure) (see, e.g., IOM, 1992). This is not an argument against evidence-based decisionmaking, only a caution that expectations should probably be modest.

Rationing of potentially beneficial services already exists—at least implicitly—in forms such as patient cost sharing, administrative mechanisms that limit access to services or providers, and various provider payment mechanisms. Although implicit rationing mechanisms have prompted varying amounts of criticism, more controversial are various options or proposals for the explicit rationing of potentially beneficial services (see, e.g., Brook and Lohr, 1986; Veatch, 1986; Morreim, 1989; Aaron and Schwartz, 1990; Daniels, 1994; Hall, 1994; Callahan, 1995). These proposals are more complex than such traditional devices as the exclusion from insurance plans of certain classes of services (e.g., long-term care) or conditions (e.g., preexisting medical problems). Such exclusions, which have been subject to continuing legislative attack, have been justified less on grounds of resource allocation than on grounds that the dynamics of a voluntary insurance market demanded them (IOM, 1993b). The discussion below focuses on proposals to ration on the basis of age or community consensus.

Age-Based Rationing

Age is one possible basis for rationing health services (see, generally, Callahan, 1987; Smeeding, 1987; Daniels, 1988; Binstock and Post, 1991; Winslow and Walters, 1992; Jecker and Schneiderman, 1994; Joint International Research Group, 1994; Callahan, 1996). For example, if you were over a specified age, open-heart surgery and similar life-prolonging interventions would not be offered or covered. (In the United States, it is probable that such interventions would still be provided for people financially able and willing to pay for them on their own.) A softer but more complex variant would be to set different limits for different age groups, perhaps covering life-prolonging treatments for those under age 85 who were conscious and had good cognitive functioning.

A less explicit approach to age-based rationing—along the lines suggested in Box 6.1—is also possible. Such an approach might be most extensively employed with the very old and also with others having a very grave prognosis.

Savings from age-based rationing have been questioned, particularly if restrictions were largely limited to the very old. Some researchers have

---

BOX 6.1
Implicit Age-Related Limitation of Care

Mr. Jones is 88, has chronic obstructive pulmonary disease and a 35 percent chance of living two months. In previous discussions about his preferences for care, he indicated that he wanted life-prolonging care. He developed severe respiratory problems and lost consciousness. His life might be slightly prolonged by aggressive treatment. Instead of explaining to his family the medical options and their likely outcome and expecting them to make the decision, Mr. Jones' physician gently describes how grave the situation is and says, "we will make him as comfortable as possible but we think he will probably die very soon." A choice of aggressive therapy is not offered. A family request for such treatment could still be accepted, but most will not consider this option.

---

pointed to evidence suggesting that the older old may already get less intensive care than younger people with equivalent health or functional status (Scitovsky, 1988; Farrow et al., 1996; Hamel et al., 1996). Scitovsky has concluded that "high-cost medical services may already be allocated to older people in their last year of life in a more rational manner than is generally assumed, with their age and functional status taken into account" (Scitovsky, 1988, p. 656). That is, the care actually provided is not "highly technical" or "center[ed] around often inappropriate cure-oriented services provided in hospitals" (Temkin-Greener, 1992, p. 699).

Without much more detailed data and analysis, it is not possible to determine the basis of apparent age-conditioned treatment intensity. It could be associated with overtreatment of younger persons or undertreatment of older persons or both.

The committee believes that public debate over age-based rationing has not really begun and may not be joined directly until the baby boom generation gets nearer the age—about the mid-fifties—when medical problems and costs begin to rise significantly. Such a debate could involve a constructive or destructive consideration of issues of justice, biological uncertainty, and potential benefits and burdens of treatments at different points in the life span.

Rationing Based on Community Consensus

A variant on rationing strategies combines evidence and clinical judgment with a public process for debating and weighing priorities. The best known example of such an approach, the so-called Oregon plan, is worth special attention because it has actually moved from the realm of theory to action and because it explicitly recognized the value of palliative care. The plan was envisioned as an "ongoing process to achieve consensus on our policy goals and the principles that will guide our health policy and as a framework in which resource allocation and reallocation can take place" (Gibson, 1993, p. 57; see also Fox and Leichter, 1991). Those involved in crafting the plan anticipated a near universal access to health insurance within the state, which would mute concerns about economic inequities.

A central element of the plan was a ranked list of health services on the basis of clinical effectiveness and social value. Services would be covered in rank order as far as revenues and judgments about budget priorities allowed. The ranking effort involved both experts and the community (e.g., through surveys and town meetings), clinical and economic data, and evidence and values (e.g., a subjective review of the ranked list by officials).

The priority-setting scheme explicitly dealt with several kinds of services involving life-threatening conditions and terminal illness. It considered essential coverage to include acute, potentially fatal conditions for which treatment could be expected to prevent death and offer full recovery (e.g., appendectomy for acute appendicitis) or to prevent death without a clear prospect of full recovery (e.g., treatment for strokes and serious burns). Essential services also included care for chronic incurable conditions for which treatment could be expected to improve life span and quality of life (e.g, treatment for diabetes and comfort care such as pain management and hospice care) (Cotton, 1992). The next highest priority of the Oregon plan included important services involving mostly nonfatal conditions. The lowest-ranking group included "fatal or nonfatal conditions of which treatment causes minimal or no improvement in quality of life, such as severe brain injury, aggressive treatment for extremely premature infants, and end stages of cancer" (Cotton, 1992).

Criticisms of the Oregon plan have involved a mix of technical, political, financial, and ethical arguments (Brown, 1991; Daniels, 1991; Eddy, 1991b; Grannemann, 1991; Cotton, 1992; Hadorn, 1992; Menzel, 1992; Azevedo, 1993; Hansson et al., 1994; Kaplan, 1994; Firshein, 1996). One criticism of this approach has been that it does not allow for differences among patients in the same diagnosis/treatment category. That is, even with over 600 categories, some patients fitting a high ranking diagnosis/treatment category may have characteristics that make them unlikely to benefit from a usually beneficial treatment whereas some patients in a low ranking category might have characteristics that give them a good chance of benefitig from a usually less effective treatment. Thus, even if evidence exists about differences in benefit based on differences in patient characteristics, the ranking scheme would not accommodate it. In addition, the analytical strategy has been criticized for potentially discriminating against those with disabilities, and concern about such discrimination was a major factor in the federal government's initial cool reaction to Oregon's request for a Medicaid waiver for the project (Menzel, 1992; Campbell, 1993).

Instead of operating on a statewide or community basis, a rationing scheme could, in principle, operate on a health plan basis with representatives of health plan members setting priorities (Medica Foundation, 1994, 1996). Such a strategy could involve hundreds of individual priority-setting exercises for different health plans. In addition to raising some of the same concerns as other rationing schemes, such an approach appears vulnerable to the same charges of overcomplexity and limits on consumer understanding that were raised for the consumer choices strategies described above.

CONCLUSION

Care at the end of life appears to be, in large measure, financed by public programs, especially Medicare. Although explicit comparisons are not available, trend data on Medicare expenditures suggest that care at the end of life has not become disproportionately more expensive and technologically intensive than other care in recent decades, although it is clear that a considerable part of Medicare spending is accounted for by those who die. Data also indicate that Medicare spending at the end of life drops with increasing age of decedents, a drop that is partially offset by increased Medicaid spending for less technologically intensive nursing home care. Except for hospice, few studies have examined the impact of Medicare or other financing practices on care at the end of life. The committee found reason to be concerned about the possible effect of several features of both the traditional Medicare program and its managed care alternatives.

The committee believes it is important to know more about the patterns and the impact on dying patients and their families of early hospital discharge, including the impact on total costs, extent of readmissions, smoothness of transition to home care (with or without hospice benefits), management of symptoms, quality of life, and family burden. The information gained from the test of the Medicare palliative care code should be helpful in evaluating the nature of hospital palliative care and its cost compared with alternatives.

Several areas of physician payment also warrant investigation. They include the fit between different patient evaluation and management codes and the time and effort required to provide palliative services in different settings. The adequacy of payment levels for nursing home and home health visits is of particular concern to the committee. The committee is also concerned that Medicare's fee-for-service program has financial incentives that do not encourage continuity of care, interdisciplinary care, or supportive care for a broad range of dying patients.

Medicare's hospice benefit might seem to overcome these difficulties, and indeed, its per diem payment, coordination with Part B physician services and with capitated managed care, and required interdisciplinary care team are illuminating and auspicious components. Hospice programs, however, cannot regularly take on care of persons without homes, family caregivers, or predictable fatal illnesses. Likewise, persons who still should receive costly drugs or supports, such as respirators or intensive care, often cannot be enrolled in hospice, and such treatments are not likely to be made more available within the hospice program.

Proposals to test new ways of financing care for those with serious chronic illness warrant serious attention. Not only is this desirable as a way of responding to the problems faced by people with less predictable prognoses but it also responds to concerns about the incentives of Medicare's current method of capitating HMOs. Seriously chronically ill persons cost much more than the Medicare capitated payment, which discourages plans from attracting such patients by developing a reputation for excellence in their care. The financing mechanism acts counter to quality. Without the testing of alternative financing strategies by the HCFA, state Medicaid programs, and health plans, it is not clear how problems with both managed care and FFS financing can be resolved.

ADDENDUM

Medicare coverage and payment provisions are complicated by the division of the program into two parts involving different services, payment methods, and beneficiary cost sharing provisions (HCFA, 1995). Medicare Part A covers mostly inpatient hospital care with limited coverage for nursing home, home health agency, and hospice care. Part B covers physician services, limited services by other professionals (e.g., chiropractors and dentists), hospital outpatient services, freestanding ambulatory surgery, physical therapy, durable medical equipment, and some other services or supplies. Beneficiaries share in the cost of their care, with the specifics varying by type of service and other conditions. For example, for 1997, the Part A hospital deductible was $760. Medicare does not cover outpatient prescription or nonprescription drugs, long-term (nonacute) care, and most routine preventive services; it covers a very limited amount of behavioral health care.

About 13 percent of Medicare beneficiaries—the dually eligible—are also covered by Medicaid. Payments of intermediate care and nursing facility care account for about one-third of all Medicaid spending. Medicaid covers required patient cost sharing for Medicare covered services for those who meet means testing criteria.

Major Features of Medicare Hospice Benefit

Eligibility

General conditions: A person must be entitled to Medicare Part A benefits and certified to have a terminal illness (defined by statute as having a life expectancy of six months or less if the illness runs its normal course).

Election and waiver statement: A person must sign a statement electing the hospice benefit and waiving the right to standard Medicare benefits for curative treatments for (or related to) the terminal condition.

Election periods: A person starts with an election period for hospice care of 90 days. Subsequent elections may be for 90, then 30 days, and finally for an indefinite period.

Revoking the benefit: If a person revokes his or her election, benefits for the election period in question are forfeited. Benefits may be reelected for the next election category, except that a person who is in the indefinite election category forfeits any further coverage for hospice care.

Coverage

General: Services are covered if reasonable and necessary for palliation or management of the terminal illness and related medical problems.

Inpatient care: Short-term inpatient care is covered if it is necessary to manage symptoms or provide respite for home caregivers.

Home care: A variety of medical and nonmedical services are available to patients at home (and sometimes in nursing homes or other institutional settings—including nursing visits, physical therapy, physician visits, medical social services, services from home health aides, counseling services (including spiritual and bereavement counseling for family members), homemaker services, outpatient drugs, and medical appliances. Continuous home care is covered if necessary to keep a patient at home during a medical crisis.

Physician Payment

Employee attending physician: These physicians are paid under the hospice daily rate for technical (e.g., lab) and administrative services and under Medicare Part B for professional services.

Outside attending physician: These physicians are paid under Medicare Part B for professional and administrative services and as part of the hospice daily rate for technical services.

Consulting physicians: These physicians are paid under Medicare Part B for professional services and under the daily rate for technical services.

Payment to Hospice

General conditions: Payment is made on a prospective per diem basis except for physician services, which are paid for on a fee-for-service basis.

Levels: Different per diem rates are set for routine home care ($94.17 in FY 1997), continuous home care ($549.65 for 24-hour care or $22.90 per hour for a minimum of 8 hours), inpatient respite care ($97.41), and general inpatient care for palliative services ($418.93).

Cap on inpatient care: For a hospice, payments are reduced if total inpatient care days exceed 20 percent of the total number of hospice care days for all Medicare patients.

Overall cap: For a hospice, total payments are limited to an amount equal to the number of Medicare patients multiplied by a statutory cap amount ($13,974 in FY 1997). (Physician services covered by Medicare Part B are not included in the cap.)

7

Legal Issues

The principle that a competent person has a constitutionally protected liberty interest in refusing unwanted medical treatment may be inferred from our prior decisions.

Cruzan v. Director, Missouri Department of Health, 497 US 261, 278 (1990)

A seriously ill or dying patient whose wishes are not honored may feel a captive of the machinery required for life-sustaining measures or other medical interventions.

Justice Sandra Day O'Connor, concurring opinion in *Cruzan*, 497 US at 28

The roles of judges, legislators, and administrative officials in influencing care at the end of life vary from the dramatic to the commonplace. On the dramatic end of the continuum are the court cases about the legality of physician-assisted suicide, which were argued before the U.S. Supreme Court as this report was being drafted. In contrast, the right of people to refuse unwanted life-sustaining and other treatments—once the subject of highly charged court cases—is now commonly accepted and enforced (if not always perfectly).

Documenting the impact of statutes, regulations, case law, and administrative actions on clinicians, patients, families, and others can be difficult. In addition, the applicability of various statutes and judicial precedents to specific patient circumstances is quite often a matter of dispute and speculation rather than straightforward matching of law to facts. Nonetheless, in the committee's view, the legal issues discussed here raise concerns either about their possible effects on compassionate and effective care for those approaching death or about the unrealistic expectations they may create or both.

This chapter considers laws relating to prescription of opioids, informed consent and advance directives, and assisted suicide. Among those with clinical, administrative, or similar involvement in end-of-life care, much of the debate about issues such as prescription regulation or informed consent is practical. For example, how can prescription laws be modified so that they do not discourage effective pain management but still respond to legitimate concerns about misuse of controlled substances? For some issues, most notably assisted suicide and euthanasia, ethical concerns may dominate legal discussions, but practical issues also arise as described later in this chapter. The focus here is primarily on how laws may affect the quality of care for dying patients.

Although the impact of malpractice litigation on medical practice is a complex and disputed question, it is discussed only briefly because the committee did not view the prospect of malpractice litigation as likely to have a significant impact on end-of-life care specifically. The committee, however, recognized concerns that physicians may engage in defensive medicine (e.g., ordering extra tests, prescribing unnecessary medications, performing hopeless CPR) because they fear being sued for a bad outcome that plaintiffs might attempt to attribute to lack of a test or procedure. Similarly, decisions might sometimes be influenced by the fear of being sued for not following a family's wishes, even if those wishes were contrary to the doctor's clinical judgment and the patient's own wishes. The committee did not find evidence that physicians were concerned about liability for failure to intervene to relieve pain or other symptoms.

In any case, many of the steps proposed in this report would tackle problems of undertreatment, overtreatment, or mistreatment of dying patients in ways that should reduce the potential for litigation and physician uncertainties and fears about being sued. At the practitioner level, these steps include changing clinicians' attitudes, knowledge, and practices so that they communicate more effectively with patients and families, engage patients and families in a process of goal setting and decisionmaking that increases trust and minimizes misunderstanding, and properly assess and treat pain and other symptoms. At the system level, they include strategies for measuring, monitoring, and improving care that seek to identify and respond to the preferences, experiences, and feelings of patients and families. If, however, these strategies fail to correct the deficits identified in Chapter 3 and if patients come to understand that the standards of care (e.g., practice guidelines) call for efforts to relieve symptoms, then litigation stemming from inattention to symptom management might become more likely—but not necessarily productive. The primary injured plaintiff would, in the case of a dying patient, likely have died, and although a family could claim injury and testify about the decedent's suffering, damages would be hard to establish. In addition, the status of practice guidelines in the courts is still evolving. Overall, the committee was doubtful that malpractice litigation could be relied upon as an instrument to improve care at the end of life.

PRESCRIPTION LAWS AND BARRIERS TO PAIN RELIEF

All patients who suffer pain—not just the dying—deserve relief through treatments that are known to be effective for most pain. Indeed, early treatment of pain as a part of a continuum of good care for those who are seriously ill may be the best approach to minimizing pain at the end of life. Other parts of this report document deficiencies in pain management and gaps in scientific knowledge. This section examines how effective pain management may be compromised by prescription drug laws that are intended to minimize drug addiction and diversion of drugs from legal to illegal sources. (Relief of dyspnea may also be affected by these laws, although this has not been the subject of much attention.) Because these laws both arise from and interact with the misperceptions and attitudes of physicians, medical boards, lawmakers, patients, and the public, reform needs to go beyond revisions in written policies to affect knowledge and values.

Anti-Diversion Policies

The Problem of Diversion and Regulatory Responses

Diversion occurs when persons with legal access to controlled substances distribute them or use them for illegal purposes or when people fradulently obtain drugs from legal sources (Cooper et al., 1992; Cooper et al., 1993).[1] Pain relief medication, for example, might be prescribed to phony patients and then sold on the streets. Alternatively, people might forge prescriptions or misrepresent their symptoms to secure prescriptions. Newspaper articles and television news reports periodically expose the problems of diverted opioids and clinician addiction. No reliable studies document the extent of opioid diversion specifically or compare it to other illegal sources (e.g., illegal imports and domestic production). A 1990 household survey estimated that 4 percent of the population over the age of 12 had used prescription analgesics, stimulants, tranquilizers, or sedatives at least once for nonmedical reasons in the preceding year, and almost 1.5 percent were currently using them (NIDA, 1991). A California estimate puts the

---

[1]Theft and other forms of illegal access are also problems but are less susceptible to control through anti-diversion regulations.

dollar value of diverted controlled substances during the mid-1980s at somewhere between $500 million and $1 billion (Marcus, 1996).

Legal and regulatory policies intended to prevent diversion include triplicate prescriptions and limits on the number of medication dosages that may be prescribed at any one time. These policies are burdensome and appear to deter legitimate prescribing of opioids (see, e.g., Cooper et al., 1992; IOM, 1995a, 1996d; Joranson, 1995a). Triplicate prescription programs require the prescribing physician to complete detailed, multiple-copy prescription forms. The forms themselves are often difficult to obtain and, if incorrectly filled out, must be completed again by the physician. The triplicate forms also become available to the state medical board, which may choose to pursue disciplinary measures on the basis of such information. Electronic forms and monitoring systems would ease the burden on physicians as well as allow easier monitoring but such systems have not been widely adopted or rigorously evaluated nor have appropriate norms to guide such oversight been developed and tested.

Some states have laws limiting the dosages a physician may prescribe to one patient at any given time. These laws force patients who suffer pain that requires frequent medication to request and renew prescriptions repeatedly. This not only inconveniences both patients and physicians but may subject patients to possible interruptions in pain management if something disrupts the timely requests and responses. Such problems are a special concern for patients who are not in a medical facility but are at home or in a care facility without an on-site physician.

The committee recognizes the problems created by illegal drug use and drug diversion and the need for law enforcement responses. It, however, knows of no evidence, anecdote, or other reason to believe that the prescription of opioids in the care of dying patients contributes in any meaningful way to drug diversion problems.

Effects on Care at the End of Life

The effect of anti-diversion policies on their intended targets is unclear. They do, however, appear to affect the rate of prescriptions and perhaps increase the use of less effective or even harmful medications (Cooper et al., 1993; Joranson and Gilson, 1994a, b; IOM, 1995a, 1996d). One study reported that when Texas introduced a multiple-copy prescription program, prescriptions for opioids to control pain were halved (Sigler et al., 1984). It is not known whether this dramatic drop resulted from declines in inappropriate prescribing and diversion or whether physicians and pharmacists became reluctant to prescribe appropriate medications. Nonetheless, the magnitude of the change makes it reasonable to expect that the regulation had some impact on patient care (Von Roenn et al., 1993; Wastila and

Bishop, 1996). Surveys of physicians—discussed further below—suggest that anti-diversion and anti-addiction policies combined with social antipathy toward real or imagined addiction discourages effective, appropriate, and legal pain prevention and management.

Options for Improvement

How can laws be constructed and interpreted in ways that minimize drug diversion without obstructing effective medical management of pain? Options include (1) replacing triplicate forms with electronic reporting of prescriptions and (2) allowing standing prescriptions for outpatients (to be monitored by home health care professionals or pharmacists). In addition to reducing regulatory barriers to effective pain prescribing practices, states could require that pain experts or palliative care specialists be represented on state medical boards to help inform board policies and interpretations. Information collected from triplicate or electronic prescriptions might also be analyzed to identify questionable prescribing practices, which could be used to guide education of physicians and pharmacists about effective and appropriate use of opioids. Another IOM committee has already recommended additional research on the effects of controlled substance regulations on patient care and scientific research (IOM, 1996d).

Anti-Addiction Policies

The creation of new addictions is a separate issue from the diversion of drugs to the black market. A collection of social forces joins with legal restrictions to create a general antipathy toward drug use that flows into the area of medical practice and undermines effective pain management. Even the terminology muddies the waters when chronic use of opioids, which produces physical dependence, is sometimes equated with addiction. For example, California law defines addicts as "habitual users," which might include patients with chronic pain who regularly and appropriately take opioids necessary to manage their pain (Marcus, 1996).

States have addressed the perceived problem of medically induced drug addiction through varied combinations of laws, regulations, and medical board disciplinary policies. Because the committee concluded that policies often reflect inadequate understanding of the mechanisms of pain and addiction, these mechanisms will be described before the policies are considered.

Mechanisms of Pain and Addiction

Efforts to devise reasonable anti-addiction policies are complicated by ignorance and confusion about the biological and psychological mechanisms of pain management and addiction (Bruera et al., 1987; WHO, 1990; Nestler et al., 1993; Von Roenn et al., 1993; Portenoy et al., 1994; Buchan and Tolle, 1995; Joranson, 1995a; Portenoy, 1996). Research indicates that addiction in patients appropriately receiving opioids for pain is very small, ranging from roughly 1 in 1,000 to less than 1 in 10,000 (Porter and Jick, 1980; Angell, 1982; Jaffe, 1985; Rinaldi et al., 1988; Portenoy and Payne, 1992; Portenoy, 1996).

The committee concluded that drug tolerance and physical dependence should be more uniformly and clearly distinguished from addiction. *Tolerance* occurs when a constant dose of a drug produces declining effects or when a higher dose is needed to maintain an effect. *Physical dependence* on opioids is characterized by a withdrawal effect following discontinuation of a drug. Such dependence is a common effect in chronic pain management, but it is not restricted to opioids. Other agents such as beta-blockers, caffeine, and corticosteroids also produce physical dependence. Further, clinical evidence suggests that patients receiving opioids can be easily withdrawn from them in favor of an alternative, effective pain control mechanism if that is clinically indicated. Typical practice is to reduce the dose by fractions, stopping administration of opioids altogether after a week or so (Doyle et al., 1993). This practice may not be relevant, however, for dying patients.

Neither physical dependence nor tolerance should be equated with addiction or substance abuse. Portenoy and Kanner (1996) proposed that "addiction is a psychological and behavioral syndrome characterized by (1) the loss of control over drug use, (2) compulsive drug use, and (3) continued use despite harm" (p. 257). This is consistent with a definition proposed by the American Medical Association: "the compulsive use of a substance resulting in physical, psychological, or social harm to the user and continued use despite that harm" (Rinaldi et al., 1988, p. 556). The federal Controlled Substances Act defines an addict as someone who habitually uses an opioid in ways that endanger public health or safety (AHCPR, 1994a).

Unfortunately, the general term *substance dependence* is often used as a synonym for addiction, perhaps because the latter is more stigmatizing. For example, the American Psychiatric Association sets out criteria for dependence rather than addiction in its *Diagnostic and Statistical Manual of Mental Disorders* (4th ed., 1995). Despite a disclaimer that the scheme focuses on "maladaptive" substance use, the discussion of substance dependence may nonetheless mislead (p. 181). A later disclaimer about distinguishing legitimate medical purposes from opioid dependence is not specific, given that, as described below, many seem to be confused about what is legitimate. The committee is particularly concerned about misinterpretation of criteria related to tolerance, withdrawal, and overuse. Tolerance and withdrawal are, in general, clinically acceptable (although not necessarily invariable or desirable) consequences of effective use of opioids to manage pain, and "overuse" as defined above may be difficult to distinguish from increasing use due to uncontrolled pain, which may result from increasing pathology, tolerance, or other sources (Weissman and Haddox, 1989). Similarly, some behaviors suggestive of addiction may be confused with those resulting from inadequately managed pain or anxiety about the reliability of pain management.

Regulatory Responses

Responses to the problem of addiction take several forms including some of those already identified in the discussion of drug diversion. Federal and state laws and regulations attempt to control the prescribing behavior of physicians, nurses, and pharmacists by criminalizing certain activities. In addition to legislatures and courts, state medical boards set policies that, although not having the official force of law, may be just as powerful in their effect. These policies dictate the standards by which physicians may be professionally disciplined. Laws and medical board policies are also intertwined, in that legislatures may place legal limitations on the extent of a medical board's powers.

Medical Board Policies.   State medical boards may establish guidelines on pain-prescribing practices that constitute official statements of board policy. Such guidelines describe acceptable medical practice and notify health care practitioners of professional boundaries. Violating them may lead to disciplinary action. The sometimes restrictive perspective of state boards could interfere with the treatment of pain. In 1987, for instance, the Washington State Medical Disciplinary Board stated that it did "not recognize repeated prescribing of controlled drugs as appropriate therapy for chronic pain" (cited in Joranson, 1995a, pp. 2–3).

Several state medical boards have issued guidelines that deal with the use of opioids to treat intractable pain.[2] In California, the nursing and pharmacy boards have also created guidelines addressing the same issue (Joranson, 1995b). These guidelines are intended not only to instruct phy-

---

[2]State medical boards that have issued guidelines regarding the use of controlled substances to treat pain (along with the year in which the guidelines were first issued) include: Utah (1987), Minnesota (1988), Massachusetts (1989), Arizona (1990), Georgia (1991), Oregon (1991), Alaska (1993), Texas (1993), Wyoming (1993), Alabama (1994), California (1994), Idaho (1995), Colorado (1996), Florida (1996), Maryland (1996), Montana (1996), North Carolina (1996), and Washington (1996) (Joranson, 1997).

sicians and other caregivers on the proper use of opioids in pain management but also to reduce physicians' fear of attracting board discipline for such use. Another way for state medical boards to improve pain control might be for the boards to educate the physicians within their states about how to comply with laws, regulations, and board-set standards. Information collected from triplicate prescription forms could be used in this educational effort.

Some state boards, however, continue to require that physicians avoid the potential for addiction and that they justify the continued prescribing of opioids (Joranson, 1995b). A survey of state medical board members conducted in 1991 showed that most would discourage the use of opioids to relieve chronic, noncancer pain; a third of them said they would investigate such a prescription as a potential violation of the law (Joranson et al., 1992). There is still, it seems, an inappropriate sense of distrust on the part of the medical boards, which this committee believes has developed, in part, on the basis of misperceptions discussed above about the nature and consequences of dependence and addiction.

Laws and Regulations.   In 1974, the federal government, through the Federal Intractable Pain Regulation, clarified the federal law that prohibits physicians from prescribing opioids to detoxify or maintain an opioid addiction (Code of Federal Regulations, Title 21 Part 1300). The regulation states that the prohibitive regulations are "not intended to impose any limitation on a physician . . . to administer or dispense narcotic drugs to persons with intractable pain in which no relief or cure is possible or none has been found after reasonable effort" (21 Code of Federal Regulations, Title 21 Sec. 1306.7[c]). The policies of the Drug Enforcement Administration are similarly explicit.

Even when antiaddiction laws exempt those with intractable pain, the protections generally do not extend to those already addicted (Joranson, 1995a). When these people become patients suffering intractable pain, physicians are not free to prescribe opioids to relieve their suffering. This problem becomes especially acute in the AIDS wards of many urban hospitals.

At the state level, a number of prescribing laws include provisions that could interfere with effective medical use of opioids. For example, in New Jersey, regulations call on physicians "periodically to either cease the medication or taper down the dosage . . . to reduce the addiction propensity for the patient" (Joranson, 1995a).

In 1988, the Commonwealth of Virginia passed the first state law addressing the need to treat pain in terminally ill cancer patients (Joranson, 1995a). The legislation—despite its positive provisions—also illustrated the misperceptions surrounding the treatment of pain. It allowed physicians to prescribe heroin to their terminally ill patients even though heroin is not legally available under federal law and has no significant advantages over other available opioids (Joranson, 1995a).

Texas was the first state to pass an Intractable Pain Treatment Act, in 1989. California followed suit in 1990 and Florida in 1994 (Joranson, 1995a).[3]

Some state pain treatment laws, (e.g., Colorado and Washington) recognize the benefits of pain control and allow physicians to prescribe controlled substances but do not address concerns about inappropriate discipline by medical boards. The Texas and California acts do address this problem by prohibiting medical board discipline of physicians who follow the provisions within the laws. Both acts also define intractable pain (following the model of the Federal Intractable Pain Regulation[4]), authorize physicians to prescribe controlled substances to treat intractable pain, and prohibit health care facilities within the states from limiting such prescriptions. California's act requires an evaluation of the patient by a specialist.

Effects on Care at the End of Life

Surveys suggest that physician apprehension about addiction and anti-addiction regulations is widespread (Cleeland et al., 1986; Portenoy, 1990; Weissman, Joranson et al., 1991; Hill, 1993; Von Roenn et al., 1993). Such apprehension is not limited to physicians within the United States. In a survey of all the governments in the world conducted by the International Narcotics Control Board (within the United Nations International Drug Control Program), 47 percent of responding governments cited health care provider reluctance due to concerns about legal sanctions as an impediment to medical use of opioids (Joranson and Colleau, 1996).

The frequency of punitive action against physicians for apparently legitimate prescribing practices is unknown, but the committee heard many

---

[3]States with intractable pain treatment policies (along with the year in which the policy was instituted) include Virginia (1988), Texas (1989), California (1990), Colorado (1992), Washington (1993), Florida (1994), Missouri (1995), Nevada (1995), Oregon (1995), and Wisconsin (1996) (Joranson, 1997).

[4]Both statutes define intractable pain as "a pain state in which the cause of the pain cannot be removed or otherwise treated and which in the generally accepted course of medical practice no relief or cure of the cause of the pain is possible or none has been found after reasonable efforts including, but not limited to, evaluation by the attending physician and surgeon and one or more physicians and surgeons specializing in the treatment of the area, system, or organ of the body perceived as the source of the pain" (Code of Federal Regulations [1988] Title 21 Sec. 1306.07[c]).

anecdotes about threatening statements by medical disciplinary boards and about physicians who find the scrutiny and requirements sufficiently burdensome that they choose not to prescribe medications needed to manage pain effectively. In addition, the earlier discussion of regulations to limit drug diversion indicate that these policies may discourage the appropriate medical use of opioids and may discourage research to develop better medications.

Options for Improvement

More states could pass carefully drawn pain treatment laws. The American Medical Association (AMA) recently adopted a resolution to create a model state law, based on the Texas and California acts (AMA, 1996a). By protecting physicians from disciplinary actions, the AMA hopes to "provide patients with the security and knowledge that intractable pain resulting from terminal illness need not persist in a chronic, unrelieved manner" (AMA, 1996a, p. 4).

Although such laws constitute an important step to promote effective pain management for patients, they may not go far enough or may imply clinical clarity that does not exist. By making positive statements about the benefit of opioid use in the control of pain, legislators hope to reduce the fear of arbitrary medical board discipline. Yet they do not, in all cases, mark a clear area of medical practice in which physicians feel free to manage their patients' pain. The more specific laws, for example those that set out detailed prescription practices, may actually afford physicians less leeway in the practice of medicine. Additionally, by carving out an area of pain treatment that is immune from medical board discipline, there may be an implication that other forms of pain treatment should be subject to disciplinary review.

Even the strongest intractable pain law is still limited by the term *intractable*. Many cases are ambiguous, and physicians may believe that they must delay opioid treatment until pain is far enough along to be called intractable. An additional problem arises when state laws define addiction without regard to pain management. As noted earlier, California defines addicts as "habitual users," which might include patients taking opioids for chronic pain. Such confusing definitions once again expose physicians to the threat of medical board discipline.

Finally, the legal affirmations in these laws of the importance of pain control do not, in themselves, correct practice patterns or improve physician training. Laws could, however, encourage patients to expect diligence in pain relief, including use of generally effective medications. Medical boards could consider disciplining physicians who fail to apply proven methods of pain control.

Overall, the committee is encouraged by recent actions to revise drug prescribing. It urges continued review of restrictive state laws, revision of provisions that deter effective pain relief, and evaluation of the effect of regulatory changes on state medical board policies, physician attitudes and practices, patients, and illegal or harmful drug use.

INFORMED CONSENT AND ADVANCE CARE PLANNING

A series of legal decisions over the past three decades has affirmed the right of people to refuse unwanted medical treatments (President's Commission, 1982; Faden et al., 1986; Appelbaum et al., 1987). As stated in an important 1960 California Supreme Court case, "Anglo-American law starts with the premise of thoroughgoing self-determination," which includes the right of individuals to refuse medical treatments (*Natanson v. Kline*, 1960). This legal reasoning reinforced a shift in emphasis in medical ethics from a dominant paternalism (i.e., action in the best interest of patients as judged by physicians) toward autonomy (i.e., patients' right to choose the course they prefer) (Childress, 1982).

One means for recognizing patient autonomy in decisionmaking is informed consent, which means that patients voluntarily accept (or refuse) a medical intervention after disclosure of its expected benefits and risks and discussion of the alternatives. For dying patients who are unconscious or in such distress that they cannot reasonably communicate their wishes when a treatment decision needs to be made, the legal concept of informed consent may have limited application.

In response, the concept of *advance care planning* was devised to allow people (whether or not they are "active patients") to specify how they want to be treated should serious illness or injury leave them without the capacity to make decisions or communicate (see, e.g., President's Commission, 1982; AARP, 1986; Emanuel and Emanuel, 1989; Annas, 1991; Burt, 1994). Documents used in advance care planning, called advance directives, take several forms, including surrogate decisionmaking arrangements and what are popularly called "living wills." For purposes of this report, advance directives refer particularly to statements intended to be legally binding.[5]

As discussed in Chapter 3, advance care planning is a broader, less legally focused concept than that of advance directives. It encompasses not

---

[5]Guardianship involves the court appointment of a decisionmaker in cases where the patient is, for some reason, incompetent to make decisions for him or herself. A guardian is usually appointed for reasons other than health care, such as financial management. State guardianship laws vary on the power of a guardian to consent to or refuse medical treatments. The committee here limits its discussion to decisionmakers appointed by patients themselves.

only preparation of legal documents but also discussions with family members and physicians about what the future may hold for people with serious illnesses, how patients and families want their beliefs and preferences to guide decisions (including decisions should sudden and unexpected critical medical problems arise), and what steps could alleviate concerns related to finances, family matters, spiritual questions, and other issues that trouble seriously ill or dying patients and their families. Impediments to advance planning and the implementation of written directives may be less a matter of law than of ordinary inertia or unwillingness to consider unpleasant matters. The rest of this section discusses resuscitation orders, living wills, designation of surrogates, and the Patient Self-Determination Act of 1991.

Do Not Resuscitate Orders

Do not resuscitate orders or DNRs are orders placed by a physician with a patient's or surrogate's consent into the patient's treatment chart. As discussed in Chapter 2, it is not unusual for severely ill patients, who may be dying from any of a variety of diseases, to suffer cardiac or respiratory arrests. The normal action when this occurs is called a "code."[6] DNRs, or "no-codes," inform hospital staff or other caregivers that, in the event of such an episode, no attempts at revival should be made. Even when attempted, success rates of cardiopulmonary resuscitation are often low, especially for elderly patients (Murphy et al., 1989). For that reason, DNRs are sometimes called DNARs or "Do Not Attempt to Resuscitate" orders.

Because DNRs are physicians' orders, they come out of the clinical rather than the legal tradition. They thus have more in common with orders for medication or lab tests than they do with such legal documents as living wills or durable powers of attorney. Additionally, many hospitals had DNR options in place before they were required to do so by law. DNRs might, however, have some legal significance, if courts take them into account when determining whether a patient's preferences have been followed. Also, because the decision by the physician to place the DNR in the chart should be made in consultation with the patient and should reflect a patient's decision to forego certain forms of life-prolonging treatment, DNRs share with living wills and durable powers of attorney a role in the process of advance care planning.

---

[6]Caregivers attempt, through the insertion of breathing tubes and a pump, or by electric shock to the heart, to revive the patient. These attempts may stabilize the patient or may result in actual damage, leaving the patient alive but in a worse condition than before the code.

Living Wills

As of 1990, 40 states and the District of Columbia allowed adults to create what is popularly called a "living will" (Strauss et al., 1990). These statutes vary in their particulars, but they generally envision that individuals may make legally binding arrangements to the effect that they shall not be sustained by medical treatment that artificially prolongs the dying process if they are in a terminal condition and can no longer make decisions.

The statutes include several safeguards against abuse. Most include a requirement that the two witnesses to the signing of the document be neither related to the patient nor involved in his or her treatment or financial support. Also, the determinations that the patient fits the statutory definition of terminal and is unable to make decisions sometimes must be made by at least two physicians. A mentally competent individual is always entitled to revoke his or her advance directive. The statutes vary on whether nutrition and hydration are considered "artificially life-sustaining" treatments. Some statutes explicitly exempt nutrition and hydration from the care a patient may choose to refuse, others give the signer the option to explicitly include them, while a third group is silent on the matter (Strauss et al., 1990).

Skeptics of living wills argue that these documents, which may be standard forms approved by the legislature of some states, provide little practical guidance in real life clinical situations, which often involve many more factors or contingencies than anticipated by standards forms (see, e.g., Brett, 1991; Lynn, 1991). Indeed, by leading patients to believe that the signing of a living will means that their preferences for an end-of-life treatment plan have been made clear, these documents could even discourage active and ongoing discussions among patients, their families, and health care professionals. In contrast, a document designating a surrogate decisionmaker could encourage such communication.

Designation of Surrogate Decisionmakers

Adults

Another legal option for advance care planning involves the designation of a surrogate to act on one's behalf in the event one becomes incompetent to make decisions about medical care. State statutes (or, in some cases, sections within the living will statutes) vary in the amount of authority a person can assign to a surrogate. For example, in California, the patient's agent, who is assigned durable power of attorney[7] for health care,

---

[7]"Durable" power of attorney differs from general power of attorney in that it does not expire when the designator loses the competence to make decisions. This is integral to health

may make all health care decisions that the patient could make for himself or herself, had he or she the capacity (California Civil Code Sec. 2500). The attorney-in-fact's duty is to follow the wishes of the power's grantor, but specific instructions need not be included in the document. In contrast, Nevada and Rhode Island that require statutory forms be used (Nevada Chapter 449 Secs. 2–8; Rhode Island Sec. 23-4.10-1). Grantors of the power of attorney choose options on the form, instructing their agents when to consent to or refuse life-sustaining treatments.

In one sense, although the statutes that provide for standard forms and checked options seem more specific, they may still lead to ambiguities of definition and decision. For example, when an agent is instructed to refuse treatment when that treatment's burdens outweigh the expected benefits, it remains up to the agent (with the help of the health caregivers and others involved) to make the determination. In fact, under the broader powers available under California's statute, the grantor and the agent may be more likely to sit down together and discuss the grantor's wishes, rather than have the grantor check a box and leave it at that.

Other states place even more limits on the powers of the agent. In New York, power of attorney may not be used to delegate medical decision-making authority, only to communicate the wishes of the grantor (Strauss et al., 1990). This inflexible provision restricts people's ability to plan ahead and may prevent humane care at the end of life.[8]

Children

Decisions regarding dying children involve special considerations (Lantos and Miles, 1989; Strain, 1994; AAP, 1995; Fleischman, 1996). Although specific state laws vary, those below a certain age are legally unable to agree to or refuse medical treatment, and so others must make decisions for them. Even so, the best interests of these patients often oblige caregivers to discuss the situation with the children in ways appropriate for their developmental level and physical condition. This discussion may go beyond the sharing of information to ask children what they want for themselves (see discussion in Chapter 3). Problems arise when those with the power to consent to treatment for children disagree with each other or with clinicians. For health care providers, parental decisionmaking may also be complicated by spousal disagreement or evidence of child abuse.

---

care decisionmaking, as it is exactly at the time of a patient's incompetence that the designated attorney-in-fact's role begins.

[8]The Conference of Commissioners on Uniform State Laws has recently proposed a Uniform Act on surrogate decisionmaking.

Parents' decisionmaking discretion is not absolute, and pediatricians view themselves as having a professional obligation to look after the best interest of their patients (AAP, 1995). In some cases, their conclusions may conflict with those of the patients' families. Some of the most difficult cases arise from parents' demands for what clinicians regard as "futile" or "inhumane" care. The possibilities for resolving conflict include sensitive conversations between the child's physician and the parents; involvement by social workers, ethicists, pastoral counsellors, or others trained in working with grief-stricken families; mediation by a hospital ethics committee; or recourse to the legal system. The latter is widely viewed as a last resort because of the burden it places on families, the stress it creates for clinicians, and the potential for negative publicity for families and institutions.

The Patient Self-Determination Act

The Patient Self-Determination Act (PSDA) was enacted by Congress in 1990 and went into effect in December 1991 (White and Fletcher, 1991; GAO, 1995b). The PSDA requires health care institutions that receive Medicare or Medicaid funds to provide written information to adult patients about state laws regarding advance directives. It also requires those institutions, among other things, to note any advance directive in a patient's file, not to discriminate between patients on the basis of whether they have an advance directive, and to educate staff and community about the availability of advance directives.

The purpose of the PSDA was to encourage greater awareness and use of advance directives so that situations of ambiguity, as illustrated by the Nancy Cruzan case, might be avoided. In that 1990 case, the United States Supreme Court recognized a competent patient's right to refuse life-sustaining treatment, but left it to the lower courts to determine whether testimony of Nancy Cruzan's previously expressed oral wishes was persuasive. In *Cruzan v. Director, Missouri Health Department*, Justice Sandra Day O'Connor suggested in a concurring opinion that written advance directives could dispel such ambiguity. That year, Congress passed the PSDA.

The law, however, appears to have had modest effects (Teno, Lynn et al., 1994; Morrison et al., 1994; Emanuel, 1995a; see also Chapter 3). There are no national studies on the rates of persons completing advance directives, but studies of discrete populations (e.g., nursing home residents or hospital patients) conducted both before and after passage of the PSDA show rates between 5 percent and 29 percent (GAO, 1995b; Yates and Glick, 1995). The SUPPORT investigators found a small increase of seriously ill patients having an advance directive since the PSDA went into effect (from one in five to one in four), but this increase did not translate into higher rates of documented resuscitation discussions or DNR orders for patients who seemed to want them (Teno, Lynn, Wenger et al., 1997).

Although it requires health care organizations to provide information, the PSDA does not specify the content of that information. Often, patients are informed of their rights regarding advance directives during admission to a hospital or long-term care facility. The information is provided on a piece of paper, one of many that crosses the table during this usually stressful time. Other problems with implementation of the PSDA exist. One study found problems in the accessibility of previously completed advance directives during subsequent hospitalizations (Morrison et al., 1995). Another study found that, of the patient charts that indicated the existence of an advance directive, only 57.5 percent actually contained a copy of the directive (Yates and Glick, 1995). The study also revealed that a mere 32 percent of medical institutions covered by the law had done any community education on advance directives. The lack of involvement of physicians, especially primary doctors, also contributes to the tendency of patients to overlook the information offered.

The committee, while recognizing the value of advance directives, questions the urgency of intensive efforts to universalize their use. In this area of decisionmaking at the end of life, the law's favorite product—the legally binding document—may sometimes stand in the way of, rather than ease, the process, especially if these documents are naively viewed as ultimate solutions to the difficulties of decisionmaking. Rather, the documents known as advance directives should be seen as a set of tools useful in the ongoing process of advance care planning. Methods must be developed for encouraging continuing conversation among patients, their families, and the health professionals involved in their care. Less legalistic ways to approach planning and decisionmaking at the end of life were discussed in Chapter 3.

PHYSICIAN-ASSISTED SUICIDE

"Physician-assisted suicide" refers to a practice by which physicians provide, but do not directly administer, the means for a patient voluntarily to hasten his or her own death. This typically is done by prescribing lethal doses of medication that the patient then ingests. "Euthanasia," in contrast, is a practice by which the means of hastening death are administered directly by the physician, for example, when a doctor injects a patient with a lethal medication.

Controversies about assisted suicide have received recent widespread attention as a result of two lawsuits challenging the constitutionality of New York and Washington laws that prohibit physician-assisted suicide. The U.S. Supreme Court heard arguments on the cases (*Vacco v. Quill*, No.

95-1858 and *State of Washington v. Glucksberg*, No. 96-110) in early 1997.[9] The litigation followed popular referenda in California and Washington in 1990 and 1991 in which proposals to legalize physician-assisted suicide were defeated. In 1992, however, Oregon voters approved a similar proposal. Oregon thus became the first jurisdiction in the United States to provide formal legal recognition of the practice of physician-assisted suicide, although court challenges delayed implementation of the law and legislative reconsideration was being discussed as this report was completed.

The committee agreed that it would not take a position on the legality or morality of assisted suicide, but it did examine some of the issues that might arise if the Supreme Court ultimately ruled either that a terminally ill person who is mentally competent and voluntarily chooses suicide has a constitutional right to self-administer lethal drugs received with the assistance of a physician or that it was constitutionally permissible for individual states, such as Oregon to permit the practice. Many of these issues were explored in friend-of-the-court briefs filed with the Court.[10]

Although proposals to legalize physician-assisted suicide typically include various safeguards or restrictions to protect patients and physicians, these provisions involve a number of ambiguities that might make them impossible or impractical to implement. For example, as noted earlier in this report, the status of being "terminally ill" has not been satisfactorily defined conceptually or in application because no boundary prognosis correlates precisely with an important clinical change and none can reliably be supported by data (Lynn et al., 1996). Subjective definitions of illness can be criticized as being so variable as to seem capricious. Already, several hospices have been challenged over terminal illness identifications, prognoses of survival, and small percentages of patients who survive for more than six months (see Chapter 6). In the case of care that is widely viewed as beneficial, the acceptance of some prognostic errors for a large population of patients is reasonable. It is harder to be so sanguine about such errors when the issue is assistance in suicide.

---

[9]On June 30, 1997 (after the initial release of this report), the Supreme Court ruled that there is no general constitutional right to physician assistance in suicide. Some of the justices, however, wrote statements that suggested that a narrowly defined right might be upheld in specific circumstances.

[10]See, for example, the briefs filed by the American Geriatrics Society, the American Medical Association, the American Nurses Association, the American Psychiatric Association et al., the Project on Death in America, and Ronald Dworkin, Thomas Nagel, Robert Nozick, John Rawls, Thomas Scanlon and Judith Jarvis Thomson. The latter was reprinted in *The New York Review of Books*, March 27, 1997, pp. 41–47. Several briefs are available at www.soros.org/death/brieftxt.html.

The criterion of voluntariness also presents problems in determining patient status and articulating boundaries (e.g., what constitutes undue influence by another party). Further, the question can be raised whether serious socioeconomic disadvantage nullifies voluntariness. If a desirable treatment would bankrupt a patient's family and, therefore, a patient chooses suicide, should a physician be authorized to assist? The dilemma between complicity with societal inequalities (by allowing assisted suicides) and magnification of them (by refusing assistance in suicides) is not readily resolvable.

Similarly, requiring that patients be mentally competent raises questions about what standards will be used, what threshold will be set, how fluctuating capacities will be handled, and what will be done about directions in advance. If competence requires very good mental functioning, then few persons known to be near death may qualify. If, however, one cannot direct suicide in advance of becoming incompetent, then people may consider preemptive suicide far in advance of death.

Proposals typically require that self-administered prescription drugs be authorized by a physician. If many physicians consider themselves ethically or otherwise precluded from doing so, pressure for more involvement of nonphysicians is likely to arise and, perhaps, to require new safeguards.

In sum, the proposed restrictions and intended safeguards in initiatives to legalize physician-assisted suicide are problematic: difficult to define, uncertain in implementation, or vulnerable to unanticipated and unwanted consequences for those they propose to protect. Resolving uncertainties would likely be a difficult process for clinicians, and the courts almost certainly would be involved in further challenges to the implementation of assisted-suicide laws.

Other questions can be posed concerning autonomy—an individual's right to exercise free choice regarding his or her life. This is the core principle that is advanced in favor of physician-assisted suicide. The committee agrees that this principle is a centrally important value. It also believes that the current serious deficiencies in the provision of care to dying people— deficiencies highlighted throughout this report—themselves compromise the autonomy principle by depriving individuals of many choices that should, and realistically can, be made available to them. As discussed in Chapter 5, substantial numbers of dying people today suffer from avoidable pain and other symptoms, and many of the arguments for physician-assisted suicide reflect fear of pain. Offering these patients just two options—either physician assistance for hastened death or continued life with untreated pain—is a highly constricted choice that undermines the principle of autonomy. Truly autonomous choice would allow for adequate relief of pain and other distressing symptoms, adequate psychological support from properly trained health care professionals, and adequate financial and personal service support for home care in preference to impersonal hospital or nursing home settings.

If, one way or another, Oregon proceeds, the committee believes that its implementation of legal physician-assisted suicide should be carefully and intensively monitored. One key objective would be to learn whether legal safeguards are truly effective. A second objective would be to determine whether general deficiencies in the care of dying people influence individual choices for physician-assisted suicide and whether legalization stimulates correction of deficiencies. If the Oregon law is implemented, advantage should be taken of the opportunity to develop a more adequate factual basis for evaluating the competing claims for and against legal recognition of physician-assisted suicide.

Individual committee members had varied views about the morality, legality, and administrability of assisted suicide. The group fully agreed, however, that the current deficiencies in the provision of care for dying people are so extensive that they may provide inappropriate incentives for people to choose hastened death if that option is made available to them without accompanying remedial measures to improve their care. The nation should not need the prod of assisted suicide to drive it to act in behalf of the dying, although this committee, realistically, believes that media coverage of the assisted suicide cases has put the issues before the public and the professions in a very attention-getting fashion.

CONCLUSION

Reliable, excellent care at the end of life is an objective that should be supported, not impeded, by public policy. Unfortunately, some laws, regulations, and policies of public/private regulatory bodies may obstruct good care, either by their specific provisions or by the fear and misunderstanding they create. Drug-prescribing laws stand out in this regard and, in the view of the committee, warrant revisions to minimize discouragement of effective pain management. Other laws and regulations reflect an overly optimistic view of the effectiveness of laws and legal documents in clarifying how people wish to be treated when dying. Legal documents have a role to play but should not deflect attention from the more significant and complex process of advance care planning as considered in Chapter 3.

Deficiencies in care of the dying were recognized well before recent assisted suicide referenda, legislative activities, and court challenges. Nonetheless, much of the recent attention to deficiencies in end-of-life care arose only when the issue of assisted suicide came before the Supreme Court. Even if assisted suicide becomes legal, both society and the professions should feel confident that no one who chooses suicide does so because care systems are deficient in meeting their needs.

8

Educating Clinicians and Other Professionals

The resident said there was "nothing to do" for this young man with head and neck cancer who was "endstage." He was restless and short of breath and he looked terrified and couldn't talk. I didn't know what do for him, so I patted him on the shoulder, said something inane and left and at 7:00 a.m. he died. The memory haunts me. I failed to care for him properly because I was ignorant.

Adapted from Charles von Gunten, *Why I Do What I Do,*
1996, p. 47

Critics have taken the medical education community vigorously to task for failing to sufficiently educate health professionals about how to provide superior, or even competent, care for dying patients.[1] On a more personal level, many physicians can recount how poorly prepared they were as students and residents to encounter dying patients and their families and how profound have been the lessons they have learned from their patients (see, e.g., ABIM, 1996b). Deficiencies in undergraduate, graduate, and continuing education for end-of-life care reflect a medical culture that defines death as failure and ignores care for dying people as a source of professional accomplishment and personal meaning. As reviewed in this chapter, major deficiencies include

* a curriculum in which death is conspicuous mainly by its relative absence;
* educational materials that are notable for their inattention to the end stages of most diseases and their neglect of palliative strategies; and
* clinical experiences for students and residents that largely ignore dying patients and those close to them.

Since this study was first considered, the committee has seen increasing

---

[1]See, e.g., Glaser and Straus, 1968; Liston, 1973; Dickinson, 1976; Mermann et al., 1991; Hill, 1995; ABIM, 1996a; and AMA, 1996b.

acknowledgement by practitioners and educators of the compelling need to better prepare clinicians to assess and manage symptoms, to communicate with patients and families, and to participate in interdisciplinary caregiving that meets the varied needs of dying patients and those close to them. Professional organizations including the American Medical Association and the American Board of Internal Medicine have launched major educational initiatives directed at both students and established clinicians, and individual medical schools are redesigning their curricula. Private foundations are supporting a number of curriculum development projects. (Appendixes C, G, and I include materials related to several of these initiatives.) The alumni bulletin of the Harvard Medical School devoted most of its Winter 1997 issue to end-of-life topics including one article on a course, Living with Life-Threatening Illness, that was developed in response to student requests and with a grant from the National Cancer Institute (Block, 1997).

These and other initiatives are promising, but persistence in their implementation, evaluation, redesign, and extension will be necessary to keep the promise from fading once initial enthusiasm subsides. In particular, the clinical elements of end-of-life care require more emphasis. For example, the committee was struck by how many schools for health professionals seem to assign end-of-life issues to ethics seminars and discussions (see, e.g., Dickinson and Mermann, 1996). Certainly, such a foothold may serve as a starting point for drawing attention to difficult clinical choices. The committee believes, however, that it is unwise and unacceptable to segregate death and dying from the rest of the clinical curriculum.

The first part of this chapter, which draws on the discussion in Chapter 3, considers the core elements of professional competence in caring for those approaching death. The rest of the chapter focuses on the undergraduate and graduate education of physicians, nurses, and social workers and also points to the importance of continuing education. The fundamental argument of the chapter is that health professions education can do better in

1.   conferring a basic level of competence in the care of the dying patient for all practitioners;
2.   developing an expected level of palliative and humanistic skills considerably beyond this basic level; and
3.   establishing a cadre of superlative professionals to develop and provide exemplary care for those approaching death, to guide others in the delivery of such care, and to generate new knowledge to improve care of the dying.

The emphasis in this chapter on professional education should not imply lack of concern about what happens in colleges, high schools, grade schools, and homes. Medical education is a powerful, transforming, and sometimes desensitizing force (Cassem, 1979; Klass, 1987; Reilly, 1987; Hafferty, 1991), but its impact is tempered by preexisting attitudes and understandings that have developed from childhood. A better understanding of the attitudes that students bring with them to professional schools and that affect their choice of health care as a profession would be useful in directing broad efforts to develop or reinforce those that support good care of dying patients. Such efforts would require the involvement of educators at every preprofessional level, parents, television producers, journalists, and others with influence over children and adolescents.

Further, although the periods of undergraduate and graduate health professions education are critical for developing the knowledge, skills, and personal qualities advocated in this report, experience in practice is also a profound teacher for the clinician who is prepared to analyze and learn. In addition, as technologies, policies, organizations, and expectations change, formal continuing education will have a role to play in helping health professionals acquire new knowledge, hone existing skills, and continually improve their abilities to care well for dying patients. The education of professionals is a life-long enterprise.

CORE COMPONENTS OF PROFESSIONAL PREPARATION FOR CARE AT THE END OF LIFE

Different people will bring to their roles as health professionals differing intellectual talents, emotional strengths, physical capacities, and other personal qualities. Just as some individuals may not be well-suited to become surgeons or pediatric nurse specialists, others may not be well-suited to specialize in palliative care. Nonetheless, the committee believed that *every health professional who deals directly with patients and families needs a basic grounding in dealing competently and compassionately with seriously ill and dying patients.* Appropriate referral is important but not sufficient.

In recent decades, those concerned with the content, quality, and certification of health professions educational programs have attempted to identify core competencies and devise formal statements of expectations for undergraduate or graduate programs in many areas of health care (Blank, 1995). A few of these statements in specialty and subspecialty areas such as anesthesiology or critical care medicine cover some aspects of end-of-life care, but none are very comprehensive in setting forth the competencies needed for consistently excellent care of very ill or dying patients (Steel, 1996). No single set of competencies will be sufficient by itself for all specialties or all health care professions, but a general listing can serve as a foundation for programs tailored to specific fields.

For this foundation, this committee identified several fundamental elements of sound professional preparation for care at the end of life. They include (1) command of relevant scientific and clinical knowledge; (2) mastery of appropriate technical, communication, interpersonal, and other skills; (3) appreciation of ethical and professional principles of care; and (4) development of organizational skills to help patients and families navigate the health care system. These four components are covered in more detail in Box 8.1, which draws from a variety of sources including the components and competencies identified by a number of organizations, clinicians, and educators (see, generally, Doyle et al., 1993; MacDonald, 1994, 1995; ABIM, 1996a; Blank, 1996a; see Appendix G for the American Board of Internal Medicine statement of clinical competencies). Although the elements listed emphasize knowledge and skills, they also reflect a concern for the attitudes, values, and feelings that shape and infuse their application in practice. For example, to the extent that students and practitioners have unexamined anxieties about death, they may unconsciously distance themselves from those who are dying and fail their patients clinically and emotionally (Howells and Field, 1982; Vargo and Black, 1984; Field and Howells, 1985).

Some specific competencies lie particularly, but not necessarily exclusively, in the realm of certain professions. For example, pharmacological management of symptoms is largely the physician's domain, although nurses, especially advanced practice nurses, may have some discretion in this area. Mobilizing community resources in behalf of patients and families is a special responsibility of social workers. Nurses play a particularly central role in coordinating interdisciplinary palliative care and attending to patient comfort. More widely shared are interpersonal and ethical competencies in end-of-life care, and many of the nonpharmacological options for preventing and managing symptoms and distress draw on the skills and sensitivities of all members of the palliative care team and, indeed, all of those who come in contact with seriously ill and dying patients.

PHYSICIAN EDUCATION

General

Despite the difficulties in bringing about curriculum reform and the many legitimate competing interests,[2] the stakes here—avoidable physical,

---

[2]The committee was, for example, aware of Renee Fox's observations about a series of reports on medical education. In her words, they have appeared at "periodic, closely spaced intervals . . . [and have] contained virtually the same rediscovered principles, the same concern over the degree to which these conceptions are being honored more in the breach than in practice, the same explanatory diagnoses [about] what accounts for these deficiencies, along with renewed dedication to remedying through essentially the same exhortations and reforms" (cited in Howell, 1992, p. 717).

BOX 8.1
Professional Preparation for End-of-Life Care

Scientific and clinical knowledge and skills, including:

- Learning the biological mechanisms of dying from major illnesses and injuries
- Understanding the pathophysiology of pain and other physical and emotional symptoms
- Developing appropriate expertise and skill in the pharmacology of symptom management
- Acquiring appropriate knowledge and skill in nonpharmacological symptom management
- Learning the proper application and limits of life-prolonging interventions
- Understanding tools for assessing patient symptoms, status, quality of life, and prognosis

Interpersonal skills and attitudes, including:

- Listening to patients, families, and other members of the health care team
- Conveying difficult news
- Understanding and managing patient and family responses to illness
- Providing information and guidance on prognosis and options
- Sharing decisionmaking and resolving conflicts
- Recognizing and understanding one's own feelings and anxieties about dying and death
- Cultivating empathy
- Developing sensitivity to religious, ethnic, and other differences

Ethical and professional principles, including:

- Doing good and avoiding harm
- Determining and respecting patient and family preferences
- Being alert to personal and organizational conflicts of interests
- Understanding societal/population interests and resources
- Weighing competing objectives or principles
- Acting as a role model of clinical proficiency, integrity, and compassion

Organizational skills, including:

- Developing and sustaining effective professional teamwork
- Understanding relevant rules and procedures set by health plans, hospitals, and others
- Learning how to protect patients from harmful rules and procedures
- Assessing and managing care options, settings, and transitions
- Mobilizing supportive resources (e.g., palliative care consultants, community-based assistance)
- Making effective use of existing financial resources and cultivating new funding sources

emotional, and spiritual suffering—are too high to dismiss proposals for changing how physicians are educated to care for patients who are approaching death. The economic, political, organizational, and other pressures now facing the medical profession, if anything, make preparation for compassionate, effective, and ethical end-of-life care more important than ever. The beneficiaries of such preparation are, most obviously, patients and families. But physicians and their colleagues will also benefit from feelings of greater competence; relief from guilt about mismanaging patients; and gratitude for being able to help patients and families experience a death that is free from preventable suffering and generally consistent with what patients and families want.

The discussion below does not probe the implications of financial and political pressures facing medical schools, residency programs, and academic health centers. These pressures include threats to cut or revamp funding for graduate medical education, proposals to restrict the number of residencies (and, possibly, the use of international medical graduates), uncertainty about resources to subsidize care for the indigent, and restructuring for participation in managed care networks (or exclusion from such networks).

Although the committee recognized these pressures, it did not consider the call for improved education in end-of-life care a disproportionate burden on schools. First, palliative care is not a special interest issue; its principles of whole-patient care and teamwork provide a model for many other areas. Second, curriculum change need not be just an expensive addition but can also be an enrichment of established educational content and formats. Third, the use of existing program models and sharing of information can reduce the curriculum development burden on any single school. Fourth, the need to look beyond the hospital setting for educational opportunities is not unique to end-of-life care, but can be considered as part of a more general effort to develop nonhospital arrangements for improved training in primary and chronic care.

Undergraduate Programs

Undergraduate medical education combines didactic and clinical experience with an extraordinary process of professional socialization. Traditionally, the first two years have been devoted to classroom instruction, generally using a lecture format. The last two years have been structured into a series of clerkships that introduce students to patients, clinical settings, and skills. This tradition derives from reforms that first began over a century ago with the objectives of strengthening medical education and reinforcing the professional stature of medicine by establishing educational standards, eliminating poor quality proprietary schools, and incorporating a strong science base into the curriculum (Flexner, 1910; Starr, 1982; Wheatley, 1988; Rothstein, 1992).

Although the traditional format still generally prevails, many schools have reshaped curricula to include new educational strategies. These strategies include case-based learning in small groups, earlier experiences with patients and simulated patients, a less abrupt division in the content of the first two and last two program years, and other innovations (Coggeshall, 1965; AAMC, 1992; Marston and Jones, 1992; Prockop, 1992; Pew Health Professions Commission, 1993; Tosteson et al., 1994). The scope of undergraduate education has also been enriched in varying degrees by the addition of more and better instruction in the behavioral and social sciences, ethics, humanities, medical informatics, and other topics beyond basic biological sciences and traditional inpatient clinical care.

The methods and objectives of these strategies for educational change are multifaceted and generally consistent with the basic concepts of palliative care and the directions proposed in this report. They include

- engaging students more directly in the learning process,
- strengthening problem-solving and reasoning skills,
- improving patient-physician communication,
- encouraging teamwork among health professionals,
- extending education into the community by placing students in the physician's office, nursing home, home, and other nonhospital settings,
- increasing the connections between scientific knowledge and clinical practice, and
- better preparing students for lifelong learning.

Not only are these methods and objectives consistent with the directions suggested here for education in end-of-life care, the care of dying patients offers some powerful opportunities for their application and, thus, for enriching education at many different points in a student's experience. Teamwork is an obvious example of such an opportunity. Similarly, efforts to improve communication skills might reasonably consider communication with patients and families about incurable diagnoses, unexpected or expected death, referral to hospice, and similar matters to represent one end of a continuum of progressively more difficult responsibilities.

The last two years of undergraduate medical education bring some special challenges. One challenge is arranging clerkships that are more reflective of modern clinical practice, which is less and less hospital-based. A second challenge is providing sufficient oversight, guidance, and feedback so that the clerkship experience is more than unguided observations of others and poorly supervised interactions with patients. With the sites of clerkships multiplying and moving out of the hospital, creating and maintaining successful partnerships between educators and practitioners can be very difficult. A third challenge is providing a more meaningful general clinical experience for students in their last undergraduate year when they are beyond their first introduction to patients and are, in many cases, already thinking about specialization.

Curriculum change is clearly a political as well as an intellectual process, especially when it comes to subtracting topics and restructuring teaching methods (AAMC, 1992; Hendrickson et al., 1993). The continuing call for many varieties of educational reform have put additional stress on an already crowded medical curriculum in which it is easier to add than to subtract topics and easier to adopt reforms than to document their effectiveness. One consequence is that the preclinical curricula are, according to one educator, "stuffed with too many courses, too many lectures, and too many faculty hobby horses that leave students at the end of two years exhausted [and] disgruntled" (Petersdorf, 1987, p. 19). Departments have turf to protect, individual faculty have habits that are entrenched, and academic administrators bear scars from previous attempts at major changes. As one anonymous educator has put it, "changing a curriculum is as easy as moving a graveyard." And as one dean described change in another context, "most deans would rather take a daily physical beating than try to make significant changes in the traditional [curriculum]" (Garrison, 1993, p. 344).

In such an environment, improved education about care at the end of life can seem like just another in a continuing stream of claims for attention to such worthy issues as nutrition, aging, race and ethnicity, informed consent, substance abuse, environmental hazards, and domestic violence. The committee rejected this perspective but acknowledged the stresses that give rise to it.

Another objection to increased educational attention to end-of-life care is that most physicians will care for few dying patients (perhaps 6 to 10 a year for the average internist) and can rely on consultants in these cases. The committee acknowledged this fact but noted that (1) broad-based education rather than early specialization is the premise of today's undergraduate curriculum, (2) physicians of all kinds—regardless of specialty—deal with patients who have serious, life-limiting illnesses, and (3) the principles and values taught in palliative care are also relevant to the care of many patients who are seriously or chronically ill but not thought to be dying. In addition, physicians in a managed care environment will likely see a broader range of patients and patient problems than in the past.

Despite the intuitive appeal of many innovative educational strategies, researchers are still trying to evaluate educational innovations, such as problem-based and small-group learning, and to understand their strengths and limitations compared with traditional lectures on abstract concepts.[3] Again, this is an issue that is generally relevant to educational reform rather than specific to calls for greater attention to the care of dying patients.

Graduate Programs

As important as undergraduate medical education is in providing a conceptual, scientific, and ethical foundation for later learning and practice, the residency years are the time when physicians really learn to care for patients and to work with other members of the health care team. Too often, in the committee's experience, the residency years bring a negative image of dying patients and a neglect of excellence in end-of-life care. Illustrative of that problem is a quote from an editorial in the *Journal for the National Cancer Institute*, which noted (without critique) that "program directors acknowledge that critically ill patients, having few or no therapeutic alternatives, can have a negative impact on House Staff and students. They urged an exposure to outpatient oncology, where treatment successes are more frequently found" (cited in MacDonald, 1995, p. 278).

Depending on the field, the residency years repeat some of the challenges of the clerkship years. Some of the key issues are: (1) developing and sustaining productive, well-supervised experiences in nonhospital settings; (2) improving experience, including participation in interdisciplinary care that is guided and evaluated according to defined objectives; (3) balancing particular institutional needs for the provision of patient care services with the educational goals of the residency experience; and (4) providing experiences with the practical realities of cost-constrained medicine tempered by seminars and other opportunities to reflect on the ethical, professional, clinical, and other implications of these realities. Residency programs are also coping with the increased emphasis on primary care that has been reinforced by cost containment and care management strategies of managed care organizations. In general, primary care physicians will likely manage more complicated conditions (with fewer referrals to specialists); thus, they will need to be better prepared to care for patients with difficult medical problems and know when to refer them to others.

---

[3]The early research on these innovations is promising but hardly conclusive (see, e.g., Albanese and Mitchell, 1993; Vernon and Blake, 1993; IOM, 1995b; Schmidt et al., 1996; Vernon and Hosokawa, 1996). The features of traditional instruction can be summarized as large, discipline-focused classes in which students are lectured on fact-oriented science and abstract knowledge, and then tested by multiple-choice examinations. In contrast, problem-based learning prefers small classes in which a teacher guides discussions on clinically related problems that emphasize concept- and problem-oriented science, often in an interdisciplinary setting.

That medical students, interns, and residents learn from nurses and other professionals how to draw blood, give injections, and otherwise provide care is a staple of educational folk culture. Some of this learning makes up for correctable deficits in formal training, and some of it appropriately reflects the depth and breadth of expertise that professionals other than physicians have gained from their education and experience. Nurses, social workers, psychologists and others can do much to broaden what physicians understand about helping families, managing emotions, providing information and reassurance, and similar aspects of care. Physicians and physician educators will not uniformly be the best sources for this kind of learning.

Education about Death and Dying

Surveys dating back to the early 1970s indicate that attention to issues of death and dying is fairly limited in the undergraduate curriculum. A 1972 survey reported that about half of the responding schools had some kind of formal program (although what this meant is not well defined), most of which were less than five years old (cited in Mermann et al., 1991). A report on another survey in the same year concluded that the area "probably represents one of the greatest failures in professional education today" (Schoenberg and Carr quoted in Mermann et al., 1991, p. 35). A 1975 survey showed a higher percentage (87 percent) of schools with some formal activity on death and dying, but for 36 percent, this activity consisted of only one or two lectures (cited in Mermann et al., 1991). These surveys suffered from a variety of methodological difficulties, but the overall picture was clear. Care for those who are dying was not an educational priority and was, in fact, hardly perceptible as an issue.

Into the early 1990s, medical education on death and dying had not changed dramatically from the 1970s (Dickinson and Mermann, 1996; AMA, 1996b). In 1994, only 5 of 126 schools offered a separate, required course on end-of-life care, although 117 said they covered it as one topic in a broader course (Hill, 1995). Most schools (66) covered the topic in an elective course, but for 40 of these schools, the elective course also covered other subjects. Seventeen schools offered elective clerkships. In 1996, the number of schools with separate required courses stood at 6 with 120 including the topic as part of a broader course.

In contrast, a 1996 review of curricula in Canadian medical schools found that all 16 schools provided specific required time for palliative care education (MacDonald, submitted for publication). The mean lecture time was almost 5 hours with another 6 hours in small-group teaching sessions. Three schools offered over 15 hours in designated palliative care instruction with two (McGill and Memorial) offering over 20 hours. Four schools, however, provided less than 5 hours. Six of the schools supported one or more full-time equivalent faculty positions (led by the University of Alberta and the University of Ottawa with six full-time faculty). A study from the United Kingdom reported a mean of 7 hours of curriculum time for palliative care (Scott and MacDonald, 1997; see also Thorpe, 1991).

In a U.S. survey that focused on student reports of their clinical training, all of the responding third-year medical students reported that they had cared for a dying patient, but 41 percent had never heard a physician talking with a dying patient, 35 percent had never discussed care for dying patients with an attending physician, and the great majority had never been present when a surgeon told a family that a patient had died (Rappaport and Witzke, 1993). Almost half of the students could not remember any consideration of death and dying in the curriculum.

At the residency program level, 1,200 residents in 55 representative internal medicine training programs were surveyed as part of an ABIM project on end-of-life patient care. "Preliminary results of this survey indicate that residents have significant difficulty in caring for patients near the end of life and conservatively rate their competency in medical knowledge, symptom and pain control assessment and management, and use of the team approach." (Blank, 1996b, p. 2). A survey by DiMaggio (1993) of psychiatric residency programs found that 56 percent of responding program directors reported that their programs offered some didactic coverage of the topic; of the residents responding, 26 percent reported participation in such lectures. As yet unpublished research based on focus groups and surveys in a number of medical schools presents similar reports of educational gaps and student or resident discomfort, uncertainty, and avoidance (Rappaport et al., 1991; Block, 1997).

The failure of residency programs to sufficiently train new physicians in care at the end of life is due, in part, to the failure of the various specialties and subspecialties to require such training. Some examples from a recent analysis of program requirements illustrate the situation (Steel, 1996). In the anesthesiology requirements, no mention of pain management is included for anesthesiology critical care. Family practice residency requirements also fail to cover pain control, and the discussion of death and dying mentions the family but not the patient. General internal medicine requirements encourage, but do not require, hospital-affiliated nursing homes and hospice programs as sites for residency training; the curriculum section does not mention pain or other symptom management. The requirements for the subspecialty of oncology do not specifically mention hospice resources.

Directions for Improvement

Fortunately, many of the proposed and partly implemented reforms in undergraduate and graduate medical education lend themselves to the incorporation of knowledge or skills relevant for end-of-life care, even if the reforms may be motivated by other concerns. For example, the case-based approach of problem-based learning can readily accommodate cases that involve dying patients or patients likely to die. Such cases can present a range of important scientific, clinical, and behavioral questions for students, many of which can be generalized to other situations.

Ethics seminars likewise provide a natural place for many difficult issues to be discussed. Indeed, their development was partly stimulated by a desire to help medical students learn to grapple with difficult "life-and-death issues." Although the committee was not aware of any systematic data on the content of ethics seminars or courses, committee experience and familiarity with course materials in a number of institutions suggested that fairly standard topics related to end-of-life care include: advance directives, informed consent, truth-telling, the principle of double-effect (i.e., that treatment to relieve distress may, as a secondary but acceptable effect, hasten death), decisions about withdrawing or not initiating certain treatments, physician-assisted suicide, and costs or resource allocation. These are important topics but cannot substitute for basic scientific and clinical knowledge about symptoms mechanisms, prevention, and relief.

From the humanities comes a different kind of contribution to the education of health professionals. In particular, fictional and true personal narratives are employed to balance, at least in part, the highly scientific and technological orientation of medical education with a fuller understanding of serious illness and the value of attentive and compassionate caring for patients and those close to them (Hunter, 1994). Literature helps students and established professionals to understand values, customs, and ethics; develop empathy and perspective; find meaning in the lives of dying patients and the experiences of caring for them; and renew and restore their spirit for a workday world often filled with distress and even tragedy (Charon et al., 1995; Hunter, Charon, and Coulehan, 1995).

One challenge in improving graduate medical education is the large number and diversity of residency experiences. Today, for example, many residents may train in institutions without strong palliative care services and consultative resources.

In this environment, formal residency requirements involving end-of-life care may be a necessary—albeit not sufficient—stimulus to change. The benefits of such changes would, of course, extend beyond the residency institution's patients.

The *Oxford Textbook of Palliative Medicine* (Doyle et al., 1993) offers general guidance on how to coordinate improved education in palliative care with other educational reforms. It suggests

- seeking to incorporate the knowledge base and concepts of palliative care in many places in the curriculum rather than trying to capture more designated courses or hours;
- helping those from other disciplines recognize opportunities to raise end-of-life issues;
- suggesting to these colleagues informative and interesting cases and other teaching materials for didactic courses, small-group learning, and other experiences;
- providing faculty role models who will inspire emulation;
- offering the best elective seminar, rotation, or other experience in the curriculum;
- capitalizing on self-paced modes of instruction, including computer programs and video materials; and
- including topics related to end-of-life care in student evaluations.

In general, educational innovations involve a mix of strategies, tools, topics, and formats. Some are most suitable for undergraduate programs and others are suitable for graduate programs; some may be woven equally well into parts of both. Schools do not have to build such a curriculum on their own. They can take advantage of general curricula designs, teaching materials, and guidance developed by others. More such material should be available in the future, in part because foundations and private organizations are sponsoring a number of initiatives intended to improve education and training in end-of-life care (see Appendix C). The array of educational strategies and tools includes the following:

- **Role models.** One argument offered by those who support the creation of a palliative care specialty is that students need role models who are skilled in all aspects of palliative care (Calman, 1988; MacDonald, 1993). As discussed further below, experienced, multidisciplinary consulting teams provide such role models, in addition to the important clinical and other expertise and instruction they may contribute to the care of patients with difficult problems. More generally, the effort to identify and create role models should extend to any facet of medical education and practice (e.g., primary care, emergency care, pediatrics, and cardiology) that touches people with life-threatening illness.
- **Patients as teachers.** Mermann et al. (1991) have discussed a course for first- and second-year students at Yale University Medical School that utilizes the authoritative voice and experience of very sick patients to describe their experiences with physicians and to inform students of what it is like to have a life-threatening illness. Each student is matched with a patient who has volunteered to be interviewed and to discuss his or her circumstances, feelings, questions, and concerns over a period of months. This

interaction is accompanied by assigned readings, faculty-led discussion, and a videotaping and discussion of students interviewing the patients.

• **Experience in following a number of patients with advanced illness and their families through the progression of the illness and seeing a palliative consultative service in action.** The idea here is similar to the approach taken in obstetrics training of requiring that students follow particular pregnant patients through delivery. The objective is not only to increase cognitive knowledge about the dying process but to encourage a better practical appreciation of the issues in planning and managing care through the course of a patient's dying and to achieve a fuller awareness of the patient's and family's experience and concerns.

• **Exposure to patient and clinician narratives, literature, and structured opportunities for personal reflection.** Just as the use of clinical teaching cases adds clinical richness and individual complexity to medical education, the use of personal narratives and literature provides compelling insights into the personal significance and interpersonal experience of caring for dying patients and those close to them and the ways in which a loved one's dying can bring richness and meaning to others as well as loss and grief. In addition to reading and writing personal narratives, students can also be prepared in advance to reflect on their experiences—for example, the first death they see as a student, the first time they witness a patient or family learning of incurable illness, or the first patient in their care who dies (Solomon, 1997). As described in the introduction to a series of personal narratives about dying and death, real stories present not only clinical and scientific medicine but "the sometimes misplaced art of medicine" (ABIM, 1996b, p. i). For example,

"Dr. S. and I had had several discussions about where he wanted to die . . . it was clear to him that the young doctors in training did not really know how to care for a dying patient. He decided that when his time was close, he would enter the hospital and teach them whatever he could. And he did . . . teaching the house staff gently to respect his decisions and his view of the relation of death to life" (Surks, 1996, pp 5-6).

"Mr. E. had recurrent angina pectoris intractable to medical management. . . . It had become common for the medical residents and cardiology fellows to avoid picking up his chart. After all, he was 'beyond therapy' and they felt uncomfortable with him . . . I asked him what his interests were. . . . As he talked about the books he had read . . . for the first time since I had known him he actually smiled and even laughed. It was obvious that there was effective therapy beyond medication . . . that had not been employed. . . . After exploring with him ways in which he could further his interest in ancient history . . . I made a pact with him . . . that unless there was some compelling reason to admit him to the hospital, I would treat him as an outpatient" (Cheitlin, 1996, p. 7).

• **Role playing.** Role playing is increasingly a part of educational curricula. For example, Tolle et al. (1989) have described role-playing sessions for residents that involve facilitators, students playing the role of a resident notifying survivors of a patient's death, and local hospice volunteers playing survivors of a patient who has died. The organizers stressed what they consider success factors for the program (which got a near 100 percent approval rating from residents): (1) scheduling the program during orientation when residents are not yet stressed with clinical work, (2) scripting the sessions to be clinically relevant, and (3) the intrinsic power of realistic simulations of an emotionally significant event.

• **Morbidity/mortality conferences, morning reports, and attending rounds.** Integrating a discussion of end-of-life issues in the day-to-day process of residency training is essential to develop and reinforce appropriate behaviors and skills (Clark, 1996). Attending physicians can be encouraged to probe students about strategies for symptom assessment and management and their effectiveness, to ask whether advanced directives or other advanced planning discussions are documented in a patient's record, to explore concerns in communicating with patients and families, and to invite students to examine and reflect on their personal responses to being with seriously ill and possibly dying patients. Because most faculty were not exposed to such discussion during their own training, incorporating it now may require major efforts in faculty development.

• **Simulated patients.** Experiences with simulated patients are intended to give students greater exposure to patient problems and to develop diagnostic and treatment management skills without prematurely exposing patients to inexperienced learners.[4] Although not suitable for many kinds of clinical problems or topics, they may be useful in helping beginning students and even advanced students or established clinicians learn about end-of-life care.

• **Hospice rotation.** Hospice rotations can involve either community-based or inpatient programs, although the latter tend to be more easily arranged (Knight et al., 1992). Gomez describes the development of a model inpatient hospice and palliative care program that was intended both to improve care for dying patients and to serve as a training site for internal medicine residents, medical students, and nurses (Gomez, 1996). The program was separated from acute care units and linked to a well-established community hospice, which provided residents the opportunity to follow

---

[4]Standardized patients are individuals who are specially trained to present consistent behavior and descriptions of symptoms. They are used primarily in teaching or evaluating diagnostic and treatment planning skills, including questioning of and listening to patients. In addition to sparing patients from serving as "teaching material," this teaching tool also allows convenient scheduling for faculty and students.

patients in other settings. The benefits of this program for residents are that it allows them to increase their technical knowledge and skills, to experience an alternative model of care focusing on patient-reported symptoms and their meticulous management, and to work closely with a diverse health care team. Ideally, the involvement of medical educators in the creation of appropriate hospice experiences for students and residents would also have a positive impact on efforts to encourage excellent symptom management and timely referrals to hospice.

•   **Intensive care.** Intensive care units can also provide experience with supportive care. As described in Chapter 4, an academic health center that served mainly as an emergency and trauma facility established a supportive care team (a clinical nurse specialist and a small rotating group of physicians) for those for whom curative, rehabilitative, or life-extending care was hopeless (Carlson et al., 1988). In addition to improving end-of-life care for these patients, the program provides residents, students, and faculty with a variety of direct educational opportunities in an acute care setting.

•   **Practice guidelines, decision support systems, and symptom assessment tools.** Chapter 5 discussed various strategies and tools for improving the quality of end-of-life care. These include evidence-based guidelines for pain management and other symptoms, decision support systems, and health status assessment tools. These strategies may be particularly valuable and reassuring to physicians in training (IOM, 1992).

•   **Teaching materials.** The American Board of Internal Medicine (ABIM) has distributed curriculum materials, including a set of personal narratives by physicians and a video (produced by others) to over 2,000 internal medicine programs in the United States. Several projects supported by the Project on Death in America will develop curriculum materials (see Appendix C). Individual faculty and institutions are also developing and sharing materials through a variety of personal and professional networks. Appendix H includes outlines for two examples of medical educational curricula on palliative care. The first was developed by the Canadian Committee on Palliative Care Education. The second was developed at Harvard University. It is important that palliative care experts work with textbook authors and publishers to incorporate material on end-stage disease and symptom management in future editions and to develop supplementary readings or other materials for existing texts. Meeting this goal will take time, but publishers are sensitive to their customers and to public pressure as indicated by increased recognition of women and minorities, regard for patient worries and preferences, concern for prevention, and consideration of issues such as drug abuse and domestic violence.

In addition to considering the place of individual educational strategies, this report encourages each medical school and residency program to work with others in the health professions, the university, and the community to develop an explicit statement on palliative care training for faculty, students, administrators, and others. The statement should

- recognize that medical students and residents need education and training in the effective and humane care of patients approaching death;
- define required and elective curriculum elements for such education and training including lectures, seminars, cases, clerkships, experiences, teaching methods, evaluation techniques, and personnel; and
- specify the scientific, clinical, interpersonal, ethical, cultural, and organizational aspects of care to be covered; and
- identify how the curriculum elements will contribute to student preparation for care of dying patients.

The last point underscores that the concern should not be narrowly with curriculum change but, more broadly, on evaluating the impact of educational strategies on practice and outcomes. As noted above, the committee understood that change is not cost-free and that educational resources need to be used wisely.

Incentives and Levers for Change

The incentives and levers for strengthening education in end-of-life care are varied. In addition to various forms of persuasive argument, a number of other, potentially more compelling means exist to secure change in medical education. Within the medical school curriculum, examination questions on symptom pathophysiology and management and other palliative care topics can focus student and faculty attention. Nationally, inclusion of such questions in licensure and board examinations would, in particular, signal the importance of the subject. The American Board of Hospice and Palliative Medicine has developed a certification examination in hospice and palliative medicine. For graduate medical education, residency program requirements and accreditation are potent means of directing attention to an issue.

For each specialty, residency review committees (RRCs) oversee the process of establishing and reviewing program requirements. The process for changing the requirements takes at least three years and more commonly lasts four or five years. As described by the ABIM, it "involves getting the language in, getting the word out to the many specialty RRCs and other professional societies and groups that are asked to comment, getting the impact statement completed to justify any new changes, and then getting the new requirements through the Accreditation Council for Graduate Medical Education for approval. From that point, the effective date for implementation is nine months to one year" (Blank, 1996b, p. 2). The lead time to get organized for the RRC process adds additional time. In sum, this approach is not quick—and appropriately so, given the significant economic and other effects on programs.

The importance of knowledge and skills in end-of-life care would be underscored if each RRC examined its specialty and subspecialty requirements to establish deficiencies and areas for improvement. As reported earlier in this chapter, a preliminary examination of requirements in several specialties suggested important gaps. Once program committees recognize that program requirements need revision, the design of those revisions would involve individual and cooperative efforts to (1) specify core competencies and formal program requirements and (2) identify how these competencies and requirements will contribute to resident preparation to care for dying patients. Changes in residency program requirements will be most effective if implemented in conjunction with changes in licensure and board examinations. Following is a discussion of whether a palliative care specialty may be necessary to provide the effort and commitment that change frequently requires.

Palliative Care as a Specialty

The criticisms of medical education and the options for improving it imply the commitment of significant energy and resources to establish objectives, correct deficiencies, design and implement innovative programs, and develop means for evaluating progress and improving programs on an ongoing basis. Given all the challenges facing medical schools, academic health centers, and universities, the sustained availability of such energy and resources can hardly be taken for granted in either the short- or the long-term. Much the same can be said about the commitment of resources in health care research, team management and participation, and other activities in an era characterized by increasingly stringent cost controls.

One strategy for drawing attention to the field of palliative care and increasing its stature in medical education and medical practice is to seek its designation as a recognized medical specialty. The United Kingdom recognized palliative medicine as a specialty in 1987, followed by Australia and New Zealand. In Canada, after some initial reluctance to pursue this strategy, an effort to win specialty recognition is under way (MacDonald, 1996). The goal is not to establish an independent field of practice like cardiology or radiology but to develop a stronger base in education and research and to provide integrated care and consulting resources for primary care physicians and specialists in other fields.

Although expertise in palliative care is not a prerequisite for deans, department chairs, individual faculty, and others to press for better education in end-of-life care, the presence of those with such expertise provides a critical reservoir of knowledge, experience, and commitment that makes it more likely that such efforts will succeed. The group of practitioners, educators, and researchers trained and experienced in palliative care is, however, fairly small and their responsibilities are quite diverse, including

- serving as consultants and role models for colleagues, students, and other members of the health care team;
- developing both scientifically based and practically useful curricula, instructional material, and other tools that furnish students and new and established practitioners with relevant knowledge, skills, and practices; and
- organizing and conducting research to extend biomedical, clinical, behavioral, and other knowledge.

In the United States, the American Board of Medical Specialties (ABMS) recognizes 24 medical specialties and approves the recognition by these boards of subspecialties.[5] Growing concern about the increasing fragmentation of medical care and its clinical, political, and economic risks has led the ABMS to establish stricter criteria for specialty recognition and to be very sparing in their application. Individual boards, such as the ABIM, have criteria for designating subspecialties. In addition to full specialty or subspecialty recognition (the latter through certificates of special competence), boards may establish certificates of added qualifications subject to approval by the ABMS.

The advantages of specialty status have been numerous, including professional stature, visibility, and power in the contest for academic resources (e.g., courses, faculty positions, residency slots), and recognition by hospitals and other organizations that credential professionals (e.g., grant hospital privileges, offer health plan contracts).[6] The case for seeking specialty recognition for palliative care has been forcefully argued in the United Kingdom, Australia, and Canada. Some groups testifying to the committee at its April 1996 public meeting noted possible benefits of a formal specialty without necessarily endorsing the step (Byock, 1996; Calder, 1996; Mahoney, 1996). The arguments for establishing a formal specialty are that it would

---

[5]Approximately 130 non-ABMS recognized boards exist. These vary in their perceived legitimacy and respectability. One report noted that 40 or so of these boards operate out of the same office in Las Vegas (ABIM, 1993).

[6]Medicare does not explicitly recognize specialty status in its resource-based fee schedule for physicians, but specialty physicians may command higher incomes by virtue of their more intensive patient management services (which are assigned higher fees) and their greater involvement in procedural services (PPRC, 1991).

- focus attention more powerfully on an existing knowledge base that is both insufficiently understood and inadequately applied and that is in need of further growth;
- recognize more explicitly and publicly that palliative care is an appropriate goal of medicine;
- conform to the value and recognition structure of medical professionals—providing credibility with peers (and perhaps patients and others) as a source of knowledge, guidance, and referral;
- attract leaders to the field; and
- nurture the development of the field and its knowledge base.

As suggested above, calls for the creation of new specialties are today greeted with considerable skepticism and reserve. Several groups testifying to the committee were mildly to strongly negative about a formal palliative care specialty (Bagley, 1996; Blank, 1996b; Felder, 1996; Viste, 1996; Volicer, 1996). The arguments against a new specialty are that it would

- imply that other specialties/health professionals need not be very concerned with prevention and relief of pain and other distress at the end of life;
- increase fragmentation of care for those with severe chronic or terminal conditions;
- demand more faculty resources during a period when faculty energies may already be approaching exhaustion;
- be confusing (i.e., create uncertainty about who should care for those severely ill but not clearly dying);
- be vulnerable to disproportionate influence by cancer care models/ personnel;
- be difficult to win acceptance in managed care environments where there is more emphasis on primary care practitioners;
- be politically suspect given concerns about oversupply of specialists and uncertainties about resources for medical schools and academic medical centers; and
- divert resources from existing specialties, many of which feel under siege from health care restructuring.

Formal specialty status is not the only way to expand the core of palliative care experts. By creating professional societies (e.g., the American Academy of Hospice and Palliative Medicine), establishing journals (e.g., the *Journal of Pain and Symptom Management*), organizing meetings and conferences, and establishing academic centers, experts in palliative care already are directing more attention to practice, research, and education in the field. Indeed, the ABIM essentially demands that such steps precede specialty recognition. The ABIM's criteria for certification of special competence are that a discipline must: have a distinct and unique body of knowledge; have clinical applicability sufficient to support a distinct clinical practice; contribute to the scholarly generation of new information and advance research in the field; have a minimum training period of 12 months; meet numerical standards for training programs, trainees, and practicing diplomates to demonstrate maturation of the discipline; and have positive value that outweighs the negative impact of certification on the field of general internal medicine or its existing subspecialties. It is not clear at this time that palliative medicine in the United States would meet all the conditions related to training programs.

The committee was initially reluctant to endorse the creation of another medical specialty for the reasons cited above. After its months of examination of the problems in care at the end of life, it concluded that the needs are so great that palliative care should become established, if not as a recognized medical specialty, then as a defined and accepted area of teaching, research, and patient care expertise.

NURSING, SOCIAL WORK, AND OTHER PROFESSIONS

Other professions, including nursing, social work, dentistry, pharmacy, physical therapy, nutrition, and pastoral counselling have not been as severely criticized as medicine for inattention to care at the end of life. In some cases such as dentistry, this may be because their direct contribution to the care of dying patients is seen as fairly limited. In other cases such as social work and nursing, educators and practitioners may be spared some criticism because caring is so central to their training and practice.

Because each health profession faces somewhat different tasks and issues in care for those who are dying, their professional education and training should reflect these differences. It is the sense of the committee that professionals whose expertise and skills are drawn on in care for dying patients would generally welcome opportunities to broaden their professional horizons, to examine how their knowledge and skills may be strengthened to more fully meet the needs of dying patients and their families, and to participate in the training and development of other health professionals. The committee encourages leaders in these other fields to take steps in this direction. The discussion below considers the fields of nursing and social work, both of which have central places in the multidisciplinary care of dying patients and those close to them.

Nursing Education

Although spared some criticism, nursing education also can be faulted for insufficiently preparing nurses to understand the physical, emotional, and spiritual needs of dying patients and their families and for failing to fully equip them to apply existing clinical knowledge and standards effectively in responding to these needs. Such critiques deserve the most careful attention by that group of professionals that Florence Nightingale defined as having special responsibility for "care of the personal health of somebody" and for seeking "to put the patient in the best condition for nature to act upon him" (Nightingale, 1859). Virginia Henderson defined the purpose of nursing as "to assist the individual, sick or well, in the performance of those activities contributing to health or its recovery, or to a peaceful death, that he would perform unaided if he had the necessary strength, will, or knowledge" (Henderson, 1961). In 1980, nursing was defined as "the diagnosis and treatment of human responses to actual or potential health problems" (ANA, 1980). These definitions illustrate the consistent orientation of nurses to providing care for the patient's well-being, regardless of the patient's diagnosis or prognosis.

The knowledge base for nursing is derived from multiple sources, including nursing science; philosophy; ethics; and physical, biomedical, social, behavioral, and economic sciences (IOM, 1983; ANA, 1995). In the last 20 years, nursing philosophy and practice have been influenced by the science of caring. Contemporary nursing practice consists of four essential features:

- "attention to the full range of human experiences and responses to health and illness without restriction to a problem-focused orientation;
- integration of objective data with knowledge gained from an understanding of the patient or group's subjective experience;
- application of scientific knowledge to the processes of diagnosis and treatment; and
- provision of a caring relationship that facilitates health and healing" (ANA, 1995).

This holistic approach to the care of all patients covers each of the dimensions of care identified in Chapter 3: physical, emotional, spiritual, and practical. Nurses are expected to have sufficient knowledge to care for patients during all life stages, including dying.

Although professional nurses, and ultimately their patients, would benefit from nurses' participation in explicit coursework about care at the end of life, attention to this topic appears to vary substantially across schools of nursing (ANA, 1996). Variation exists in the availability of courses, their content, the degree to which end-of-life issues are integrated into basic nursing coursework, and the preparation of the faculty. Some topics related to critical care, pain management, pediatrics, and other specialized areas may be concentrated in advanced curricula, but general nursing curricula should address differences in dying patients related to clinical condition, family circumstances, mental status, and other factors that may call for different nursing strategies.

Corner (1993) identified four career stages—nurse student, new graduate, experienced nurse, and advanced professional—that should be considered in developing educational programs to improve care for dying patients. For the last three categories, continuing education is needed to accommodate technological developments, career shifts, and changing ethical or legal positions. Moreover, to the extent that cost pressures on hospitals and nursing homes continue to reduce the presence of professional nurses, the training and supervision of lower-level personnel who provide nursing care becomes an increasing concern (IOM, 1996c).

Studies of nursing curricula are limited but suggest that nursing students may get little supervised experience with dying patients, minimal guidance in handling their personal reactions to dying patients and grieving families, and little education about symptom assessment (see, e.g., Degner et al., 1991; Frommelt, 1991; Corner, 1993; Coolican et al., 1994; Kingma, 1994; Ross and MacDonald, 1994; Dukes et al., 1995). One theme in critiques of nursing education in end-of-life care is the need for updating the curriculum. For example, nursing programs have been criticized for using outdated models of death education (Coolican et al., 1994; Kingma, 1994). A Canadian review argued that educators need to pay more attention to the problems that nurses face in caring for patients dying at home—keeping current, being isolated, dealing with bureaucracies, and working collaboratively (Ross and MacDonald, 1994).

Improvements in the preparation of nurses can—with modifications appropriate to the objectives, knowledge bases, and formats of nursing education—follow many of the same paths identified for medical educators. That is, clinical knowledge, interpersonal skills, ethical awareness, and other aspects of effective care for dying patients can often be integrated and coordinated with case-based learning, role playing, experiences in different sites, and similar elements that are commonly included in general curriculum reform initiatives.

One of the most difficult problems that nurses face is dealing with patients and families that are being neglected or inappropriately managed by physicians. To the extent that physician education and practice shifts toward a more collaborative approach, nurses will be in a better position to apply their skills and understandings to improve what physicians learn and how they care for patients. To take advantage of such shifts and encourage them, it makes good strategic sense for nurses and nurse educators to promote collaborative educational and training experiences in medical schools, residency programs, and physician continuing education activities.

Social Work Education

Social workers have been described as the hub of interdisciplinary efforts to provide comprehensive medical and support services to patients facing death (Blackman, 1995a). As the health care professionals who focus solely on the psychosocial aspects of death and dying, they consider patient and family adjustment to life-threatening illness and offer them help in making decisions about treatment and obtaining resources that will support the best quality of life possible for dying patients and those close to them. As more care has shifted from institutional settings to homes and as survival with serious illness is extended, social workers have helped to coordinate an increasingly broad range of services to people and families coping with complex medical regimens and periodic physical or emotional crises (Sheldon, 1993; Loscalzo and Zabora, 1996).

Psychological screening, assessment, counseling, referral, and practical assistance with financial and other problems are key responsibilities for social workers. Their role clearly focuses on some of the problems—such as caring for the family and collaborative care—that physicians and, to a lesser extent, nurses have been criticized for neglecting. For cancer patients and their families in the United States, about 75 percent of their supportive counseling is provided by social workers (Coluzzi et al., 1995). Social work is often organized around a model that identifies the social and psychological tasks that patients and families confront at the end of life. Social workers should be educated and trained to help with such difficult tasks as:

- maintaining a meaningful quality of life during illness and the approach of death;
- coping with disfigurement and loss of function;
- confronting existential and spiritual questions;
- making decisions about end-of-life care; and
- planning for survivors' lives after the loss of their loved one.

Social workers are trained in baccalaureate and graduate programs, some of which focus on the health field, others of which are more general. Clinical social workers—who counsel individuals and have graduate degrees—must be licensed by the state. Although they do not provide medical services, social workers in the health care arena need a sound understanding of the medical problems their patients are facing. Some professional organizations, social service agencies, universities, and other organizations sponsor a broad range of continuing education and multidisciplinary training opportunities for social workers.

Nonetheless, specialized course work that focuses on the dying process, bereavement, ethical and legal considerations, and related end-of-life issues appears to be quite limited. Also, as is true for other health professionals, social workers who want to improve their skills in end-of-life care face a dearth of postgraduate training opportunities.

For social workers, like nurses, collaborative educational and training experiences in conjunction with medical schools, residency programs, and physician continuing education activities may help all participants improve their competency in the psychosocial dimensions of care at the end of life and their ability to participate effectively in multidisciplinary patient care. Such specialized, multidisciplinary training is not widely available. This undoubtedly reflects the traditional avoidance in health professions education of emotional reactions, spiritual concerns, bereavement, and other issues for which scientific knowledge, operational concepts and terms of references, and testable hypotheses have been scarce. As education and research agendas change, social workers and other health professionals will benefit from greater scientific understanding in these areas.

Even for social workers who do not specialize in health care, encounters with dying and death are not uncommon but training to deal with these complex, highly charged situations is limited. A few examples of such situations include: domestic violence, community violence, substance abuse, homelessness, and natural disasters (e.g., earthquakes, floods). Social work training tends to focus on clinical approaches to crisis support and intervention rather than on the longer-term emotional aspects of dying, death, and bereavement in these contexts.

Social workers's training should also prepare them to help family caregivers and survivors, an often forgotten group. Spouses, parents, and children (especially wives, mothers, and daughters) are often primary caregivers for people dying over periods of months and even years. For nontraditional families, support for caregivers in this context may be particularly demanding. Death marks an end and a beginning for families and friends, who both mourn their loss and face the often difficult process of reconstructing life on terms very different from before.

CONTINUING PROFESSIONAL EDUCATION

Learning is a lifelong process for medical and other professionals in health care. Health professions education may thus be seen as a continuum in which the professional degree marks the midpoint and in which education and reeducation continue "until the professional life of the practitioner is finished" (Coggeshall, 1965, pp. 39-40). To the extent that health professions schools and residency programs strengthen the attention to end-of-life care in undergraduate and graduate programs, the foundation for continuing education programs should likewise be strengthened.

The basic options for continuing education programs to improve how health professionals care for those approaching death are mostly familiar ones. They include consultation, clinical demonstration, lectures and rounds, courses and conferences, journals, self-learning programs, and reflective practice (Scott and MacDonald, 1997). The last item—reflective practice—draws from academic nursing the concept of learning through reflection (see, e.g., Atkins and Murphy, 1993). Such learning may involve chart reviews, practice audits, patient feedback, and interactive consultations and may be incorporated in processes of continuous quality improvement discussed in Chapter 5.

General strategies for lifelong learning are changing as university-based and other video conference capacities expand and as the Internet and similar electronic media make resources for self-learning more sophisticated and far-reaching. Distance learning options in palliative care have already been developed in Australia (cited in Scott and MacDonald, 1997).

In general, research on the effectiveness of continuing education programs in influencing attitudes, extending knowledge, or enhancing technical skills is limited, and relatively little relates to care for dying patients. Multidisciplinary continuing education—designed to reflect model end-of-life care—may not attract those with the physician's traditional distrust of such education (Scott and MacDonald, 1997). A survey of general practitioners in one English community suggested another possible problem when it found that the majority of those responding favored didactic education in end-of-life care and expressed discomfort about the prospect of experiential education (MacLeod and Nash, 1991). Further, if educational programs do not suggest how new knowledge or skills can be put to immediate use, they may also fail to attract participants.

As mentioned in Chapter 1 and described further in Appendix C, established physicians are the focus of the education initiative being undertaken by the American Medical Association with the participation of many other groups. This initiative recognizes the difficulties of changing the culture of medicine but argues that it can be successfully altered without challenging it in a confrontational and accusatory fashion. Instead, it will concentrate on supportive training of established physicians including preparing them to go back to their communities to train others.

CONCLUSION

On the basis of its experience, literature review, public meetings, and other sources, the committee agreed that the criticisms of medical school education in end-of-life care are merited. Dying is too important a part of life to be left to one or two required lectures or to be set aside on grounds that medical educators are already swamped with competing demands for time and resources. Moreover, educators and clinicians should understand, first, that end-of-life care is not just an ethics issue but a subject for scientific and clinical attention and, second, that it focuses not only on facts and technical skills but also on relationships and emotions, including those of the clinician.

Despite some increase in coverage of care for dying patients, it appears that relevant instruction, clinical experience, and assessments of student attitudes, knowledge, and skills are still limited, even as they pertain to patients who die in hospitals. Clinicians in training are not systematically prepared to assess the clinical and psychosocial factors that indicate what extent of curative, life-prolonging, and palliative care is appropriate for a patient or how it is to be initiated and managed through the course of illness. Attention to skills in communication and shared decisionmaking (including listening skills) remains a weakness. Students receive little interdisciplinary training and are not coached in using a team approach to caring for dying patients and their families. The potential for learning from the other health professions appears to be undervalued. Students are also not directed to explore and reconsider their own and their profession's attitudes toward death or to reflect on what constitutes a good death.

A number of models for curricula are available, including teaching cases and other materials, and more are being developed. Many involve objectives and methods that are consistent with widely endorsed steps designed to integrate scientific and clinical knowledge, improve problem-solving and interpersonal skills, and extend community-based learning. Thus, the effort implied by the committee's recommendations should not prove excessive, nor should the demand for new curriculum time be unreasonable. Moreover, the process of designing curriculum elements related to effective and compassionate care at the end of life is likely to prove helpful in refining and reinforcing other objectives and strategies related to improved interpersonal, teamwork, and reasoning skills. Nonetheless, focusing attention on end-of-life care also requires that the leverage points of professionalism—such as licensure examinations and residency requirements—be employed.

The committee believes that most of the goals of improved end-of-life care can be achieved by persistent pursuit of the other goals and strategies adopted by those committed to the field and by the adoption, by the appropriate parties, of other recommendations stated in this report. In the United States, professional, social, and perhaps political momentum for change has been created in the last three years, and it seems reasonable to allow its effects to be more fully felt. Seeking specialty status and maintaining the bureaucratic apparatus to sustain such status inevitably absorbs resources already in scarce supply. Nonetheless, to accomplish the goals for education, research, and improved care set forth in this report probably requires the equivalent of specialty recognition.

In order to promote and monitor the initiatives already under way to improve health professionals' education and to consider what additional steps may need to be taken, the committee encourages the Institute of Medicine to organize, within the next one to three years, a symposium on the education of health professionals in care at the end of life. The objective would be to assess progress and identify directions for further efforts to ensure that physicians, nurses, social workers, and others have the attitudes, knowledge, and skills to care well for those approaching death.

9
Directions for Research to Improve Care at the End of Life

More light!

Goethe, last words, 1832

Goethe's dying words were not a plea for more research on the end of life, but they are fitting nonetheless. From the cellular to the social level, much remains to be learned about how people die and how reliably excellent and compassionate care can be achieved. Important, unanswered questions exist about the fundamental physiological mechanisms of the symptoms that cause so much suffering among dying patients and about the kinds of interventions that will relieve these symptoms. Basic epidemiological information on how people die is limited, and the influence of attitudes and beliefs on people's experience of dying and on caregiving practices is little charted. In addition, a better understanding of the reasons for the inadequate application of existing knowledge would help in identifying organizational, economic, and other incentives for the provision of accessible, effective, and affordable care at the end of life.

Deficiencies in knowledge and its use have important consequences. Hundreds of thousands of Americans face death each year experiencing severe symptoms and distress, including pain, fatigue, shortness of breath, nausea, wasting, delirium, anxiety, and depression. Although complete relief of such distress cannot be expected, relatively limited investments in cancer and pain research have already had important benefits, as described below. Furthermore, in this era of evidence-based medicine, the outcomes of clinical research are increasingly being used to determine what care is covered by public and private health insurance. In various ways, then, a lack of research on palliative therapies may translate into lack of resources to care for dying patients.

235

The shortage of scientific knowledge reflects a lack of clinical interest in high-quality palliative care, interest that would serve as a powerful stimulus to research. The committee argues that caring for dying patients can be personally rewarding and intellectually challenging. It demands that clinicians learn and apply a wide variety of skills and knowledge. For example, effectively balancing the benefits and adverse effects of multiple drug therapy in a metabolically compromised patient is clearly a complex and exacting task. *Dying patients are not people for whom "nothing can be done" either now or in the future.* Basic biomedical research into the pathophysiology of symptoms and mechanisms of symptom relief—following the model used in pain research—provides a promising foundation for improved patient care and a tighter focus for clinical research on care of patients likely to die.

This chapter focuses on directions for extending the knowledge base for effective, reliable care at the end of life. Unlike other chapters, this chapter uses certain technical terms that may not be understandable to some readers; it does so in an effort to underscore research gaps and opportunities. The following sections consider a symptom-based strategy for biomedical research, directions for behavioral and health services research, ethical issues in research involving dying patients, some important methods issues in end-of-life research, and barriers to research and consequent opportunities for leadership from the nation's research establishment. Although the committee recognized the methodological, ethical, and economic difficulties that can complicate end-of-life research, it did not believe that these problems are insurmountable if leaders recognize the relevance and promise of symptom and other research intended to help reduce suffering at the end of life. Such leadership would help attract more bright young trainees who could readily master the techniques required for the conduct of that research, both in the laboratory and at the bedside.

A SYMPTOM-BASED STRATEGY FOR
BIOMEDICAL RESEARCH

Earlier chapters of this report have described the symptoms that cause significant distress for many dying patients. Although deficits in the use of existing knowledge need to be corrected, it is also important to extend the base of knowledge about the pathophysiology of symptoms and the mechanisms for symptom relief and prevention. Pain is the most widely noted and feared symptom and has been the subject of an active and productive research strategy. This report particularly challenges the biomedical research community and its supporters to direct new intellectual energy to better understanding and countering the mechanisms of other physical and emotional consequences of advanced diseases (and treatment side effects), particularly fatigue, wasting, shortness of breath, nausea, confusion, anxiety, and depression.

Successful biomedical research depends on the interaction of basic scientists and clinical colleagues. Medical advances in managing pain and in understanding and treating chemotherapy-induced nausea reflect such interaction (MacDonald, 1995; Max, 1996). The committee concluded that progress in understanding and managing other symptoms would be advanced by applying and extending the research strategies that have been developed to investigate pain.

The committee also concluded that although palliative care research has received little emphasis in the past 20 years, modest investments appear to have paid substantial dividends in the prevention and relief of symptoms experienced by cancer patients. Advances resulting from cancer research—some of which benefit those who die of cancer as well as long-term survivors—have occurred in several areas (see, e.g., Holland and Rowland, 1990; Breitbart and Holland, 1993; Doyle et al., 1993; AHCPR, 1994a; Gavrin and Chapman, 1995; Portenoy and Kanner, 1996). These include

- managing cancer pain;
- managing nausea and vomiting associated with the use of chemotherapeutic drugs;
- using chemotherapy, radiation therapy, surgery, and other procedural interventions to palliate symptoms in selected cases;
- managing psychiatric symptoms by pharmacological and behavioral techniques;
- addressing special social and developmental issues (e.g., school, play) for children with cancer; and
- incorporating quality-of-life measures in cancer clinical trials.

Several of the above advances have improved symptom control and psychosocial well-being without adding substantial costs for care. For example, the conclusion that opioids and many other symptom-controlling drugs can be effectively administered subcutaneously when oral administration is not effective or feasible has simplified the care of patients and avoided the use of more expensive intravenous or intramuscular therapies (Bruera et al., 1988). Patients and families can readily learn to administer hypodermic injections, thus enabling them to spend longer periods at home with reduced costs and improved quality of life.

Directions for Pain Research

The discussion below begins by presenting pain as a model for symptom research. It then suggests how this model might be applied in three other areas: cachexia-anorexia syndrome, dyspnea, and cogntive/emotional symptoms. Although the physiological details will vary for different symptoms, the general strategy for directing research resources appears broadly applicable.

Pain as a Model for Symptom Research

Based on the committee's experience and investigations for this study, pain appears to be the only major symptom where a constellation of basic scientists and clinicians have worked together to understand the pathophysiology of the symptom and to develop logical therapeutic interventions on the basis of research observations. The most extensive body of work supported by NIH involves pain. In 1995, building on several years of work, 10 units of NIH announced an initiative "to stimulate and foster a wide range of basic and clinical studies on pain" (NIH, 1995, p. 1). Among the topics and areas mentioned for investigation, one singled out effectiveness of "biobehavioral pain management in terminally ill and dying patients" (NIH, 1995, p. 9), but many other topics (e.g., relationship to other symptoms, pain assessment strategies, comparison of different prevention and alleviation strategies) also should have some relevance for this patient population.

In FY 1996, according to one estimate, NIH spent about $70 million on pain research out of an approximate total budget of $12 billion (John Retzlaff, NIH, personal communication, May 27, 1997). One researcher has suggested that this relatively modest public investment "primed the pump" for a substantial research investment by industry, which for many years had confined its work to anti-inflammatory drugs and short-acting opioids (Mitchell Max, personal communication, September 17, 1996 and March 18, 1997). For example, NIH-funded research into the relationship between opioid blood levels and pain relief led industry to develop sustained-release opioid tablets, skin patches, and patient-controlled analgesic infusion pumps. Other research on the pain-inhibiting neurotransmitters has also led to new pain treatments (Max et al., 1992; Wall and Melzack, 1994; Yaksh and Malmberg, 1994). In another previously neglected clinical area, pain related to nerve injury, NIH-supported development of animal models and clinical trial methods in pain have recently stimulated many companies to synthesize candidate compounds and initiate clinical trials. A similar industrial "second wave" of research might be predicted if public-supported research into other symptoms can suggest a physiological rationale for treatment and show that clinical trials can separate active from inactive treatments.

The many successes of clinical pain research in the past two decades—ranging from spinal opioid therapy for surgical and cancer pain to sumitriptan for migraine—rest on a foundation of basic neuroscience that could be applied to many other symptoms. Thousands of researchers have been studying specialized nerve endings and connecting circuits in the spinal cord and brain that give rise to pain and other sensations. Dozens of neuro-scientific techniques that have been developed to study pain and opioid effects could be adapted to the study of other symptoms. These techniques include mapping of neurotransmitters, identifying the changes in cellular and gene activity triggered by these impulses, developing animal models, and three-dimensional imaging of the brain activity triggered by symptoms (Hunt et al., 1987; Draisci et al., 1991; IOM, 1991; Kandel et al., 1991; Capechhi, 1994; Takahashi et al., 1994).

In the field of pain, many additional promising investigative avenues can be identified. These include:

- improving techniques for drug delivery (Storey et al., 1990; Berti and Lipsky, 199; Cleary, 19975; Coluzzi, 1997).
- introducing nonsteroidal anti-inflammatory drugs, which selectively affect the inflammatory components of pain and do not interfere with other essential body activities mediated by prostaglandins (Akarasereenont et al., 1994; Hayllar and Bjarnason, 1995).
- introducing more refined, receptor-specific opioids. Pain inhibition may be mediated by an opioid receptor type that does not influence sedation, bowel function, or respiratory function (Bigelow and Preston, 1995; Breitbart, 1996; Portenoy, 1996).
- identifying novel analgesics that influence nonopioid systems in the central nervous system (Eide et al., 1995; Rang and Urban, 1995; Nelson et al., in press). Particularly noteworthy is the recent discovery of multiple excitatory systems that maintain and enhance particularly severe forms of chronic pain. Current laboratory studies on animal models and initial clinical trials suggest that new types of nonopioid analgesics can successfully influence these pain-stimulating systems.
- strengthening developmental pharmacology intended to maximize benefits and minimize harms by taking into account patient differences in age, race, gender, weight, metabolic status, and other relevant factors.
- identifying prognostic factors to help guide preventive strategies and linking symptoms to quality of life measures to help guide care priorities (Donnelly and Walsh, 1995b).
- improving knowledge of the clinical features and treatment of pain arising in the viscera. Recent work in animal models suggests that visceral pain has some mechanisms that are distinct from other types of pain and that could provide opportunities for therapies. These mechanisms include the sensitivity of primary visceral afferents to kappa opioids (Sengupta et al., 1996) and transmission in the posterior funiculus of the spinal cord, an

area readily accessible to surgical or electrical interventions (Al-Chaer et al., 1996).

Promising Leads for Research on
Cachexia-Anorexia-Asthenia Syndrome

Palliative care experts have identified the symptom complex of cachexia-anorexia-asthenia as a major complaint of patients, who rank the symptoms first or second in prevalence in many cancer studies (Bruera, 1993; Portenoy et al., 1994; Seale and Cartwright, 1994; Donnelly and Walsh, 1995b). In addition to cancer, this syndrome is common in many other illnesses, including AIDS, advanced congestive heart failure, and chronic obstructive pulmonary disease. It is also common in children with chronic lethal conditions (e.g., congenital anomalies) who are not actively dying. It creates dependency on others, with consequent emotional and fiscal cost. Moreover, cachexia can actually result in the death of many patients when sufficient protein to maintain vital body functions is lost.

Those clinicians and scientists who are not familiar with the concepts of preventable suffering and palliative care may assume that wasting, loss of appetite, and weakness are inevitable in the dying process. Some studies, however, suggest that these symptoms are amenable to treatment that affects patient's quality of life and, perhaps, survival time. Observations indicate that cachexia-anorexia may involve a cytokine cascade induced by the disease process or occurring in reaction to it (Grunfeld and Feingold, 1996; Mitch and Goldberg, 1996; Jaskowiak and Alexander, 1997; Moldawer and Copeland, 1997).[1] The specific influence of cytokines may vary from disease to disease. For example, in cancer patients, tumor products may play an important causal role with cytokines acting in an indirect supportive mode (Todorov et al., 1996; Tisdale, 1997). As research findings on the relative influence of cytokines and chemical products induced by disease processes emerge, interference with this process should allow patients to have an improved quality of life as they die and may prolong life for some. As with pain, when the pathophysiology of the symptom complex is more clearly understood, specific interventions can be formulated and tested. Starting points for research should include

- more precise descriptive terminology for the cachexia-anorexia-asthenia complex and the creation of working groups to create a "common language" for research studies;

---

[1]Cytokines are hormone-like proteins that are secreted by various kinds of cells and that are involved in immune responses, cell-to-cell communication, and metabolism. Interferons and interleukins are cytokines.

- development of a standard symptom assessment format for studies on cachexia-anorexia-asthenia, similar to what is available for pain;
- an assessment of the costs of the cachexia-anorexia-asthenia complex; and
- investigation of particular therapy options based on fuller understanding of pathophysiology and the experience of symptoms as reported by patients and families.

In recent years, it has been demonstrated, for the first time, that the trajectory of anorexia and weight loss can be altered using hormonal agents (Bruera et al., 1990; Loprinzi et al., 1990). More specific interfering agents, acting directly on cytokines, are now available in the laboratory. The promise is that such agents may improve appetite and add weight in cachectic patients. The cytokine cascade, which contributes to the cachexia-anorexia syndrome, is becoming better understood, leading researchers to investigate inhibitors of cytokines or of agents that interfere with cytokine receptor expression and function (Plata-Salaman, 1995; Erickson and Hubbard, 1996; Laviano, 1996; Meydani, 1996). Cytokines are induced by cancer tissue and, under certain circumstances, may act as tumor inhibitors. The complex interaction of cytokine production ↔ cytokine inhibition can be studied in animal tumor models. In addition, cytokines may act indirectly by inducing the production of other chemicals that directly influence nutrient metabolism. Identification of these substances may produce additional therapeutic leads. Another promising lead relates to the study of specific nutrients, for example, omega-3 fatty acids and branched-chain amino acids (Endres et al., 1989; Downer et al., 1993; Karmali, 1996). Finally, growth hormone or IGF-1 therapy may enhance well-being in some patients with chronic wasting (LeRoith, 1997).

Relative to other pharmaceutical interventions, the current drugs available for the control of cachexia-anorexia range from modest in cost (short-term use of corticosteroids) to moderately expensive (progestational agents). The cost of more specific interventions remains to be determined. Overall, given the number of patients affected, the costs of their dependency, the distress caused by the syndrome, and the intriguing findings of recent research, this is a priority area for collaborative investigation.

Directions for Research on Dyspnea

Dyspnea can be defined as "subjective difficulty or distress in breathing," often experienced as shortness of breath (Stedman's Medical Dictionary, 1995). Frequently occurring in combination with other symptoms, dyspnea is a common source of suffering for patients in the last months of life. Dyspnea can result from malignancy metastatic to the lungs or pleura, from heart failure, from chest wall weakness due to neuromuscular disease, or from primary pulmonary disease.

Until recently, if the cause of dyspnea could not be reversed, help for dyspneic patients was limited (Davis, 1994). Several lines of research now suggest that resigned acceptance should not govern the thinking on dyspnea. Promising areas for further investigation include (1) opioids; (2) respiratory stimulants; (3) oxygen therapy; and (4) support for respiratory muscles.

Opioids already have a role in controlling dyspnea similar to their use in the management of cancer pain. They moderate the reflexive drive to breathe and thereby decrease patient awareness of dyspnea; they may also improve breathing efficiency and exercise endurance (Doyle et al., 1993). Questions that warrant investigation include:

- How does morphine influence the pathophysiology of dyspnea?
- Are some opioids more effective than others for relieving dyspnea? Which have the optimal therapeutic margin? Do nebulized opioids have a role? Some pilot studies suggest that inhaled morphine relieves the dyspnea of metastatic disease in the lung (Davis, 1994). Would it show similar effects for congestive heart failure? Is there evidence for a specific effect on pulmonary receptor sites?
- If, as it appears to be, allowing a degree of opioid-induced hypercapnia (high levels of arterial carbon dioxide pressure) may be effective in relieving dyspnea, what levels of arterial carbon dioxide are safest and as free as possible of undesirable effects, such as clouding of consciousness?
- Is processing of the sensation of dyspnea in the brain organized in a way that would potentially allow one to relieve the perception of shortness of breath without suppressing the automatic drive to breathe?

Respiratory stimulants also warrant investigation in dyspnea therapy. Several agents, including phosphodiesterase inhibitors, progestational agents, and methylphenidate have stimulatory effects on respiratory centers in the medulla (Aubier et al., 1983; Mikami et al., 1989). Such effects prompt the question: Will these agents help to improve respiratory activities in chronically ill patients, or will the stimulatory effect on the respiratory center undesirably increase the perception of dyspnea?

Oxygen is clearly indicated in patients who are hypoxic (oxygen-deficient). Investigators might explore whether there is a role for oxygen therapy in nonhypoxic patients under any circumstances.

Support for respiratory muscles is another area for therapeutic investigation. Patients with advanced chronic illness often have the cachexia-anorexia syndrome and have lost a great deal of somatic protein. Their diaphragm and the external accessory respiratory muscles may be particularly vulnerable to wasting and fatigue. One pertinent research question, then, is whether improvement in patient nutrition, with consequent improvement in respiratory muscle content and strength, might limit dyspnea. Another question is whether newer techniques of ventilatory support might assist failing respiratory muscles and relieve the dyspnea.

Cognitive and Emotional Symptoms

In the arena of cognitive and emotional symptoms, a concerted effort to develop a multidisciplinary biomedical and psychological research strategy that focuses on the dying patient could bring progress in a number of important areas, including delirium and milder confusional states, depression, anxiety, sleep disorders, hallucinations, and suicidal ideation (see, e.g., Holland and Rowland, 1990; Breitbart and Holland, 1993; Hyman and Nestler, 1993; Breitbart et al., 1995). The biology of these symptoms as they affect patients with advanced life-threatening illnesses has been little examined; even their prevalence is not well charted.

For example, few studies of the prevalence of depression have investigated patients with far advanced disease (see, e.g., Hinton, 1972; Bukberg et al., 1984; Chochinov et al., 1994). The same holds true for delirium, which is common in advanced cancer patients and is important as a source of distress to families and health care personnel as well as patients (see, e.g., Lipowski, 1987; Fainsinger and Young, 1991; Bruera et al., 1992; Smith et al., 1995). Similarly, scientific study of the biology and importance of cognitive and emotional symptoms is limited for patients with severe congestive heart failure, chronic obstructive pulmonary disease, and diabetes (see, e.g., Littlefield et al., 1990; Leedom et al., 1991; Cowley and Skene, 1994; Hawthorne and Hixon, 1994).

Certainly, some anxiety and depression are understandable responses to serious illness and loss. This contributes to disagreement about the nature and prevalence of clinical depression in the population of patients who are dying (Bukberg et al., 1984; Kathol et al., 1990; Chochinov et al., 1994). Others disagreements involve diagnostic criteria, treatment strategies, and assessments of the benefits and burdens of particular therapeutic agents.

General directions for biomedical research in cognitive and emotional symptoms in patients approaching death include some elements, primarily methodological, common to those proposed above for other symptoms. Directions for research include

- use of uniform descriptive terminology and classification schemes where they now exist and development of such terminology and taxonomies of disorders where they do not now exist;

- • development, use, and refinement of reliable, valid, and practical symptom assessment tools and measures for studying the prevalence and severity of psychological symptoms in patients with advanced disease and for evaluating interventions appropriate for such patients;
- • studies of the prevalence of neuropsychiatric symptoms and syndromes in patients with different diseases and circumstances (e.g., age, sex, care setting) and the distress created by these symptoms as reported by patients and families;
- • examination of the relative contributions to diminished mental functioning and patient well-being of specific disease processes and the side-effects of therapeutic interventions to treat a disease or relieve some of its symptoms;
- • investigation of the biochemical, immunological, neurobiological, and other physiological effects of the stresses imposed on patients and those close to them by life-threatening illnesses;
- • assessment of the costs of different neuropsychiatric syndromes and symptoms as they affect patients with advanced disease; and
- • comparison of alternative pharmacological and nonpharmacological therapy options (singly and in combination) including novel uses or combinations of existing therapies.

Social science and health services research, some directions for which are outlined below, offer additional opportunities for understanding and reducing the cognitive and emotional toll of advanced disease. In all areas, researchers need to consider (1) the extent to which different psychological symptoms coexist and interact with each other and with physical symptoms and (2) the patient and the family as a unit for purposes of assessing and managing symptoms, especially psychological symptoms (Breitbart et al., 1995).

SOCIAL, BEHAVIORAL, AND HEALTH SERVICES RESEARCH

A stronger foundation of scientific and clinical knowledge about symptom mechanisms and effective therapies for the dying patient is important but insufficient to guide improvements in care at the end of life. More needs to be understood about the extent and severity of physical, emotional, financial, and other adversities experienced by people dying from common diseases; about the possibility of spiritual growth and other valued experiences at the end of life; and about the attitudinal, organizational, legal, cultural, and other factors that impede the application of existing knowledge and principles of care. This kind of understanding will help in developing strategies that will make it easier for individuals and organizations to provide good care than to fail to do so.

Some research needs are so basic that it is surprising they still exist. For example, as Chapter 2 made clear, even elementary descriptive and epidemiological knowledge about how and where people die is very limited. Likewise, more is assumed than is known about what people want as they approach death; what is meaningful to their families and others close to them; and how the care and support that is valued can be effectively and efficiently organized. For example, although interdisciplinary care allows people with special training and experience to help patients with the many different burdens created by life-threatening illness, the benefits and costs of particular configurations of interdisciplinary expertise must still be evaluated. Similarly, continuity of care is widely viewed as desirable, but firm knowledge of how and to what extent it makes a difference is surprisingly limited (Donaldson, 1997). Evidence is beginning to accumulate about the contributions of continuous quality improvement strategies, but their value in end-of-life care is essentially anticipated rather than demonstrated. Chapter 5 identified the need for better conceptualization and measurement of outcomes meaningful to dying people and those close to them and described a number of the challenges of developing reliable, valid, and practical information to guide patient care and provide accountability.

Chapter 6 noted only limited information is available on the cost of dying in different ways, at different ages, in different places, and with different care. Research on the impact of different kinds of financial incentives is virtually nonexistent as it involves dying patients. Many welcome, while others worry about, the growth of managed care and for-profit health care institutions, but the consequences for dying patients are almost entirely unexamined. Demonstration projects testing the effects on end-of-life care of alternative practitioner and provider payment mechanisms are virtually unknown.

The next section identifies some methods issues that particularly complicate social, behavioral, and health services research. Following that is a discussion that suggests directions for future research. Although this discussion is not comprehensive or specific enough to direct particular projects, it provides a framework to be debated and refined.

Methods Issues in End-of-Life Research

No methods issues may be unique to research on care of the dying, but the mix of problems and the pivotal nature of certain problems create particular difficulties concerning the amount and quality of research in this field. Further, as pointed out in Chapter 5, many of the questions that face researchers also arise for administrators, clinicians, policymakers, and others attempting to measure, monitor, and improve the quality of end-of-life care and manage resources. Although some research questions may be addressed using the gold standard of clinical research, the randomized controlled trial, improvements in care may well require careful but innovative use of nonrandomized and sometimes uncontrolled settings. Methods to interpret and apply these research strategies, which may overlap with the methods of continuous quality improvement, merit further development.

For purposes of identifying patients, organizing services, and evaluating outcomes, one fundamental step would be the development of clearer concepts, definitions, and markers of the "last phase of life" as it has meaning in physiological, clinical, psychological, social, and cultural terms. Markers of the last phase of life may variously include (1) formal diagnoses; (2) easily observed physical signs and symptoms; (3) more subtle indicators from patient history, physical examinations, and tests; (4) scores generated by prognostic models; (5) acknowledgement by patients, families, or clinicians; or, (6) for some purposes, retrospective identification following death of a time or clinical juncture before death (e.g., one week before death, last hospitalization).

Although the research, policy, ethical, and cultural merits, limitations, and implications of different markers of the dying phase need attention, an inescapable difficulty is that the anchor of end-of-life studies requires decisions about a prospectively uncertain end point. Will research questions be tied to timing relative to expected death (e.g., when a patient is predicted to have a 10 percent chance of living six months) or to timing relative to a particular event (e.g., when a patient receives a specific diagnosis or enrolls in hospice care)? Another complication is that the ultimate end point—death—varies somewhat with treatment itself as illustrated in some of the illustrative cases presented in Chapters 3 and 4.

For economic analyses, most cost accounting involves a fixed period of time or an episode of hospitalization. Here, at least for some purposes, studies count costs from a certain stage of illness through to death or for a particular period of time. How an analyst is to account for variation related to the starting point (e.g., when a diagnosis is made, which may be early or late in the course of some diseases) or the effect of treatment decisions (e.g., when the patient receives therapies that both relieve symptoms and prolong life) has not been worked out. Strategies that involve multiple data collection points add flexibility and information but are burdensome and expensive. For example, much end-of-life research requires interviews with patients or surrogates, as well as, perhaps, interviews with caregivers and reference to patient records. Such research is expensive and complicated. Thus, alternatives and trade-offs need to be explored.

Researchers also face complexities in studying patients with multiple symptoms that may interact with each other. Such interactions are not well described or understood. Similarly, researchers may find it difficult to distinguish symptoms caused by the patient's illness from those resulting from treatments.

Yet another problem with studies of people near the end of life involves missing or potentially distorted data. Many patients in these studies die without being questioned; others cannot be questioned directly about their symptoms, concerns, or attitudes because their illness or treatment or both have left them confused, weak, or unconscious. Their condition may also change frequently, which limits continued informed consent and participation in some studies. Missing data requires examination of possible imputation or substitution strategies, for example, using surrogates, but little research or analysis is available to guide choices.

In addition to the problem of whether a patient is functioning cognitively, issues related to diversity in language, religion, ethnicity, and other cultural attributes arise. How, for example, do and should measurement instruments and strategies take into account such diversity among patients and families?

Another challenge is that patient care occurs under many different financing arrangements and in myriad locations, many of which involve fragmentary and poorly developed record systems. Data systems for the nation's thousands of health insurance plans ordinarily do not distinguish between individuals who died and those no longer in the plan for reasons such as retirement or switch to another health plan so tracking people across time to determine outcomes can be difficult. In addition, current systems for measuring and monitoring the quality of care include very little that is directly related to care at the end of life. Many physical, emotional, and social issues of central concern (e.g., symptoms, counseling, satisfaction, impoverishment, meaningfulness) are not ordinarily part of patient data systems. Priorities for the development, testing, and refinement of reliable, valid, and practical quality measurement tools include not just the experience of symptoms but their burden as felt by patients. The point of citing such difficulties is not to discourage research but to encourage a realistic understanding of its challenges.

Directions for Investigation

As a starting point for establishing priorities and formulating a research agenda, the committee suggests a number of important areas for investigation. These investigations would draw on the expertise of epidemiologists, psychologists, economists, sociologists, anthropologists, health services researchers, and others. The list is only suggestive of the array of knowledge necessary to improve care at the end of life and the rich arenas for research by those in the behavioral and social sciences, humanities, epidemiology, and related fields.

Epidemiology of Dying and Death

Although refinements in the reliability, validity, completeness, and time-liness of "vital statistics" on the cause of death are a continuing objective, those interested in improving care at the end of life have a particular interest in better information on where people die and what paths they follow through different settings. Data on numbers, causes, and places of deaths and basic demographic characteristics (e.g., age, race) are routinely gathered by government, but information on dying pathways must come from special studies. In the absence of integrated, comprehensive, computer-based patient records, such studies will generally be small-scale and limited to a few institutions or communities and will thus present problems of generalizability. Nonetheless, a better descriptive understanding of common pathways during dying is possible for different settings of care.

An additional set of questions focuses on variations in the clinical pathways of dying—including the duration and pattern of the dying process (e.g., steady decline or relative stability marked by crises); symptom prevalence and level of distress; functional and cognitive impairments; and variation within and across populations of patients by diagnosis, demographic, and other characteristics. Because most people who die are older adults, much research should focus on this large population. Other populations are important but may be difficult to study. Little is known about the experiences of special populations such as younger people with preexisting physical and mental disabilities; children at various ages; people without insurance; those in the inner city and very rural areas; and religious, ethnic, and other minorities. Given the special sorrows and stresses created by life-threatening illness in children, the developmental aspects of illness and patient care involving neonates, infants, children, and adolescents need attention.

Delivery, Financing, and Improvement of Health and Other Services

As in much health services research, a useful descriptive step is mapping the nature and extent of variation in end-of-life care across clinicians and care settings. The more ambitious task is to investigate whether and how differences in outcomes and costs relate to differences in the clinical problems, characteristics, and preferences of dying patients; the settings and processes of care; and the mechanisms of structuring and financing care. Such research will help clarify the barriers to organizational excellence (or adequacy) in care at the end of life. To the extent that clinician attitudes, skills, and knowledge—for example, misplaced concern about addiction, ignorance of pharmacological and nonpharmacological strategies for symptom relief, disinterest in dying patients—contribute to inadequate care, then a broad range of techniques for changing attitudes, increasing knowledge, and modifying behavior may be employed. Modest amounts of research from other areas provide some hints about the effectiveness of different strategies (e.g., distributing information is usually ineffective as a sole strategy).

A series of questions can be raised about strategies for identifying problems, structuring accountability, and improving care. For example, are patient or family reports on care more reliable and useful than satisfaction measures in identifying problems and improving care? How well-suited are different quality measures for internal and external quality assessment? Can guidelines for clinical practice, decision-support tools, performance feedback, and similar strategies improve clinical practice and care outcomes? If certain structures and processes can be linked to better outcomes, can they—at least for some purposes—be used as reliable and valid but less costly proxies for outcomes?

Chapters 3, 4, and 5, which outlined the dimensions of care at the end of life and the arrangements for providing and evaluating care, suggested many questions. For example, will new criteria intended to guide hospice referrals for noncancer patients be practical to apply and will they affect levels of hospice use? What happens during the actual practice of home care for dying patients, and what are the effects of different care processes and structures (e.g., home care within or outside a hospice program)? The same general questions can be asked about care at the end of life in nursing homes. Hospital care is becoming somewhat better understood, but documented interventions to improve care remain elusive. Beyond the health care system, do the administrative boundaries separating social, medical, and other services create difficulties, and if so, how might these boundaries be redesigned?

With cost pressures encouraging health care managers to reduce staffing levels and reassign responsibilities from more highly to less highly trained personnel (e.g., from RNs to LPNs or aides), researchers need to investigate the impact of shifts in caregiving personnel on very sick and dying patients. Are patients suffering pain and other symptoms waiting longer for attention? What is happening to the interpersonal aspects of care and to the extent and quality of symptom assessment, management, and charting in patient records?

Similarly, the extent and impact of cost-driven shifts in the site of care for dying patients, which has been scarcely considered, warrants investigation to identify the benefits and burdens for patients and families as well as the impact on organizations delivering and financing care. Other important questions involve the characteristics and effects of different ways of managing transitions from one care setting to another and alternative methods for coordinating care for people with serious, progressive disease. In addition, it would be useful to learn about how strategies to prevent and relieve symptoms affect costs of care over the trajectory of serious illness.

As noted in Chapter 6, only the most global estimates of the cost of care at the end of life are available, and these estimates are largely limited to costs for older individuals covered by Medicare. Future research may be limited by losses in Medicare's administrative database as certain information on interventions and diagnoses is lost in capitated care. Such information is important for analyzing the impact of different financing mechanisms on the behavior and choices of practitioners and patients, the availability and quality of services, the clinical outcomes for patients, the perceptions of patients and those close to them, and the level and distribution of costs across different parties. One critical question is whether some financing arrangements pose particular threats to patient well-being, trust, and access to care. In this regard, it would be useful to learn about the patterns of enrollment, disenrollment, and continued enrollment by seriously ill patients in different types of managed care and in traditional health care plans.

Caregiver Experience and Bereavement

Palliative care is noteworthy in its concern for the patient in the context of the family (including nontraditional families). Many factors affect the physical, emotional, and practical experiences of those close to the patient and the types of interventions that will be practical and effective. Some issues—anticipatory grief, bereavement, anxiety—warrant research along the lines described in the earlier discussion of biomedical research on cognitive and emotional symptoms in patients. The efficacy and appropriateness of pharmacological therapies for grieving survivors remain important issues, but the role of different forms of social support and the relationship between caregiver experience and social and demographic characteristics also warrant further exploration.

Culture, Communication, Perceptions, and Decisionmaking

Changes in how people die have challenged clinical, cultural, and ethical norms and understandings about care at the end of life, as have changes in the ethnic, religious, linguistic, and social composition of the American population. The increasing racial and ethnic diversity in the United States has led those committed to improved end-of-life care to try to learn more about how perceptions, preferences, and behaviors vary and how communication and care strategies can respect differences in the context of organizational systems designed to provide reliable, excellent, and efficient care. This interest also reflects a recognition that—in addition to a strong basic science and clinical knowledge base—better support for patients and families will depend on a better understanding of the cultural, emotional, affective, and nonrational aspects of perception of symptoms, attitudes, behavior, and decisionmaking.

A modest body of research has accumulated in certain areas such as clinician, family, or surrogate awareness and acceptance of patient preferences; variation and stability in patient preferences about end-of-life care; communication of bad prognoses and treatment uncertainties; attitudes about assisted suicide; and measurement of attitudes and anxieties about dying and death. This research has laid out a range of questions for further investigation including: legal and other problems facing members of nontraditional families when their loved ones are not competent to make decisions; links between desire for assisted suicide and difficulties experienced or expected in receiving appropriate palliative care; and patient and family willingness or desire to rely more on clinicians to make certain important decisions about end-of-life care. Puzzled by patients reporting both high levels of pain and moderate or high levels of satisfaction with care, pain researchers have identified the determinants of patient and family satisfaction with pain treatment as an important research issue (APS, 1995).

As indicated in Chapter 8, the effectiveness of educational strategies in changing health professionals' knowledge, attitudes, and behavior is an important area for investigation. Research on the value of case-based learning, role playing, and similar strategies is generally promising, but overoptimistic claims should be avoided. Also relevant is research on strategies for using guidelines for clinical practice to educate clinicians and change their practices. For example, can academic detailing, computer-based decision support tools, and similar approaches improve the extent to which clinicians apply existing guidelines on pain management to the care of dying patients?

The role of the mass media in influencing knowledge, attitudes, and decisions about end-of-life care is just beginning to be explored. To the extent that the media can be interested in presenting a more balanced and realistic view of dying, research would be useful in designing programs that will attract public attention, improve understanding, and encourage people to behave in ways that allow a more comfortable dying.

ETHICAL ISSUES IN RESEARCH ON DYING PATIENTS

Ethical issues in research on care at the end of life require special consideration because patients with advanced chronic illness are a vulnerable population that tends to be particularly dependent on health workers. Variable degrees of cognitive failure such as dementia or fluctuating delirium are common and may limit a patient's ability to offer a truly informed consent. Moreover, patients may exhibit changing patterns of illness that will call upon investigators to constantly renegotiate informed consent and ensure that strict adherence to the protocol does not interfere with the patient's overall care. Patients with life-threatening illness and their families may be desperate as they sense that options have collapsed around them.

The ethical issues involved in enrolling and maintaining vulnerable subjects in clinical and other research have been the subject of much discussion. A variety of institutional mechanisms have been devised to provide for consideration of such ethical questions and oversight of research involving human subjects (President's Commission, 1982; Cassel, 1988; Annas, 1991; Kass et al., 1996; Vanderpool, 1996). More generally, the principles of research ethics must be applied within a compassionate environment by wise, charitable, and virtuous investigators.

Notwithstanding legitimate concerns, ethical risks should not be overstated. By its nature, research involving symptom-relief strategies may be associated with fewer adverse effects than many trials of agents intended to cure or significantly retard the advance of life-threatening illnesses; these latter trials are commonly regarded as acceptable. Restricting patients suffering from advanced illness from clinical trials may deprive them of improved treatments for symptoms. In addition, to deprive palliative care patients of the opportunity to make their own decisions about participation deprives them of the special meaning of doing something to benefit future generations. Altruism is an important value for some people faced with irreversible illness.

Concern about research that potentially exploits specially vulnerable subjects led to strict limits on research in nursing homes (Cassel, 1988). In recent years, these concerns have been reevaluated, and more flexible guidelines are now commonly observed. Although it is true that seriously ill patients or nursing home residents may, by virtue of their illness or the fact of institutionalization, be uniquely dependent on caregivers and thus vulnerable to exploitation, the committee believes that is possible to create standards for consent and oversight that protect the subjects but still allow them the right to participate in studies. Research may be ethically conducted if certain principles are followed and certain questions appropriately answered. The broadest principles rely on the fundamental precepts of respecting persons, doing good, avoiding harm, and treating people justly (Beauchamp and Childress, 1994). More specific considerations include the following (MacDonald, 1993; Vanderpool, 1996):

• *Purpose.* Trials with the objective of improving patient quality of life using low-risk interventions usually will not present ethical dilemmas. In contrast, participation in Phase 1 drug trials, where the chance of benefit is small, can present serious ethical concerns. Nevertheless, in these situations, if the purposes of the patient, family, and physician are consonant and clearly understood, ethical dilemmas may be resolved.

•   *Patient competence.* Informed consent can only be given by competent patients, and research on those who cannot give consent (e.g., unconscious emergency department patients) has raised serious concerns and prompted the development of guidelines on the conduct of research for such patients. Cognitive defects are common in patients with advanced chronic illness, many of whom are elderly. Screening tools for competence may be needed for research involving such patients.

•   *Double agency.* Health professionals engaged in research are acting as double agents in that their research may help the research subject but also create benefits for society at large, advance basic knowledge, enhance careers, and improve the competitive position of sponsors. However, the current medical milieu commonly places health professionals in patient care settings in the role of double agents with responsibilities not only to patients, but to the patient's family, and to their own colleagues, departments, institutions, medical faculties, and, most problematic of all, the state or private health agencies. Although this double-agency status must be accepted, the resolution of the dilemmas it may create can generally be resolved by making clear that the patient's well-being is the top priority.

•   *Industry priorities and research directions.* Given limited resources for research, the research activities of many health professionals are undoubtedly influenced by the support available from the pharmaceutical industry. This may limit or skew the direction of palliative care research because most large firms appear to be less interested in drugs that interfere with the pathophysiology of symptoms but do not affect the overall disease trajectory. Thus, some promising lines of scientific investigation may be neglected. Earlier in this chapter, the committee suggested a symptom-based research strategy following the pain model. Better understanding of the pathophysiology of other symptoms may particularly attract manufacturers interested in identifying new uses of existing drugs such as opioids.

In sum, that ethical questions deserve attention does not automatically preclude the conduct of research on end-of-life issues. For researchers, inducing harm out of proportion to potential benefit is a risk that must be carefully considered with the patient, primary caregivers, and appropriate family members and evaluated within the context of established institutional review processes and policy guidelines.

RESEARCH LEADERSHIP

Box 9.1 lists a number of factors that have contributed to the dearth of

---

BOX 9.1
Limiting Factors in Research to Improve Care at the
End of Life

Developmental Issues

- Limited political constituency and advocacy base
- Weak governmental and commercial funding for research that is not aimed at curing disease
- Lack of links between basic science and palliative care researchers
- Low academic priority of end-of-life care
- Minimal ties to established academic units
- Absence of recognized medical specialty and multi-institutional research groups

Ethical Concerns

- Patient ability to provide informed consent
- Potential interference with care
- Potential added burden of suffering

Methodological-Logistical Problems

- Small population base in clinical and organizational studies
- Changing patient health status and prognostic uncertainties
- Conceptual disagreements (e.g., definition of palliative therapy)
- Absence of internationally recognized systems for classifying, assessing, or measuring most symptoms, outcomes, and quality-of-life variables relevant to end-of-life care
- Competing demands for time from direct patient care
- Lack of investigator training in appropriate research techniques
- Lack of methodologies adapted to the special problems presented by end-of-life research

---

SOURCE: Adapted from MacDonald, 1993.

---

research on the experience of dying patients and on interventions to improve, prevent, or relieve symptoms and improve patients' quality of life while dying. In the committee's view, underlying many of these obstacles is the shared view of many researchers, educators, and practitioners that dying is a failure, that end-of-life care is unrewarding, and that scientific research in the area is uninteresting. Within academic health centers, the same structural and leadership factors that lead to inattention to end-of-life care in the curriculum contribute to the lack of research in the area.

The neglect of research also reflects economic forces that drive research funding priorities. One apparent impediment is that a number of effective approaches to symptom relief use morphine and other drugs that are available generically, which may make them less interesting to industry-supported researchers. However, as the introduction of new longer-acting oral morphine formulations demonstrates, it is possible to market profitable versions of generic drugs such as morphine. Such profitable drugs may, however, create affordability problems for patients or for hospice programs operating on a fixed per diem payment. Also, if health care organizations do not see palliation as important to their institutional well-being, they will be tempted to cut costs by skimping on palliative care including pharmaceuticals.

Unfortunately but unsurprisingly, dying patients do not form an energetic, ongoing constituency to advocate for more research. As observed earlier, their survivors tend to be exhausted and grieving and, after a time, they are expected to put their lives back together and move on. In addition, hope inclines people—especially patients, families, and clinicians—to focus on curing disease rather than on developing more effective interventions to comfort those approaching death. These dynamics can deflect advocacy groups that champion research to prevent or cure various diseases from vigorously and publicly promoting palliative research to help those who will, inevitably, die of these causes. By devoting at least a portion of their resources to promoting symptom-focused and other research to reduce suffering for those with advanced progressive illness, these advocacy groups could play an important role in creating public demand for improved care. It is also critical for those in leadership roles in research, clinical practice, education, and public policy to advocate for dying people who cannot advocate for themselves or those who will follow them.

The major public funder of biomedical research is the National Institutes of Health (NIH).[2] NIH is an enterprise that is structured around research on organ systems, driven by investigator interests, and focused on mechanisms of disease. This stance has attracted fairly generous funding, even in recent years when other government health programs have faced reduction or elimination of funding. In the future, however, the issue of research priorities will get more attention. Also, the controversy over assisted suicide may prompt policymakers to propose research mandates that do not have much scientific potential to produce results that help dying patients.

Certainly, research on the pathophysiology of symptoms, mechanisms

---

[2]In an effort to understand the scope of government biomedical research on end-of-life issues, the committee met with representatives of the National Institutes of Health (NIH). As this report was going to press, NIH staff were organizing a conference for September 1997 to consider directions for NIH-sponsored research on symptom management in palliative care settings.

of symptom relief, and the dying pathways and experiences of patients with different diseases has not been a priority at NIH, and such research is even difficult to identify in its databases. For example, in material provided to the committee, the National Cancer Institute identified 15 active research protocols (as of summer 1996) potentially relevant to this committee's work, but most of them appeared to involve side effects of therapies intended primarily to prolong life (e.g., managing chemotherapy side effects, coping with radiation treatment for prostate cancer, alleviation of platinum-induced peripheral neuropathy) (Varricchio et al., 1996). In some cases, such research may be generalizable to relief of symptoms induced by disease or by treatments to palliate symptoms (e.g., bowel symptoms related to opioid therapy for pain), but the extent to which this is the case needs explicit investigation.

One promising development has been the work by patient groups, clinicians, health services researchers, and others to encourage biomedical researchers and public and private research sponsors to include quality-of-life measures in clinical trials (Johnson and Temple, 1985; Moinpour et al., 1989; Nayfield et al., 1991; Varricchio et al., 1996). Quality-of-life measures, however, often emphasize physical activities and return to work with less attention to "issues that are documented to be relevant to terminally ill persons such as hope, loneliness, depression, anger and anxiety about what is happening to the patient and to family and friends" (McMillan and Mahon, 1994, p. 438). Thus, although the committee believes that the introduction of quality-of-life measures in clinical trials is an important step, research specifically focused on the quality of life for dying patients is also needed.

The committee could not locate any specific data on the number of patient deaths occurring within NIH clinical trials and other research programs, but it expected that clinical trials on heart disease, cancer, stroke, and AIDS—major causes of death in the U.S. adult population—record thousands of deaths. Little or no systematic data are collected on how these patients die and what their symptoms and needs are. Although the number of deaths in trials involving neonates, infants, children, and adolescents is smaller, the same dearth of information applies.

Because resources are limited and priorities must be set, those advocating specific studies related to end-of-life care must be able to argue the case for these studies. They will generally need to address several core questions (IOM, 1992, 1995c) including

• How significant is the clinical problem—its prevalence (current, estimated future) burden of illness (e.g., morbidity, quality of life), economic burden, and variability in treatments or outcomes across regions or population subgroups?

- What is the likelihood that research results will affect decisions and outcomes?
- Will the research constructively supplement conclusions from other research?

To help in setting research priorities as well as increasing knowledge to guide both scientific and clinical research, the committee strongly encourages NIH and other biomedical research groups to consider the inclusion of data collection protocols that would gather more information on people who die from the diseases being investigated in clinical trials. This information would provide a clearer picture of patients' experience during the months before they died of conditions such as congestive heart failure, chronic obstructive pulmonary disease, and end-stage renal disease. Such protocols could be added to all clinical trials of potentially fatal illnesses, much as the National Cancer Institute added quality-of-life measures to its cooperative protocols some years ago. Such data would provide guidance for decisions about priorities for symptom research based on the burden of distress and suffering as well as on scientifically promising questions for investigation.

Public resources for health services research and other topics outside biomedicine are more limited. One major sponsor of such research, the Agency for Health Care Policy and Research (AHCPR), has faced funding threats and political controversy in its efforts to promote evidence-based medicine and guidelines for clinical practice.[3] The committee saw the research supported by this agency as a valuable national resource (see, also, IOM, 1995c). Its limited resources notwithstanding, the committee also believed the agency can play an important leadership role in directing attention to end-of-life issues in health services research. The NIH should be encouraged to work with other federal agencies, such as the AHCPR, the Department of Veterans Affairs, and the Food and Drug Administration to consider developing cross-cutting initiatives or to nurture and coordinate pain and other symptom research and research on the effectiveness of other interventions frequently used at the end of life. The initial objectives would be (1) to promote more sharing of ideas and concepts among researchers from different disease fields and disciplines, (2) to provide a focal point for proposals by those researchers interested in symptoms, quality of life for dying patients, and related issues, and (3) to urge investigators and staff to

---

[3]For example, NIH staff noted that although they sought advice from the Agency for Health Care Policy and Research (AHCPR) about alternative end points for clinical trials, AHCPR's resources were so limited that it could not support its own research agenda in the area.

consider creative, economical ways of incorporating questions on end-of-life issues in a wider range of studies. (One example is a study sponsored by the National Heart, Lung, and Blood Institute that looked at risk factors and prognoses for cardiovascular diseases for people over age 65 and included an ancillary study that looked at behaviors and burdens of caregivers for those with severe disease (Schulz et al., 1997). Other longer-term objectives would be to encourage interdisciplinary research and to develop career tracks for researchers interested in these topics and to attract researchers to areas not previously identified as being "interesting." The committee recognized that these kinds of initiatives are difficult to create and sustain but believed that policymakers and research leaders can devise creative ways to support focused biomedical research that will ultimately help people have a better quality of life while dying.

CONCLUSION

Progress in a clinical field is dependent on its research base. Deficiencies in basic scientific and clinical knowledge affect both the availability of effective palliative therapies and the reimbursement of palliative services. The recruitment of excellent young professionals to an area of medical care depends in some part on the opportunities in the field for posing and resolving stimulating questions. This chapter has highlighted a number of exciting areas of inquiry that could build on findings that are accumulating in fields such as pain and immunology research. A major challenge to the field of palliative medicine is to work with colleagues in other fields to generate and conduct research in these and related areas. A broader task is to cultivate understanding of the potential benefits of such research among government and industry sponsors of research, to develop stronger ties with patient advocacy groups, and to promote public demand for knowledge that will improve the quality of life for people who are dying.

10

Conclusions and Recommendations

Our lives are time travel, moving in one direction only. We accompany one another as long as we can; as long as time grants us.

Joyce Carol Oates, *A Letter to My Mother*, 1996

We go toward something that is not yet.

Paul Tillich, *The Eternal Now*, 1959

Dying is at once a fact of life and a profound mystery. Death comes to all, yet each person experiences it in ways that are only partly accessible to the family member or physician, the researcher or philosopher. In principle, humane and skillful care for the dying is a social obligation as well as a personal offering from those directly involved. In reality, both society and individuals fall short of what is reasonably, if not simply, achievable.

Evidence and experience both indicate that much dying is far harder than it should be. Like the mythic king Tantalus, who reached for fruit and water just beyond his grasp, the dying person has too often been destined to seek but not find a pain-free and peaceful death. Such a fate need not be; better deaths are possible now.

This is not to claim that dying and death can be made easy, although certain illnesses tend to bring less-difficult deaths than others; nor is it to suggest that caring well for those approaching death can be made an exact science or flawless art. Caring well involves a frequently stressful, imperfect effort to balance science with sentiment, honesty with hope, patterns of care with room for exceptions.

This report has identified ways in which clinicians, educators, and communities do not care adequately for those approaching death. It has pointed to steps that can improve care at the end of life and sustain improvements through difficult times. It has also highlighted the reasons for believing that professionals, policymakers, and the public are ready to support such steps. These reasons range from the examples of well-known men and women facing death with grace to the focus on deficiencies in care stimulated by the debate over assisted suicide. In sum, the timing appears right to press for a vigorous societal commitment to improve care for the dying. Such a commitment would motivate and sustain local and national efforts to strengthen and apply the existing knowledge base, reform procedures and policies that impede good care for the dying, and stress the caring functions of health delivery systems.

TODAY AND TOMORROW

The preceding chapters have profiled important aspects of dying in America. They have noted that three-fourths of those who die are elderly and that most people who die are covered by Medicare or other federal, state, or local programs for older, disabled, or impoverished people. Compared to earlier times, death now comes more often in old age from a chronic or progressive disease. Most deaths occur in institutions, mainly hospitals and, to a lesser extent, nursing homes. The proportion of people who die at home is, however, increasing. Only a minority of all deaths involve people cared for by formal hospice programs, and the majority of these involve cancer diagnoses. All patients can potentially benefit from good palliative care, but hospice programs as organized and financed in the United States are most applicable to those with relatively predictable prognoses.

Although specifics may vary according to the nature of a person's disease and his or her personal circumstances, care for dying people and those close to them has several broad dimensions: physical, psychological, spiritual, and practical. Each of these dimensions is intertwined in the key processes of care, which include determining and communicating diagnosis and prognosis, establishing goals and plans, and fitting palliative and other care to these goals. The way care is organized, financed, monitored, and regulated affects how these processes are carried out in different settings for different kinds of patients.

The twenty-first century will bring new realities as well as continuing problems and opportunities in care at the end of life. It will undoubtedly deliver improvements in what medical science can do to prevent and relieve distress for those approaching death, but demographic, economic, and other trends will strain systems that already find it difficult to deliver what clinical knowledge currently allows—and what compassion should grant.

The committee focused primarily on trends and expectations relevant to care for dying patients during the next 10 to 20 years. One of these expectations is that policymakers and others will need to prepare during this period for the final demographic consequences of the post-World War II baby boom. The oldest members of the baby boom generation will reach age 65 in the year 2011, and the youngest members will do so nearly 20 years later. Barring dramatic unexpected developments, older adults will constitute a larger proportion of the population than today, and the absolute numbers of dying patients will be much larger. In the face of an ever-increasing population with chronic conditions, the current system, with its emphasis on acute curative care, will fail to provide needed long-term chronic care and palliative and support services. Although health care and social service providers have a long lead time compared with the educators and communities who had to scramble to provide schooling for the baby boom generation, the difficulties that policymakers are having with Social Security and Medicare do not bode well for the nation's ability to cope with an aging population.

In addition, continuing increases in longevity will mean that the proportion of those dying past age 75 will increase. The impact on the health care system and society on larger numbers of people dying in older old age will depend in part on their health status in the years before death. The "compression of morbidity hypothesis," for which the evidence is ambiguous, posits that an increase in healthier life styles means that people will experience disabling conditions for a smaller proportion of the years before death than today. Even if this does occur, the overall impact of the larger proportion of older people and their longer life span will still pose enormous challenges for social and health care systems.

Demographic politics are likely to be complex in coming years. On the one hand, the so-called senior lobby should be strengthened by the "baby boom" cohort. The "baby boomers," throughout their childhood, youth, and early middle age, have drawn public attention to their needs and concerns. On the other hand, the burden on the smaller working-age population of supporting its elders raises the specter of a generational backlash (even though younger people could also be burdened if the social support available to their aging parents is reduced). Such a backlash could take many forms, including means-testing Social Security benefits or less sympathy for supportive services for frail elderly people, those with serious disabilities, and people who are dying.

Cultural trends add further complexity to demographic politics. Immigrants, who tend to be young and have more children than native-born Americans, have been a major source of growth in the total U.S. population (NRC, 1997). Nonhispanic Caucasians—now a majority—are a decreasing proportion of the U.S. population. Thus, the large elderly population in the first decades of the next century will be dependent on a smaller and more culturally diverse population of younger people.

As described in preceding chapters, health care in the United States is undergoing major changes. The use of hospital services has dropped significantly, and further declines are likely, particularly in those areas with continued relatively high rates of use. Hospital care will likely be less available to dying patients, potentially including some who could benefit from such care as well as many who will do better with alternatives.

Despite indications that health care spending increases have moderated from years past, the pressure to cut health care costs does not appear to be abating. In particular, given the bleak financial picture for Medicare and the significant portion of spending accounted for by beneficiaries in their last year of life, these constraints may be manifested in some degree of age-based rationing. That is, older people could be denied services simply because of their age, without regard to their life expectancies, function, or expected benefit from care. Decreased access to advanced technologies intended to prolong life could be a highly visible issue, although it is relatively unimportant for the great majority of those dying at an advanced age.

If successful, increased efforts to shift Medicare beneficiaries into various forms of managed care will test these entities, whose enrollment now is overwhelmingly concentrated in younger, healthier age groups. Potential problem areas include payment, contracting, and utilization review mechanisms that limit access to clinicians and care teams experienced in palliative care, patient scheduling norms that limit time for careful clinician-patient communication, marketing strategies intended to discourage enrollment or encourage disenrollment by seriously ill people, drug formularies that exclude or restrict important medications, and bureaucratic hurdles that discourage people from seeking care or preclude them from receiving requested services. One characteristic of many managed care organizations is an emphasis on moving more responsibility for diagnosis and patient management to primary care clinicians, including nurse practitioners, nurses, and other nonphysicians. How well this will work for seriously ill and elderly patients is not yet clear. A major role for nurses and other health care professionals is, however, already well tested in hospice, social health maintenance organizations, and other settings that care for patients dying of advanced progressive diseases, particularly cancer, and for frail elderly people.

As well as focusing attention on competing ethical and policy values, this prospect of constrained resources underscores the need for more valid and reliable tools for assessing health status, measuring outcomes, and linking them to health interventions. Considerable progress is being made in this arena. In addition, improved computer-based information and decision support systems promise several benefits. At the level of the individual, they will help patients, families, and clinicians in making more informed decisions about care at the end of life. At the system or societal level, they will strengthen structures and processes of accountability involving health care providers, purchasers, patient/consumers, and public officials.

Moreover, advanced information and communications technologies may make health care more accessible for some who face geographic or other barriers to care. Although the potential for practical, effective, and affordable "medicine at a distance" is more promised than proved, telemedicine could help bring palliative and other expertise and services to homes, nursing homes, and other places where they are not very available today (IOM, 1996e). People who have chronic and advanced illnesses but do not qualify for hospital inpatient care could benefit.

FINDINGS AND RECOMMENDATIONS

Although the committee found many problems, it also found much that was good and improving in care for those approaching death. It was impressed by the principles, aspirations, and practices being advanced by the field of palliative medicine and being implemented or attempted through interdisciplinary care teams in varied settings, including hospices, hospitals, nursing homes, and private homes. More effort is now being devoted to understanding differences in people's paths toward death and developing programs that are flexible enough to accommodate these differences. In addition to dedicated professionals, many volunteers contribute their time and energy to provide emotional and practical support to dying patients and those close to them. People from a variety of backgrounds have also joined together to direct the attention of policymakers and ordinary citizens to the need to remove barriers to good care created by laws, regulations, organizational practices, and lack of supportive community resources.

Care for the dying should also benefit from ongoing efforts to improve continuity of care, strengthen information systems, prevent health problems, and create accountability for the quality of care. The developing fields of outcomes measurement can make important contributions to the care of the dying by teaching us how to conceptualize and measure quality of life and well-being for those approaching death. Quality improvement strategies are helping to identify and remedy system problems that impede good care. The committee is encouraged by the growing interest in end-of-life issues as recently evidenced by the publication of books and articles for lay and professional audiences, the commitment of foundation resources to support research and education, and the organization of conferences, working groups, and other initiatives sponsored by professional societies and others.

Deficiencies in Care at the End of Life

Notwithstanding these positive features, the committee concluded that very serious problems remain. Indeed, in this committee's view, if physician and hospital performance in infection control were as poor as it is, for example, in pain management, the ensuing national outcry would create an immediate demand for responses from clinicians, managers, and educators.

The committee identified four broad deficiencies in the current care of people with life-threatening and incurable illnesses. *First,* too many people suffer needlessly at the end of life both from errors of omission—when caregivers fail to provide palliative and supportive care known to be effective—and from errors of commission—when caregivers do what is known to be ineffective and even harmful. As reported in Chapter 3, studies have repeatedly indicated that a significant proportion of dying patients and patients with advanced disease experience serious pain, despite research identifying a range of effective pharmacological and other options for relieving most pain. Other symptoms are less well studied, and more research on symptom prevalence and management is needed, but the information available to the committee suggested similar care problems. Deficiencies in the application of existing knowledge to prevent and manage pain and other distressing symptoms stem from an unfortunate mix of ignorance about effective pharmacological and other interventions, misplaced concern about opioid addiction, and inadequate attention to people's quality of life while dying. These problems are reinforced by care systems that are not structured to provide the clinical expertise, reliability, continuity, and emotional support needed by people approaching death. Cultural biases and fears about illness, disability, and death may also contribute to avoidance of dying patients and those close to them.

In perverse counterpoint to the problem of undertreatment, the aggressive use of ineffectual and intrusive interventions may prolong and disfigure the period of dying. Some of this care is knowingly accepted; some is provided counter to patients' wishes; much is probably provided and accepted with little knowledge or consideration of its probable benefits and burdens. Medical culture still tolerates and even rewards the misapplication of life-sustaining technologies while slighting the prevention and relief of suffering.

Second, legal, organizational, and economic obstacles conspire to obstruct reliably excellent care at the end of life. Despite some reforms, outdated and scientifically flawed drug-prescribing laws, regulations, and interpretations by state medical boards still frustrate and intimidate physicians who wish to relieve their patients' pain. Addiction to appropriately prescribed opioids is virtually nonexistent whereas their underprescription for pain is well documented. Organizational structures often interfere with the coordination and continuity of care and impede the further development and application of palliative care strategies in patient care, professional education, and research.

Financial incentives also discourage health care practitioners and providers from rearranging care so that it serves dying patients well. Traditional financing mechanisms—including arrangements based on discounted fees—provide incentives for the overuse of procedural services and the under-provision of the assessment, evaluation, management, and supportive services so important for people with serious chronic or progressive medical problems. Medicare hospice benefits have helped fill gaps for a small segment of dying patients, but many more have conditions that do not readily fit the current hospice model or requirements. Alternatives to fee-for-service financing in combination with restrictive administrative practices pose different potential hazards that are largely unstudied as they affect seriously and incurably ill people.

Third, the education and training of physicians and other health care professionals fails to provide them with the knowledge, skills, and attitudes required to care well for the dying patient. Many deficiencies in practice stem from fundamental prior failures in professional education. Despite encouraging signs of change, most clinicians-in-training experience and learn too little of the caring that helps people to live well while dying. Undergraduate, graduate, and continuing medical education do not sufficiently prepare health professionals to recognize the final phases of illnesses, construct effective strategies for care, communicate with patients and those close to them, and understand and manage their own emotional reactions to death and dying.

Fourth, current knowledge and understanding are inadequate to guide and support the consistent practice of evidence-based medicine at the end of life. In addition to existing knowledge not being well used, we still know too little about how people die; how they want to die; and how different kinds of physical, emotional, and spiritual care might better serve the dying and those close to them. Biomedical and clinical research have emphasized the development of knowledge that contributes to the prevention, detection, or cure of disease and to the prolongation of life. Research on the end stages of diseases and the physiological bases of symptoms and symptom relief has been less well supported. Epidemiological and health services research has likewise not provided a strong base for understanding the degree to which people suffer symptoms (except, perhaps, cancer pain), experience death alone rather than in the company of those who care, comprehend diagnostic and prognostic information, and achieve a dying that is reasonably consistent with their preferences, community norms, and palliative care principles. Methods development is important to define and measure outcomes other than death (including patient and family perceptions) and to monitor and improve the quality of care for those approaching death.

More generally, it seems that this nation has not yet discovered how to talk realistically but comfortably about the end of life, nor has it learned how to value the period of dying as it is now experienced by most people.

For most of human history, death came fairly quickly in childhood or at adult ages that today seem relatively young. As the twentieth century ends, most people in economically advanced countries live fairly healthy lives into older age but then experience progressive disability for some time before they die. Except what can be inferred from newspaper obituary pages, this reality is largely shunned by the news, information, and entertainment media as distasteful or uninteresting. One result is an unhelpful combination of public fear, misinformation, and oversimplification that views misery as inescapable, pain as unavoidable, and public spending as misdirected for people who are approaching death.

Recommendations and Future Directions

The committee developed seven recommendations directed at different decisionmakers and different deficiencies in care at the end of life. These recommendations and a brief explanation follow. Each applies generally to people approaching death, including those for whom death is imminent and those with serious, eventually fatal illnesses who may live for some time.

RECOMMENDATION 1: **People with advanced, potentially fatal illnesses and those close to them should be able to expect and receive reliable, skillful, and supportive care.** Educating people about care at the end of life is a critical responsibility of physicians, hospitals, hospices, support groups, public programs, and media. Most patients and families need information not only about diagnosis and prognosis but also about what support and what outcomes they should reasonably be able to anticipate. They should, for example, not be allowed to believe that pain is inevitable or that supportive care is incompatible with continuing efforts to diagnose and treat. They should learn—before their last few days of life—that supportive services are available from hospices and elsewhere in the community and that those involved in their care will help arrange such services. Patient and family expectations and understanding will be aided by advance care planning that considers needs and goals, identifies appropriate surrogate decisionmakers, and avoids narrow preoccupation with written directives. To these ends, health care organizations and other relevant parties should adopt policies regarding information, education, and assistance related to end-of-life decisions and services. For those who seek to build public understanding of dying as a part of life and to generate public demand for reliable and effective supportive services, one model can be found in the perspectives, spirit, and strategies that have guided efforts to promote effective prenatal care and develop mother- and family-oriented arrangements for childbirth.

RECOMMENDATION 2:   Physicians, nurses, social workers, and other health professionals must commit themselves to improving care for dying patients and to using existing knowledge effectively to prevent and relieve pain and other symptoms. Most patients depend on health care professionals to prevent and manage the varying physical and psychological symptoms that accompany advanced illness. To meet their obligations to their patients, practitioners must hold themselves and their colleagues responsible for using existing knowledge and available interventions to assess, prevent, and relieve physical and emotional distress. Unrelieved pain and other symptoms are the most evident problems that practitioners can readily avoid for the great majority of patients, but problems with communication, appropriate regard for patient and family wishes, and timely referral to palliative care specialists or teams are other areas in need of improvement. When good practice is hindered by organizational, financial, or legal impediments, health professionals have the responsibility as individuals and members of larger groups to advocate for system change.

RECOMMENDATION 3:   Because many deficiencies in care reflect system problems, policymakers, consumer groups, and purchasers of health care should work with health care providers and researchers to

a. strengthen methods for measuring the quality of life and other outcomes of care for dying patients and those close to them;

b. develop better tools and strategies for improving the quality of care and holding health care organizations accountable for care at the end of life;

c. revise mechanisms for financing care so that they encourage rather than impede good end-of-life care and sustain rather than frustrate coordinated systems of excellent care; and

d. reform drug prescription laws, burdensome regulations, and state medical board policies and practices that impede effective use of opioids to relieve pain and suffering.

Although individuals must act to improve care at the end of life, systems of care must be changed to support such action. System change requires the involvement of public and private purchasers of care, regulators, and others whose policies and practices may create incentives for inappropriate care and barriers to excellent care.

Better information systems and tools for measuring outcomes and evaluating care are critical to the creation of effective and accountable systems of care and to the effective functioning of both internal and external systems of quality monitoring and improvement. Reliable and valid information about quality of care should be available to patients, purchasers, and accrediting organizations, but organizations also need to audit their structures and processes for problem areas and commit themselves to improving care on an ongoing basis. Problem areas include insufficient numbers and types of properly trained personnel, nonexistent or inadequate protocols for symptom assessment and management, and poor procedures for evaluating the need for patient transfers or referrals and for carrying out such transfers without harm to patients. The committee supports the development of guidelines for clinical practice that assist clinicians in preventing and relieving symptoms and in managing the end stages of specific diseases.

Policymakers and purchasers need to consider both the long-recognized deficiencies of traditional fee-for-service arrangements and the less thoroughly understood strengths and limitations of alternatives, including various kinds of capitated and per case payment methods that apply in diverse ways to individual practitioners, interdisciplinary care teams, specific institutions, networks of providers, or integrated systems of care. Particularly in need of attention are the levels of payment for home and nursing home visits by physicians, the interpretation of evaluation and management codes, the lack of diagnosis- or condition-related adjustments in hospice payments for both home and inpatient care, and other financing incentives that may discourage hospices or health plans from enrolling sicker patients. In addition, reimbursement methods and related incentives should encourage continuity of care that supports patients all the way through death and reduces disconnected and episodic care. Health care professionals and organizations also need to formulate ethical guidelines to guard against possible conflicts of interest in capitated and other care systems.

The problems with laws relating to prescribing practices are twofold. One problem is outdated, scientifically flawed laws and regulations themselves. The other problem is clinician, regulator, and public misunderstanding of the appropriate use of opioids. State medical societies, licensing boards, legislative committees, and other groups should cooperate to review state laws, regulations, board practices, and physician attitudes and practices to identify problem areas and then devise revisions in those statutes and regulations that unduly burden clinical management of pain. Regulatory review and revision should be accompanied by educational efforts to increase scientifically and clinically based knowledge and correct misperceptions about the appropriate medical use of opioids and about the biological mechanisms of opioid dependence, addiction, and pain management. Legal change should help—but cannot be relied upon alone—to correct undertreatment.

RECOMMENDATION 4:   Educators and other health professionals should initiate changes in undergraduate, graduate, and continuing education to ensure that practitioners have the relevant attitudes, knowledge, and

skills to care well for dying patients. Dying is too important a part of life to be left to one or two required (but poorly attended) lectures, to be considered only in ethical and not clinical terms, or to be set aside on the grounds that medical educators are already swamped with competing demands for time and resources. Every health professional who deals directly with patients and families needs a basic grounding in competent and compassionate care for seriously ill and dying patients. For clinicians and others to be held truly accountable for their care of the dying, educators must be held accountable for what they teach and what they implicitly and explicitly honor as exemplary practice. Textbooks and other materials likewise need revision to reflect the reality that people die and that dying patients are not people for whom "nothing can be done." As described in Chapter 8, a number of promising curriculum models exist, and others are being developed and tested.

RECOMMENDATION 5: **Palliative care should become, if not a medical specialty, at least a defined area of expertise, education, and research.** The objective is to create a cadre of palliative care experts whose numbers and talents are sufficient to (a) provide expert consultation and role models for colleagues, students, and other members of the health care team; (b) supply educational leadership and resources for scientifically based and practically useful undergraduate, graduate, and continuing medical education; and (c) organize and conduct biomedical, clinical, behavioral, and health services research. More generally, palliative care must be redefined to include prevention as well as relief of symptoms. Attention to symptoms should begin at earlier points during the trajectory of an illness because early treatment may well contribute to lessening pain at the end of life. The model for palliative care stresses interdisciplinary, comprehensive, and continuing care of patients and those close to them.

RECOMMENDATION 6: **The nation's research establishment should define and implement priorities for strengthening the knowledge base for end-of-life care.** The research establishment includes the National Institutes of Health, other federal agencies (e.g., the Agency for Health Care Policy and Research, the Health Care Financing Administration, the National Center for Health Statistics), academic centers, researchers in many disciplines, pharmaceutical companies, and foundations supporting health research. Their active support and involvement is necessary to advance basic and clinical research on the physiological mechanisms and treatment of symptoms common during the end of life, including neuropsychiatric problems. To extend understanding of quality-of-life issues in the treatment of advanced disease, those supporting clinical trials should encourage the collection of more information on the quality of life of those who die while enrolled in such trials. A further step is to support more research on the physiological mechanisms and treatment of symptoms common during the end of life, including neuropsychiatric problems. Pain research appears to supply a good model for this enterprise to follow. In addition, pathways need to be developed to further the dissemination and replication of proven health care interventions and programs. Demonstration projects to test new methods of financing and organizing care should be a priority for the Health Care Financing Administration. To encourage change in the attitudes and understandings of the research establishment, the committee urges the National Institutes of Health and other public agencies to take the lead in organizing a series of workshops, consensus conferences, and agenda-setting projects that focus on what is and is not known about end-stage disease and symptom prevention and treatment and that propose an agenda for further research. For the Agency for Health Care Policy and Research, the committee encourages support for the dissemination and replication of proven health care interventions and programs through clinical practice guidelines and other means.

RECOMMENDATION 7:   A continuing public discussion is essential to develop a better understanding of the modern experience of dying, the options available to dying patients and families, and the obligations of communities to those approaching death. Individual conversations between practitioners and patients are important but cannot by themselves provide the supportive environment for the attitudes and actions that make it possible for most people to die free from avoidable distress and to find the peace or meaning that is significant to them. Although efforts to reduce the entertainment and news media's emphasis on violent or sensational death and unrealistic medical rescue have not been notably successful, a modicum of balance has recently been provided by thoughtful analyses; public forums; and other coverage of the clinical, emotional, and practical issues involved in end-of-life care. Regardless of how the current, highly publicized policy debate over physician-assisted suicide is resolved, the goal of improving care for those approaching death and overcoming the barriers to achieving that goal should not be allowed to fade from public consciousness. Much of the responsibility for keeping the public discussion going will rest not with the media but with public officials, professional organizations, religious leaders, and community groups.

Finally, the committee agreed that it was not prepared to take a position on the legality or morality of physician-assisted suicide. The issue should not, in any case, take precedence over those reforms to the health care system that would improve care for all dying patients. The goal of those who favor legalizing physician-assisted suicide is to promote patient autonomy, but true autonomy is not possible when significant numbers of people have the limited choice between suicide or continued suffering. If the laws permitting physician-assisted suicide are implemented at the state level, careful monitoring of their consequences for the quality of care and the public's trust in health care will be very important.

CONCLUDING THOUGHTS

Improving care at the end of life will require many changes in attitudes, policies, and actions. Such changes will involve a multitude of people and institutions that have a role in making and implementing decisions about patient care or in structuring the environments in which such decisions are reached and realized. Clearly, what patients and their families know, expect, and desire is important. Health care professionals play critical roles in diagnosis, communication, guidance and direction, treatment, negotiation, and advocacy for patients at many levels. Decisions by health plan managers, institutional administrators, and governmental officials shape and often impede the ability of patients, families, and clinicians to construct a care plan that serves the dying person well.

In general, changes in systems of care—not just individual beliefs and actions—are necessary if real gains are to be made in helping people live well despite fatal illness. Such widespread changes depend in part on a stronger social consensus on what constitutes appropriate and supportive care for those approaching death. Widely publicized—albeit not necessarily typical—instances of patient and family powerlessness to stop what they see as futile and painful treatments reflect a lack of such consensus. Paradoxically, this lack of consensus also is evident when patients or families demand treatments that practitioners see as useless, counterproductive, or even inhumane. It similarly reveals itself in a health care delivery and financing system that still rewards life-prolonging interventions (even when they will be ineffectual) and slights palliative and supportive services for those for whom life-extending treatment is neither helpful nor desired.

Freud may have been right that "our unconscious does not believe in its own death; it behaves as if immortal" (Freud, 1915, in Freud, 1959, p. 304). The committee was optimistic, nonetheless, that this society would cultivate the conscious intelligence and spirit to recognize the reality of death and the likelihood that it will bring distress. It likewise was optimistic that people would work together to create humane systems of care that assure the consistent use of existing knowledge to prevent and relieve suffering and that support efforts to provide people the right care at the right time in the right way. The analyses, conclusions, and recommendations presented here are offered with optimism that we can, individually and together, "approach" death constructively and create humane care systems that people can trust to serve them well as they die.

References

AAMC (Association of American Medical Colleges). *ACME-TRI Report: Educating Medical Students.* Washington, D.C.: AAMC, 1992.

AAP (American Academy of Pediatrics), Committee on Bioethics. Informed Consent, Parental Permission, and Assent in Pediatric Practice. *Pediatrics* 97:314–317, 1995.

Aaron, H.J. *Serious and Unstable Condition: Financing America's Health Care.* Washington, D.C.: Brookings Institution, 1991.

Aaron, H.J., and Schwartz, W.B. *The Painful Prescription: Rationing Hospital Care.* Washington, D.C.: Brookings Institution, 1984.

Aaron, H.J., and Schwartz, W.B. Rationing Health Care: The Choice Before Us. *Science* 247:418–422, 1990.

AARP (American Association of Retired Persons). *A Matter of Choice: Planning Ahead for Health Care Decisions.* Washington, D.C.: AARP, 1986.

AARP. *Images of Aging in America: Final Report.* Washington, D.C.: AARP, 1995.

ABIM (American Board of Internal Medicine). *Final Report of the Advisory Committee on Recognizing New and Emerging Disciplines in Internal Medicine.* Philadelphia: ABIM, 1993.

ABIM. *Caring for the Dying: Identification and Promotion of Physician Competency: Educational Research Documents.* Philadelphia: ABIM, 1996a.

ABIM. *Caring for the Dying: Identification and Promotion of Physician Competency: Personal Narratives.* Philadelphia: ABIM, 1996b.

Abrahm, J.L., Callahan, J., Rossetti, K., and Pierre, L. The Impact of a Hospice Consultation Team on the Care of Veterans with Advanced Cancer. *Journal of Pain and Symptom Management* 12(1):23–31, 1996.

ACP (American College of Physicians). *Home Care Guide for Advanced Cancer: When Quality of Life is the Primary Goal of Care,* P.S. Houts, ed. Philadelphia: ACP, 1995.

Addington-Hall, J., and McCarthy, M. Audit Methods: Views of the Family after the Death. In *Clinical Audit in Palliative Care,* I. Higginson, ed. New York: Radcliffe Medical Press, 1993.

272

Agich, G.J. Actual Autonomy and Long-Term Care Decision Making. Pp. 113–136 in *Long-Term Care Decisions: Ethical and Conceptual Dimensions*, L.B. McCullough and N.L. Wilson, eds. Baltimore: Johns Hopkins University Press, 1995.

AGS (American Geriatrics Society). Measuring Quality of Care at the End of Life: A Statement of Principles. *Journal of the American Geriatrics Society* 45:526–527, 1997.

AHCA (American Health Care Association). *Facts and Trends: The Nursing Facility Sourcebook*. Washington, D.C.: AHCA, 1995.

AHCPR (U.S. DHHS PHS Agency for Health Care Policy and Research). *Clinical Practice Guideline Number 9: Management of Cancer Pain*. Rockville, Maryland: AHCPR Publication No. 94-0592, 1994a.

AHCPR. *Clinical Practice Guideline Number 10: Unstable Angina: Diagnosis and Management*. Rockville, Maryland: AHCPR Publication No. 94-0602, 1994b.

AHCPR. *Clinical Practice Guideline Number 11: Heart Failure: Evaluation and Care of Patients with Left-Ventricular Systolic Dysfunction*. Rockville, Maryland: AHCPR Publication No. 94-0612, 1994c.

Ahorony, L., and Strasser, S. Patient Satisfaction: What We Know About and What We Still Need to Explore. *Medical Care Review* 50:49–79, 1993.

Ajemian, I. The Interdisciplinary Team. Pp. 17–28 in *Oxford Textbook of Palliative Medicine*, D. Doyle, G.W.C. Hanks, and N. MacDonald, eds. Oxford: Oxford University Press, 1993.

Akarasereenont, P., Mitchell, J.A., Thiemermann, C., and Vane, J.R. Relative Potency of NSAIDs as Inhibitors of Cox-1 or Cox-2. *British Journal of Pharmacology* 110:183, 1994.

Al-Chaer E., Lawand, N.B., Westlund, K.N., and Willis, W.D. Pelvic Visceral Input into the Nucleus Gracilis Is Largely Mediated by the Postsynpatic Dorsal Column Pathway. *Journal of Neurophsyiology* 111:968–980, 1996.

Albanese, M.A., and Mitchell, S. Problem-Based Learning: A Review of Literature on Its Outcomes and Implementation Issues. *Academic Medicine* 68:52–81, 1993.

Allen, A. The Invisible Hand: Greed, Ethics, and the New Value of Dying. *The Washington Post Magazine*. November 17, 1996:13–17, 28–32, 1996.

AMA (American Medical Association). *Report of the Board of Trustees: Treatment of Intractable Pain* (Resolution 204, I-95). AMA Board of Trustees Report 26-A-96. Chicago: 1996a.

AMA. *Report of the Council on Medical Education: Medical Education for End-of-Life Care*. CME Report 4-I-96. Chicago: 1996b.

AMDA (American Medical Directors Association). *Depression: Clinical Practice Guidelines; Heart Failure: Clinical Practice Guideline; Pressure Ulcers: Clinical Practice Guideline; Urinary Incontinence: Clinical Practice Guideline*. AMDA: Columbia, Maryland, 1996.

American Medical News. Caring about Care at the End of Life (editorial), p. 17. May 12, 1997.

American Pain Society Quality of Care Committee. Quality Improvement Guidelines for the Treatment of Acute Pain and Cancer Pain. *Journal of the American Medical Association* 274(23):1874–1880, 1995.

ANA (American Nurses Association). *Nursing: A Social Policy Statement*. Kansas City, Missouri: 1980.

ANA. *Nursing's Social Policy Statement*. Washington, D.C., 1995.

ANA. *Written Testimony Before the IOM Committee on Care at the End of Life*. Washington, D.C., April 1996.

Angell, M. The Quality of Mercy. *New England Journal of Medicine* 306:98–99, 1982.

Annas, G.J. Ethics Committees: From Ethical Comfort to Ethical Cover. *Health Care Review* 21(3):18–21, 1991.

Annas, G. The Health Care Proxy and the Living Will. *New England Journal of Medicine* 324(17):1210–1213, 1991.

Annas, G. How We Lie. *Hastings Center Report* 25(6 Suppl.):S12–S14, 1995.

APA (American Psychiatric Association). *Diagnostic and Statistical Manual of Mental Disorders,* 4th Edition. Washington, D.C.: American Psychiatric Association. 1994.

Appelbaum, P.S., Lidz, C.W., and Meisel, A. *Informed Consent: Legal Theory and Clinical Practice.* New York: Oxford University Press, 1987.

APS (American Pain Society), Quality of Care Committee. Quality Improvement Guidelines for the Treatment of Acute Pain and Cancer Pain. *Journal of the American Medical Association* 274:1874–1880, 1995.

Aries, P. *Western Attitudes Toward Death: From the Middle Ages to the Present.* Baltimore: Johns Hopkins University Press, 1974.

Aries, P. *The Hour of Our Death.* New York: Alfred A. Knopf, 1981.

Aroskar, M.A. Bathing: On the Boundaries of Health Treatment: Case Commentary. In *Everyday Ethics: Resolving Dilemmas in Nursing Home Life,* R.A. Kane and A.L. Caplan, eds. New York: Springer, 1990.

Atkins, S., and Murphy, K. Reflection: A Review of the Literature. *Journal of Advanced Nursing,* 18(8):1188–1192, 1993.

Au, E., Loprinzi, C.L., Dhodapkar, M., et al. Regular Use of a Verbal Pain Scale Improves the Understanding of Oncology Inpatient Pain Intensity. *Journal of Clinical Oncology* 2751–2755, 1994.

Aubier, M., Murciano, D., Viires, N., et al. Diaphragmatic Contractility Enhanced by Aminophylline: Role of Extracellular Calcium. *Journal of Applied Physiology* 54:460–464, 1983.

Audet, A.M., Greenfield, S., and Field, M. Medical Practice Guidelines: Current Activities and Future Directions. *Annals of Internal Medicine* 113(9):709–714, 1990.

Avorn, J., and Soumerai, S. Improving Drug-Therapy Decisions through Educational Outreach: A Randomized Controlled Trial of Academically Based "Detailing." *New England Journal of Medicine* 308:1447–1463, 1983.

Azevedo, D. Rationing: America: From De Facto to Explicit? *Medical Economics* :184–199, 1993.

Baer, N.A. Cardiopulmonary Resuscitation on Television: Exaggerations and Accusations. *New England Journal of Medicine* 334(24):1604–1605, 1996.

Bagley, B. *Statement Before the IOM Committee on Care at the End of Life on Behalf of the American Academy of Family Physicians.* Washington, D.C., April 29, 1996.

Baines, B., Barnhart, C., Haefemeyer, J., et al. Completion of Advance Directives in the Outpatient Setting: A Process Improvement Project. Presented at the Conference on End-of-Life Health Care in Managed Care Systems. Center for Biomedical Ethics, University of Minnesota, Minneapolis, November 1–2, 1996.

Baines, B., Gendron, B.A., Lindstedt, R.N., et al. The Care Options Program: Providing Appropriate End-of-Life Care for the Non-Hospice Terminally Ill Patient. Presented at the Conference on End-of-Life Health Care in Managed Care Systems. Center for Biomedical Ethics, University of Minnesota, Minneapolis, November 1–2, 1996.

Barry, M.J., Mulley, A.G., Jr., Fowler, F.J., and Wennberg, J.E. Watchful Waiting vs. Immediate Transurethral Resection for Symptomatic Prostatism: The Importance of Patients' Preferences. *Journal of the American Medical Association* 259:3010–3017, 1988.

Bascom, P.B., and Tolle, S.W. Care of the Family when the Patient Is Dying. *Western Journal of Medicine* 163(3):292–296, 1995.

Batalden, P., and Buchanan, E.D. Industrial Models of Quality Improvement. In *Providing Quality Care: The Challenge to Clinicians,* N. Goldfield and D. Nash, eds. Philadelphia: American College of Physicians, 1989.

Beauchamp, T.L., and Childress, J.F. *Principles of Biomedical Ethics,* 4th Edition. New York: Oxford University Press, 1994.

Beck-Friis, B., Norberg, H., and Strang, P. Cost Analysis and Ethical Aspects of Hospital-Based Home-Care for Terminal Cancer Patients. *Scandinavian Journal of Health Care* 9(4):259–264, 1991.

Benjamin, A.E. An Historical Perspective on Home Care Policy. *Milbank Memorial Fund Quarterly* 71(1):129–166, 1993.

Berger, M.M., Marazzi, A., Freeman, J., and Chiolero, R. Evaluation of the Consistency of Acute Physiology and Chronic Health Evaluation (APACHE II) Scoring in a Surgical Intensive Care Unit. *Critical Care Medicine* 20(12):1681–1687, 1992.

Bernard, J.S., and Schneider, M. *The True Work of Dying: A Practical and Compassionate Guide to Easing the Dying Process.* New York: Avon Books, 1996.

Bernardin, Joseph Cardinal. Death as a Friend. *New York Times,* pp. 112, 114–115, December 1, 1996.

Bernat, J.L. How Much of the Brain Must Die in Brain Death? *Journal of Clinical Ethics* 3(1):21–26, 1992.

Bernstein, K., and Jensen, H.B. Managing Change in Developing Communication Systems for Integrated Care: The Funen Model. In *Proceedings of Medical Informatics Europe 1994,* P. Barahona, M. Veloso, and J. Bryant, eds. Lisbon: European Federation of Medical Informatics.

Berti, J.J., and Lipsky, J.J. Transcutaneous Drug Delivery: A Practical Review. *Mayo Clinic Proceedings* 70:581–586, 1995.

Berwick, D.M. Continuous Improvement as an Ideal in Health Care. *New England Journal of Medicine* 320(1):53–56, 1989.

Berwick, D.M. The SUPPORT Project: Lessons for Action. *Hastings Center Report* 25(6 Suppl.):S21–S22, 1995.

Berwick, D.M. Harvesting Knowledge from Improvement (Editorial). *Journal of the American Medical Association* 275(11):877–878, 1996.

Berwick, D.M., Godfrey, A.B., and Roessner, J. *Curing Health Care: New Strategies for Quality Improvement.* San Francisco: Jossey-Bass, 1990.

Bigelow, G.E., and Preston, K.L. Opioids. In *Psychopharmacology: The Fourth Generation of Progress,* F.E. Bloom and D.J. Kupfer, eds. New York: Raven Press, 1995.

Binstock, R.H., and Post, S.G., eds. *Too Old for Health Care?: Controversies in Medicine, Law, Economics, and Ethics.* Baltimore: Johns Hopkins University Press, 1991.

Bishop, C., and Skwara, K.C. Recent Growth of Medicare Home Health. *Health Affairs* 12(3):95–110, 1993.

Blackhall, L.J., Murphy, S.T., Frank, G., et al. Ethnicity and Attitudes Toward Patient Autonomy. *Journal of the American Medical Association* 274(10):820–825, 1995.

Blackman, R.A. Helping the Terminally Ill Face Death with Dignity. *Quality Letter* March:19–23, 1995a.

Blackman, R.A. Program Reaps Unexpected Cost Benefits: Options Program Cuts Demand for Care While Improving Quality of Life for Terminally Ill Patients. *Healthcare Demand Management* 1(1):13–16, April 1995b.

Blalock, H.M. *Social Statistics,* Rev. 2d ed. New York: McGraw Hill Book Company, 1979.

Blank, L. Defining and Evaluating Physician Competence in End-of-Life Patient Care: A Matter of Awareness and Emphasis. *Western Journal of Medicine* 163(3):297–301, 1995.

Blank, L. Defining Clinical Competence and Strategies for Evaluation. In *Care for the Dying: Identification and Promotion of Physician Competency: Educational Resource Document.* Philadelphia: ABIM, 1996a.

Blank, L. *Statement Before the IOM Committee on Care at the End of Life on Behalf of the American Board of Internal Medicine.* Washington, D.C., April 29, 1996b.

Blendon, R.J. The Public's View of the Future of Health Care. *Journal of the American Medical Association* 259:3587–3593, 1988.

Blendon, R.J., Szalay, U.S., and Knox, R. Should Physicians Aid Their Patients in Dying?: The Public Perspective. *Journal of the American Medical Association* 267:2658–2662, 1992.

Block, S. Learning about End-of-Life Care: Recent Data. Presentation at Medical Education for Care Near the End of Life National Consensus Conference, Washington, D.C., May 16, 1997.

Block, S. and Billings, J.A. Patient Requests for Euthanasia and Assisted Suicide in Terminal Illness: the Role of the Psychiatrist. *Psychosomatics* 36:445–457, 1995.

Block, S., Billings, J.A., and Peterson, L. My Patients, My Self. *Harvard Medical Alumni Bulletin* 70(3):37–42, 1997.

Bloom, B.S., Knoor, R.S., and Evans, A.E. The Epidemiology of Disease Expenses: The Costs of Caring for Children with Cancer. *Journal of the American Medical Association* 253:2393–2397, 1985.

Bluebond-Langer, M. *The Private Worlds of Dying Children.* Princeton, N.J.: Princeton University Press, 1978.

Blumenthal, D. Quality of Health Care: Part 1: Quality of Care—What Is It? *New England Journal of Medicine* 335:891–894, 1996.

Blumenthal, D., and Scheck, A.C. *Improving Clinical Practice: Total Quality Management and the Physician.* San Francisco: Jossey-Bass, 1995.

Bock, S.J., and Boyette, M. *Stay Young the Melatonin Way.* New York: Plume, 1995.

Bonica, J.J. Treatment of Cancer Pain: Current Status and Future Need. Pp. 589–616 in *Proceedings of the Fourth World Congress on Pain;* Seattle, Washington, August 31–September 5, 1984. Vol. 9, *Advances in Pain Research and Therapy.* New York: Raven Press, 1985.

Bonica, J.J. Cancer Pain. Pp. 400–460 in *The Management of Pain,* 2d Edition, Vol. 1, J.J. Bonica, ed. Philadelphia: Lea and Febiger, 1990.

Bookbinder, M., Coyle, N., and Thaler, H. Implementing National Standards for Cancer Pain Management. *Journal of Pain and Symptom Management* 12(6):334–347, 1996.

Braveman, P., Olivia, G., Grisham Miller, M., et al. Adverse Outcomes and Lack of Health Insurance Among Newborns in an Eighty-County Area of California: 1882–1986. *New England Journal of Medicine* 321(8):508–513, 1989.

Breitbart, W. Pharmacotherapy of Pain in AIDS. *A Clinical Guide to AIDS and HIV,* pp. 359–378, G.P. Wormser, ed. Philadelphia: Lippincott-Raven Publishers, 1996.

Breitbart, W. Pain in AIDS. *Proceedings of the 8th World Congress on Pain,* Progress in Pain Research Management, Vol. 8, pp. 1–38, T.S. Jensen, J.A. Turner, and Z. Wiesenfeld-Hallin, eds. Seattle: IASP Press, 1997.

Breitbart, W., Bruera, E., Chochinov, H., and Lynch, M. Neuropsychiatric Syndromes and Psychological Symptoms in Patients with Advanced Cancer. *Journal of Pain and Symptom Management* 10:131–141, 1995.

Breitbart, W., and Holland, J.C., eds. *Psychiatric Aspects of Symptom Management in Cancer Patients.* Washington, D.C.: American Psychiatric Press, 1993.

Breitbart, W., McDonald, M.V., Rosenfeld, B., et al. Pain in Ambulatory AIDS Patients. I: Pain Characteristics and Medical Correlates. *Pain* 68:315–321, 1996.

Breitbart, W., Rosenfeld, B.D., Passik, S.D., et al. The Undertreatment of Pain in Ambulatory AIDS Patients. *Pain* 65:243–249, 1996.

Brescia, F.J., Portenoy, R.K., Ryan, M., et al. Pain, Opioid Use, and Survival in Hospitalized Patients with Advanced Cancer. *Journal of Clinical Oncology* 10:149–155, 1992.

Breslow, D.M. Creative Arts for Hospitals: The UCLA Experiment. *Patient Education and Counseling* 21:101–110, 1993.

Brett, A. Limitations of Listing Specific Medical Interventions in Advance Directives. *Journal of the American Medical Association* 266(6):825–828, 1991.

Brim, O.G., Jr., Friedman, H.E., Levine, S., and Scotch, N.A, eds. *The Dying Patient*. New York: Russell Sage Foundation, 1970.

Brock, D.B., and Foley, D.J. Demography and Epidemiology of Dying in the U.S., with Emphasis on Deaths of Older Persons. In *A Good Dying: Shaping Health Care for the Last Months of Life*. Briefing book for symposium sponsored by The George Washington University Center to Improve Care of the Dying and the Corcoran Gallery of Art, April 30, 1996.

Brody, H., Campbell, M.L., Faber-Langendoen, K., and Ogle, K.S. Withdrawing Intensive Life-Sustaining Treatment: Recommendations for Compassionate Clinical Management. *New England Journal of Medicine* 336(9):652–657, 1997.

Brook, R.H., and Lohr, K.N. Will We Need to Ration Effective Health Care? *Issues in Science and Technology* Fall:68–77, 1986.

Brook, R.H., Chassin, M., Park, R., et al. A Method for Detailed Assessment of the Appropriateness of Medical Technologies. *International Journal of Technology Assessment in Health Care* 2:53–63, 1986.

Brook, R.H., McGlynn, E.A., and Cleary, P.D. Quality of Health Care: Part 2: Measuring Quality of Care. *New England Journal of Medicine* 335:966–970, 1996.

Brown, G. *Statement Before the IOM Committee on Care at the End of Life on Behalf of the Hospice of the Blue Grass*. Washington, D.C., April 29, 1996.

Brown, L. *Politics and Health Care Organization: HMOs as Federal Policy*. Washington, D.C.: Brookings Institution, 1983.

Brown, L.D. The National Politics of Oregon's Rationing Plan. *Health Affairs* 10(2):67–77, 1991.

Brown, R.S., Clement, D.G., Hill, J.W., et al. Do Health Maintenance Organizations Work for Medicare? *Health Care Financing Review* 15(1):7–23, 1993.

Bruera, E. Research in Symptoms Other than Pain. Pp. 87–92 in *Oxford Textbook of Palliative Medicine*, D. Doyle, G.W.C. Hanks, and N. MacDonald, eds. Oxford: Oxford University Press, 1993.

Bruera, E., Brenneis, C., and MacDonald, R.N. Continuous Sc Infusion of Narcotics for the Treatment of Cancer Pain: An Update. *Cancer Treatment Reprint* 71(10):953–958, 1987.

Bruera, E., Brenneis, C., Michaud, M., Bacovsky, R., Chadwick, S., Emeno, A., and MacDonald, N. Use of the Subcutaneous Route for the Administration of Narcotics in Patients with Cancer Pain. *Cancer* 2(62):407–411, 1988.

Bruera, E., and MacDonald, S. Audit Methods: The Edmunton Symptom Assessment System. In *Clinical Audit in Palliative Care*, I. Higginson, ed. New York: Radcliffe Medical Press, 1993.

Bruera, E., Macmillan, K., Hanson, J., et al. A Controlled Trial of Megestrol Acetate on Appetite, Caloric Intake, Nutritional Status, and Other Symptoms in Patients with Advance Cancer. *Cancer* 66:1279–1282, 1990.

Bruera, E., Miller, M.J., McCallion, J., et al. Cognitive Failure in Patients with Terminal Cancer: A Prospective Study. *Journal of Pain Symptom Management* 7:192–195, 1992.

Bruera, E., Schoeller, T., and MacEachern, T. Symptomatic Benefit of Supplemental Oxygen in Hypoxemic Patients with Terminal Cancer: The Use of the N of 1 Randomized Controlled Trial. *Journal of Pain and Symptom Managment* 7:365–368, 1992.

Brunetti, L.L., Carperos, S.D., and Westlund, R.E. Patients' Attitudes Towards Living Wills and Cardiopulmonary Resuscitation. *Journal of General Internal Medicine* 6(4):323–329, 1991.

Buchan, M.L., and Tolle, S.W. Pain Relief for Dying Persons: Dealing with Physicians' Fears and Concerns. *Journal of Clinical Ethics* 6(1):53–61, 1995.

Buckingham, R.W. *The Handbook of Hospice Care.* Amherst, New York: Prometheus Books, 1996.

Buckman, R. Communication in Palliative Care: A Practical Guide. Pp. 47–61 in *Oxford Textbook of Palliative Medicine,* D. Doyle, G.W.C. Hanks, and N. MacDonald, eds. Oxford: Oxford University Press, 1993.

Bukberg, J.B., Penman, D., and Holland, J.C. Depression in Hospitalized Cancer Patients. *Psychosomatic Medicine* 46:199–212, 1984.

Bunker, J.P. Surgical Manpower: A Comparison of Operations and Surgeons in the United States and in England and Wales. *New England Journal of Medicine* 282:135–144, 1970.

Burt, R.A. Apparent Impact of Laws Affecting Dying, Decisionmaking, and Appropriate Care. In *Summary of Committee Views and Workshop Examining the Feasibility of an Institute of Medicine Study of Dying, Decisionmaking, and Appropriate Care.* IOM Committee for a Feasibility Study on Care at the End of Life, M.J. Field, ed. Washington, D.C.: Institute of Medicine, 1994.

Byock, I.R. *Statement Before the IOM Committee on Care at the End of Life on behalf of the Academy of Hospice Physicians.* Washington, D.C., April 29, 1996.

Byock, I. *Dying Well: The Prospect for Growth at the End of Life.* New York: Riverhead Books, 1997a.

Byock, I. Why Do We Make Dying So Miserable? *The Washington Post,* January 22, 1997b.

Calder, K. *Statement Before the IOM Committee on Care at the End of Life on Behalf of the American Alliance of Cancer Pain Initiatives.* Washington, D.C., April 29, 1996.

Callahan, D. *Setting Limits: Medical Goals in an Aging Society.* New York: Simon and Schuster, 1987.

Callahan, D. Allocating Health Resources. *Hastings Center Report* 18:14–20, 1988.

Callahan, D. Frustrated Mastery: The Cultural Context of Death in America. *Western Journal of Medicine* 163(3):226–230, 1995.

Callahan, D. Controlling the Costs of Health Care for the Elderly: Fair Means and Foul. *New England Journal of Medicine* 335(10):744–746, 1996.

Calman, K.C. Palliative Medicine: On the Way to Becoming a Recognized Medicine. *Journal of Palliative Care* 4(1–2):12–4, 1988.

Campbell, C.S. Gridlock on the Oregon Trail. *Hastings Center Report* 23(4):6–7, 1993.

Campbell, M.L. Breaking Bad News to Patients. *Journal of the American Medical Association* 271:1052, 1994.

Campbell, M.L. Program Assessment through Outcomes Analysis: Efficacy of a Comprehensive Care Team for End-of-Life Care. *AACN Clinical Issues* 7:159–167, 1996.

Campbell, M.L., and Frank, R.R. Experience with an End-of-Life Practice at a University Hospital. *Critical Care Medicine* 25:197–202, 1997.

Capecchi, M.R. Targeted Gene Replacement. *Scientific American* 270(3):52–59, 1994.

Caplan, A.L. The Morality of the Mundane: Ethical Issues Arising in the Daily Lives of Nursing Home Residents. In *Everyday Ethics: Resolving Dilemmas in Nursing Home Life,* R.A. Kane and A.L. Caplan, eds. New York: Springer, 1990.

Caralis, P.V., Davis, B., Wright, K., and Marcial, E. The Influence of Ethnicity and Race on Attitudes Toward Advance Directives, Life-Prolonging Treatments, and Euthanasia. *Journal of Clinical Ethics* 4:155–165, 1993.

Carlson, R.W., Devich, L., and Frank, R.R. Development of a Comprehensive Supportive Care Team for the Hopelessly Ill on a University Hospital Medical Service. *Journal of the American Medical Association* 259(3):378–383, 1988.

Carper, J. *Stop Aging Now!* New York: Harper-Collins, 1995.

Carter, R. *Helping Yourself Help Others: A Book for Caregivers.* New York: Random House, 1994.

Cassel, C. Ethical Issues in the Conduct of Research in Long Term Care. *Gerontologist* 28(Suppl.):90–96, 1988.

Cassel, C. Attitudes of Physicians Towards Caring for the Dying Patient. In *Summary of Committee Views and Workshop Examining the Feasibility of an Institute of Medicine Study of Dying, Decisionmaking, and Appropriate Care.* IOM Committee for a Feasibility Study on Care at the End of Life, M.J. Field, ed. Washington, D.C.: Institute of Medicine, 1994.

Cassel, C. Letter to Colleagues about New Medicare Palliative Care Code. Milbank Memorial Fund, New York, July 20, 1996.

Cassell, E.J. *The Nature of Suffering and the Goals of Medicine.* New York: Oxford University Press, 1991.

Cassem, E. Difficult Deliberations about Care at the End of Life. In *Summary of Committee Views and Workshop Examining the Feasibility of an Institute of Medicine Study of Dying, Decisionmaking, and Appropriate Care.* IOM Committee for a Feasibility Study on Care at the End of Life, M.J. Field, ed. Washington, D.C.: Institute of Medicine, 1994.

Cassem, N. Internship, Liberty, Death and Other Choices. *Harvard Medical Alumni Bulletin* 53(6):46–48, 1979.

Cella, D.F., and Tulsky, D.S. Measuring Quality of Life Today: Methodological Aspects. *Oncology-Huntington* 4(5):29–38, 1990.

Chambers, C.V., Diamond, J.J., Perkel, R.L., and Lasch, L.A. Relationship of Advance Directives to Hospital Charges in a Medicare Population. *Archives of Internal Medicine* 154(5):541–547, 1994.

Chang, R.W.S. Individual outcome prediction models for intensive care units. *Lancet* 2:(8655):143–146, 1989.

Chang, R.W.S., Lee, B., Jacobs, S., et al. Accuracy of Decisions to Withdraw Therapy in Critically Ill Patients: Clinical Judgment Versus a Computer Model. *Critical Care Medicine* 17(11):1091–1097, 1989.

Charon, R., Banks, J.T., Connelly, J.E., et al. Literature and Medicine: Contributions to Clinical Practice. *Annals of Internal Medicine* 122:599–606, 1995.

Chassin, M.R., Kosecoff, J., Park, R.E., et al. *Indications for Selected Medical and Surgical Procedures: A Literature Review and Ratings of Appropriateness: Coronary Angiography.* R-3201/1-CWF/HF/HCFA/PMT/RWJ. Santa Monica, California: RAND Corporation, 1986.

Cheitlin, M.D. The End of Therapy Is not the End of Treatment. In *Caring for the Dying: Identification and Promotion of Physician Competency: Personal Narratives.* Philadelphia: ABIM, 1996.

Chernow, B. *The Pharmacologic Approach to the Critically Ill Patient,* 3d Edition. Baltimore: Williams & Wilkins, 1994.

Cherny, N.I., and Catane, R. Professional Negligence in the Management of Cancer Pain: A Case for Urgent Reforms. *Cancer* 76(11):2181–2185, 1995.

Cherny, N.I., Coyle, N., and Foley, K.M. Suffering in the Advanced Cancer Patient: Part I: A Definition and Taxonomy. *Journal of Palliative Care* 10(2):57–70, 1994.

Childress, J.F. *Who Should Decide?: Paternalism in Health Care.* New York: Oxford University Press, 1982.

Childress, J.F. The Place of Autonomy in Bioethics. *Hastings Center Report* 20(1):12–17, 1990.

Chlebowski, R.T., Palomares, M.R., Lillington, L., Grosvernor, M. Recent Implications of Weight Loss In Lung Cancer Management. *Nutrition* 12:S43–S47, 1996

Chochinov, H.M., et al. Depression and the Desire for Death Among the Terminally Ill. Presented at the American Psychiatric Association Meeting, Washington, D.C., May, 1992.

Chochinov, H.M., Wilson, K.G., Enns, M. and Lander, S. The Prevalence of Depression in the Terminally Ill; Effects of Diagnostic Criteria and Symptom Threshold Judgments. *American Journal of Psychiatry* 151: 537–540, 1994.

Choron, J. *Death and Western Thought*. New York: MacMillan, 1963.

Christakis, N.A. Timing of Referral of Terminally Ill Patients to an Outpatient Hospice. *Journal of General Internal Medicine* 9(6):314–320, 1994.

Christakis, N.A. *Prognostication and Death in Medical Thought and Practice*. Ann Arbor, Michigan: University Microfilms, 1995.

Christakis, N.A. Predicting Patient Survival Before and After Hospice Enrollment. In *A Good Dying: Shaping Health Care for the Last Months of Life*. Briefing book for symposium sponsored by The George Washington University Center to Improve Care of the Dying and the Corcoran Gallery of Art, April 30, 1996.

Christakis, N.A., and Escarce, J.J. Survival of Medicare Patients After Enrollment in Hospice Programs. *New England Journal of Medicine* 335(3):172–178, 1996.

Christensen, K. Continuous Quality Improvement and Advance Treatment Planning. Presented at End of Life Health Care in Managed Care Systems Conference. Center for Biomedical Ethics, University of Minnesota, Minneapolis, November 1–2, 1996.

Citron, M.L., Johnson-Early, A., Fossieck, B.E., Jr., et al. Safety and Efficacy of Continuous Intravenous Morphine for Severe Cancer Pain. *American Journal of Medicine* 77:199–204, 1984.

Clark, H. Relevant Teaching Strategies: Attitudes, Behaviors, and Communications Skills. In *Care for the Dying: Identification and Promotion of Physician Competency: Educational Resource Document*. Philadelphia: ABIM, 1996.

Clauser, S.B. Recent Innovations in Home Health Care Policy Research. *Health Care Financing Review* 16(1):1–6, 1994.

Cleary, J. Double Blind Randomized Study of the Treatment of Breakthrough Pain in Cancer Patients: Oral Transmucosal Fentanyl Citrate Versus Placebo. *Proceedings of the American Society for Clinical Oncology* 16:52A (Abstract No. 179), 1997.

Cleary, P.D., and McNeil, B.J. Patient Satisfaction as an Indicator of Quality Care. *Inquiry* 25:25–26, 1988.

Cleary, P.D., Edgman-Levitan, S., Roberts, M., et al. Patients Evaluate Their Hospital Care: A National Survey. *Health Affairs* 10(4):254–267, 1991.

Cleeland, C.S. Measurement of Pain by Subjective Report. Pp. 391–404 in *Drug Treatment of Cancer Pain in a Drug-Oriented Society*, Vol. 11: *Advances in Pain Research and Therapy*. C.S. Hill, Jr. and W.S. Field, eds. New York: Raven Press, 1989.

Cleeland, C.S., Cleeland, L.M., Dar, R., and Rinehardt, L.C. Factors Influencing Physician Management of Cancer Pain. *Cancer* 58(3):796–800, 1986.

Cleeland, C.S., Gonin, R., Hatfield, A., et al. Pain and Its Treatment in Outpatients with Metastatic Cancer. *New England Journal of Medicine* 330:592–596, 1994.

Cobbs, E.L., and Barry, Z. *Statement Before the IOM Committee on Care at the End of Life on Behalf of the Washington Home and Hospice*. Washington, D.C., April 29, 1996.

Coderre, T.J., Katz, J., Vaccarino, A.L., and Melzack, R. Contribution of Central Neuroplasticity to Pathological Pain: Review of Clinical and Experimental Evidence. *Pain* 52:259–285, 1993.

Coddington, D.C., Moore, K.D., and Fischer, E.A. *Making Integrated Health Care Work*. Englewood, Colorado: Center for Research in Ambulatory Health Care Administration, 1996.

Coggeshall, L.T. *Planning for Medical Progress Through Education*. Evanston, Illinois: Association of American Medical Colleges, 1965.

Cohen, M.H., Anderson, A.J., Krasnow, S.H., et al. Continuous Intravenous Infusion of Morphine for Severe Dyspnea. *Southern Medical Journal* 84:229–234, 1991.

Cohen, S.B., Carlson, B.L., and Potter, D.E.B. Health Care Expenditures in the Last Six Months of Life. *Health Policy Review* (American Statistical Association Section on Health Policy) 1(2):1–13, 1995.

Cohen, S.R., and Mount, B.M. Quality of Life in Terminal Illness: Defining and Measuring Subjective Well-Being in the Dying. *Journal of Palliative Care* 8(3):40–45, 1992.

Cohen, S.R., Mount, B.M., Strobe, M.G., et al. The McGill Quality of Life Questionnaire: A Measure of Quality of Life for People with Advanced Disease. *Palliative Medicine* 9:207–219, 1995.

Colombotos, J. and Kirchner, C. *Physicians and Social Change.* New York: Oxford University Press, 1986.

Coluzzi, P. A Titration Study of Oral Transmucosal Fentanyl Citrate for Breakthrough Pain in Cancer Patients. *Proceedings of the American Society for Clinical Oncology* 15:41a, 1997.

Coluzzi, P.H., Grant, M., Doroshow, J.H., et al. Survey of the Provision of Supportive Care Services at the National Cancer Institute-Designated Cancer Centers. *Journal of Clinical Oncology* 13(3):756–764, 1995.

Connell, C. Art Therapy as Part of a Palliative Care Programme. *Pallitive Medicine* 6:18–25, 1992.

Coolican, M.B., Stark, J., Doka, K.J., and Corr, C.A. Education About Death, Dying, and Bereavement in Nursing Programs. *Nurse Education* 19(6):35–40, 1994.

Cooper, J.R., Czechowicz, D.J., Petersen, R.C., and Molinari, S.P. Prescription Drug Diversion Control and Medical Practice. *Journal of the American Medical Association* 268(10):1306–1310, 1992.

Cooper, J.R., Czechowicz, D.J., and Molinari, S.P., eds. *Impact of Prescriptioin Drug Diversion Control Systems on Medical Practice and Patient Care.* NIDA Research Monograph 131. Rockville, Maryland: NIDA, 1993.

Corner, J. The Nursing Perspective. Pp. 781–790 in *Oxford Textbook of Palliative Medicine,* D. Doyle, G.W.C. Hanks, and N. MacDonald, eds. Oxford: Oxford University Press, 1993.

Cotton, P. 'Basic Benefits' Have Many Variations, Tend to Become Political Issues. *Journal of the American Medical Association* 268(16):2139–2141, 1992.

Covinsky, K.E., Goldman, L., Cook, E.F., et al. The Impact of Serious Illness on Patients' Families. *Journal of the American Medical Association* 272:1839–1844, 1994.

Covinsky, K.E., Landefeld, C.S., Teno, J., et al. Is Economic Hardship on the Families of the Seriously Ill Associated with Patient and Surrogate Care Preferences? *Archives of Internal Medicine* 156:1737–1741, 1996.

Cowley, A.J., and Skene, A.M. Treatment of Severe Heart Failure: Quantity and Quality of Life. *British Heart Journal* 72(3):226–230, 1994.

Coyle, N., Adelhardt, J., Foley, K.M., and Portenoy, R.K. Character of Terminal Illness in the Advanced Cancer Patient: Pain and Other Symptoms During the Last Four Weeks of Life. *Journal of Pain and Symptom Management* 5(2):83–93, 1990.

Cranford, R., and Dondera, E. *Institutional Ethics Committees.* Ann Arbor, Michigan: Health Research Press, 1982.

Culler, S.D., Callahan, C.M., and Wolinsky, F.D. Predicting Hospital Costs Among Older Decedents over Time. *Medical Care* 33(11):1089–1105, 1995.

Daniels, N. *Am I My Parents' Keeper?: An Essay on Justice between the Young and Old.* New York: Oxford University Press, 1988.

Daniels, N. Is the Oregon Rationing Plan Fair? *Journal of the American Medical Association* 265(17):2232–2235, 1991.

Daniels, N. Four Unsolved Rationing Problems: A Challenge. *Hastings Center Report* 24(4):27–29, 1994.

Dar, R., Beach, C.M., Barden, P.L, and Cleeland, C.S. Cancer Pain in the Marital System: A Study of Patients and Their Spouses. *Journal of Pain and Symptom Management* 7(2):87–93, 1992.

Davies, N.E., Davies, G.H., and Sanders, E.D. William Cobbett, Benjamin Rush and the Death of General Washington. *Journal of the American Medical Association* 249:912–915, 1983.

Davis, C.L. The Therapeutics of Dyspnea. *Cancer Surveys* 21:85–98, 1994.

Degner, L.F., Gow, C.M., and Thompson, L.A. Critical Nursing Behaviors in Care for the Dying. *Cancer Nursing* 14(5):246–253, 1991.

Della Penna, R. *Statement Before the IOM Committee on Care at the End of Life on Behalf of Kaiser Permanente.* Irvine, California, November 23, 1996.

DeSpelder, L.A., and Strickland, A.L. *The Last Dance: Encountering Death and Dying.* Mountain View, California: Mayfield, 1996.

Diamond, G.A. Future Imperfect: The Limitations of Clinical Prediction Models and the Limits of Clinical Prediction. *Journal of the American College of Cardiology* 14(3 Suppl. A):12A–22A, 1989.

Dickinson, G. Death Education in U.S. Medical Schools. *Journal of Medical Education* 51:34–36, 1976.

Dickinson, G.E., and Mermann, A.C. Death Education in U.S. Medical Schools, 1975–1995. *Academic Medicine* 71(12):1348–1349, 1996.

Diem, S.J., Lantos, J.D., and Tulsky, J.A. Cardiopulmonary Resuscitation on Television: Miracles and Misinformation. *New England Journal of Medicine* 334(24):1578–1582, 1996.

Die Trill, M., and Holland, J. Cross-Cultural Differences in the Care of Patients with Cancer: A Review. *General Hospital Psychiatry* 15:21–30, 1993.

Dietrick-Gallagher, M., Polomano, R., and Carrick, L. Pain as a Quality Management Initiative. *Journal of Nursing Care Quality* 9:30–42, 1994.

DiMaggio, J.R. Educating Psychiatry Residents About Death and Dying: A National Survey. *General Hospital Psychiatry* 15(3):166–170, 1993.

Donabedian, A. *Explorations in Quality Assessment and Monitoring, 3 vols.* Vol. 1, *The Definition of Quality and Approaches to Its Assessment.* Vol. 2, *The Criteria and Standards of Monitoring.* Vol. 3, *The Methods and Findings of Quality Assessment and Monitoring: An Illustrated Analysis.* Ann Arbor, Michigan: Health Administration Press, 1980, 1982, 1985.

Donabedian, A. Evaluating the Quality of Medical Care. *Milbank Memorial Fund Quarterly* 44:166–203, 1966.

Donaldson, M. Provider Continuity. Prepared for Conference on Measuring Care at the End of Life, August 27–28, 1996, updated March 1997.

Donnelly, S., and Walsh, D. The Symptoms of Advanced Cancer. *Seminal Oncology* 22(2 Suppl.):67–72, 1995a.

Donnelly, S., and Walsh, D. The Symptoms of Advanced Cancer: Identification of Clinical and Research Priorities by Assessment of Prevalence and Severity. *Journal of Palliative Care* 11:27–32, 1995b.

Donovan, M., Dillon, P., and McGuire, L. Incidence and Characteristics of Pain in a Sample of Medical-Surgical Inpatients. *Pain* 30:69–87, 1987.

Dougherty, C.J. The Common Good, Terminal Illness, and Euthanasia. *Issues in Law & Medicine* 9(2):151–166, 1993.

Doukas, D.J., and Gorenflo, D.W. Analyzing the Values History: An Evaluation of Patient Medical Values and Advance Directives. *The Journal of Clinical Ethics* 4(1):41–45, 1993.

Downer, S., Joel, S., and Allbright, A. A Double Blind Placebo-Controlled Trial of Medroxyprogesterone Acetate (MPA) in Cancer Cachexia. *British Journal of Cancer* 67(5):1102–1105, 1993.

Doyle, D., Hanks, G.W.C., and MacDonald, N., eds. *Oxford Textbook of Palliative Medicine.* Oxford, England: Oxford University Press, 1993.

Draisci, G., Kajander, K.C., Dubner, R., et al. Up-Regulation of Opioid Gene Expression in Spinal Cord Evoked by Experimental Nerve Injuries and Inflammation. *Brain Research* 560:186–192, 1991.

Dukes, C.S., Turpin, B.A., and Atwood, J.R. Hospice Education about People with AIDS as Terminally Ill Patients: Coping with a New Epidemic of Death. *American Journal of Hospice and Palliative Care* 12(1):25–31, 1995.

Durlak, J.A. Changing Death Attitudes through Death Education. Pp. 243–260 in *Death Anxiety Handbook: Research, Instrumentation, and Application,* R.A. Neimeyer, ed. Washington, D.C.: Taylor & Francis, 1994.

Durlak, J.A., and Riesenberg, L.A. The Impact of Death Education. *Death Studies* 15:39–58, 1991.

Eddy, D. Rationing by Patient Choice. *Journal of the American Medical Association* 265:105–108, 1991a.

Eddy, D. Oregon's Methods: Did Cost-Effectiveness Analysis Fail? *Journal of the American Medical Association* 266(15):2135–2141, 1991b.

Eddy, D. *Clinical Decision Making: From Theory to Practice: A Collection of Essays from JAMA.* Boston: Jones and Bartlett Publishers, 1996.

Eide, P.K., Stubhaug, A., Oye, I., and Breivik, H. Continuous Subcutaneous Administration of the N-methyl-D-aspartic Acid (NMDA) Receptor Antagonist Ketamine in the Treatment of Post-Herpetic Neuralgia. *Pain* 61:221–228, 1995.

Eisenberg, J. *Doctors' Decisions and the Cost of Medical Care: The Reasons for Doctors' Practice Patterns and the Ways to Change Them.* Ann Arbor, Michigan: Health Administration Press Perspectives, 1986.

Ellis, R.P., Pope, G.C., Iezzoni, L.I., et al. Diagnosis-Based Risk Adjustment for Medicare Capitation Payments. *Health Care Financing Review* 17(3):101–128, 1996.

Emanuel, E.J. Cost Savings at the End of Life: What Do the Data Show? *Journal of the American Medical Association* 275(24):1907–1914, 1996.

Emanuel, E.J., and Emanuel, L.L. Four Models of the Physician-Patient Relationship. *Journal of the American Medical Association* 267(16):2221–2226, 1992.

Emanuel, E.J., and Emanuel, L.L. The Economics of Dying: The Illusion of Cost Savings at the End of Life. *New England Journal of Medicine* 330(8):540–544, 1994.

Emanuel, L.L. Advance Directives for Medical Care: A Case for Greater Use. *Archives of Internal Medicine* 324:889–895, 1991.

Emanuel, L.L. What Makes A Directive Valid? *Hastings Center Report* 24(6 Suppl.):S27–S29, 1994.

Emanuel, L.L. Advance Directives: Do They Work? *Journal of the American College of Cardiology* 25(1):35–38, 1995a.

Emanuel, L.L. Structured Deliberation to Improve Decisionmaking for the Seriously Ill. *Hastings Center Report* 25(6 Suppl.):S14–S18, 1995b.

Emanuel, L.L., Danis, M., Pearlman, R.A., et al. Advance Care Planning as a Process. *Journal of the American Geriatrics Society* 43:440–446, 1995.

Emanuel, L.L., and Emanuel, E.J. The Medical Directive: A New Comprehensive Advance Care Document. *Journal of the American Medical Association* 261:3288–3293, 1989.

Emma, L. *Statement Before the IOM Committee on Care at the End of Life on Behalf of HealthCare Partners Medical Group.* Irvine, California, November 23, 1996.

Enck, R.E. *The Medical Care of Terminally Ill Patients.* Baltimore, Maryland: Johns Hopkins University Press, 1994.

Endres, S., Ghorbani, R., Kelley, V.E., et al. The Effect of Deitary Supplementation with n-3 Polyunsaturated Fatty Acids on the Synthesis of Interleukin-1 and Tumour Necrosis Factor by Mononuclear Cells. *New England Journal of Medicine* 320:265–271, 1989.

Englehardt, H.T. *The Foundations of Bioethics.* New York: Oxford University Press, 1986.

Englehardt, H.T. Market Rationing, or Why a Two-Tier System of Health Care Is Morally Unavoidable. Unpublished paper. May 6, 1991.

Erickson, K.L., and Hubbard, N.E. Dietary Fish Oil Modulation of Macrophage Tumoricidal Activity. *Nutrition.* 12:S34–S38, 1996.

Esserman, L., Belkora, J., and Lenert, L. Potentially Ineffective Care: A New Outcome to Assess the Limits of Critical Care. *Journal of the American Medical Association* 274(19):1544–1551, 1995.

Etzioni, A. *The Spirit of Community: Rights, Responsibilities, and the Communitarian Agenda.* New York: Crown Publishing Group, 1991.

Expert Advisory Group. *Consultative Document: A Policy Framework for Commissioning Cancer Services.* London: Her Majesty's Stationery Office, 1994.

Experton, B., Li, Z.L., Branch, L.G., et al. Does Managed Care Manage Vulnerable Populations? Hospital Readmission of the Frail Elderly by Payor/Provider Type. Presented at the annual Meeting of the Association for Health Services Research, Chicago, 1996.

Experton, B., Li, Z.L., Branch, L.G., et al. The Impact of Payor/Provider Type on Health Care Utilization and Expenditures Among the Frail Elderly. *American Journal of Public Health* 87(2):210–216, 1997.

Experton, B., Ozminkowski, R.J., Branch, L.G., and Li, Z.L. A Comparison of Payor/Provider Type of the Cost of Dying Among the Frail Elderly. *Journal of the American Geriatrics Society* 44:1098–1107, 1996.

Fade, A., and Kaplan, K. Managed Care at the End of Life Decisions. *Trends in Health Care, Law & Ethics* 10: 239–242, 1995.

Faden, R.R., Beauchamp, T.L., and King, N.M. *A History and Theory of Informed Consent.* New York: Oxford University Press, 1986.

Fainsinger, R., and Young, C. Cognitive Failure in Terminally Ill Patients. *Journal of Pain Symptom Management* 6:492–494, 1991.

Farley, D.O., Carter, G.M., Kallich, J.D., et al. Modified Capitation and Treatment Incentives for End Stage Renal Disease. *Health Care Financing Review* 17(3):129–142, 1996.

Farrow, D.C., Hunt, W.C., and Samet, J.M. Temporal and Regional Variability in the Surgical Treatment of Cancer Among Older People. *Journal of the American Geriatric Society* 44:559–564, 1996.

Felder, M. *Statement Before the IOM Committee on Care at the End of Life on Behalf of the American Association of Health Plans.* Washington, D.C., April 29, 1996.

Ferrell, B.A. Cost Issues Surrounding the Treatment of Cancer-Related Pain. *Journal of Pharmacological Care Pain Symptom Control* 1:9–23, 1993.

Ferrell, B.A. *Statement Before the IOM Committee on Care at the End of Life on Behalf of City of Hope National Medical Center.* Irvine, California, November 23, 1996.

Ferrell, B.A., Ferrell, B.R., and Osterwell, D. Pain in the Nursing Home. *American Journal of Nursing* 95(7):43–45, 1990.

Ferrell, B.R., Cronin Nash, C., and Warfield, C. The Role of Patient-Controlled Analgesia in the Management of Cancer Pain. *Oncology Nursing Forum* 18(8):1315–1321, 1992.

Ferrell, B.R., and Griffith, H. Cost Issues Related to Pain Managment. *Journal of Pain and Symptom Management* 9(4):221–234, 1994.

Field, D., and Howells, K. Medical Students' Self-Reported Worries about Aspects of Death and Dying. *Death Studies* 10:147–154, 1985.

Firshein, J. Oregon Rationing Experiment Faces Hard Times. *Lancet* 347(9008):1110, 1996.

Fleischman, A.R., Nolan, K., Dubler, N.N., et al. Caring for Gravely Ill Children. *Pediatrics* 94:433–439, 1994.

Fleischman, A.R. *Statement Before the IOM Committee on Care at the End of Life on Behalf of the American Academy of Pediatrics.* Washington, D.C., April 29, 1996.

Flexner, A. *Medical Education in the United States and Canada: A Report to the Carnegie Foundation for the Advancement of Teaching.* Boston: D.B. Updike, Merrymount Press, 1910.

Foley, K.M. The Treatment of Cancer Pain. *New England Journal of Medicine* 313(2):84–95, 1985.

Foley, K.M. Pain Assessment and Cancer Pain Syndromes. Pp. 148–165 in *Oxford Textbook of Palliative Medicine,* D. Doyle, G.W.C. Hanks, and N. MacDonald, eds. Oxford: Oxford University Press, 1993.

Foley, K.M. Epidemiology of Death: The How, Why, Where and Symptoms of Dying. In *Summary of Committee Views and Workshop Examining the Feasibility of an Institute of Medicine Study of Dying, Decisionmaking, and Appropriate Care.* IOM Committee for a Feasibility Study on Care at the End of Life, M.J. Field, ed. Washington, D.C.: Institute of Medicine, 1994.

Foley, K.M. Pain Relief into Practice: Rhetoric Without Reform. *Journal of Clinical Oncology* 13:2149–2151, 1995.

Foreman, J. 70% would pick hospice, poll finds. *Boston Globe,* October 4, 1996.

Fowler, F.J. The Proceedings of the Conference on Measuring the Effects of Medical Treatment. *Medical Care* 33(4 Suppl.), 1995.

Fowler, F.J., Cleary, P.D., Patrick, D.., and Benjamin, K.L. Methodological Issues in Measuring Patient-Reported Outcomes: The Agenda of the Working Group on Outcomes Assessment. *Medical Care* 32:JS65–JS76, 1994.

Fox, D.M., and Leichter, H.M. Rationing Care in Oregon: The New Accountability. *Health Affairs* 10(2):7–27, 1991.

Fox, D.M., and Leichter, H.M. State Model: Oregon: The Ups and Downs of Oregon's Rationing Plan. *Health Affairs* 12(2):66–70, 1993.

Fox, R.C. The Medicalization and Demedicalization of American Society. Pp. 9–22 in *Doing Better and Feeling Worse: Health in the United States.* New York: W.W. Norton & Company, 1977.

Freud, S. *Collected Papers, Vol. I,* J. Riviere, trans. New York: Basic Books, 1959.

Fries, J.F., Koop, C.E., Beadle, C.E., et al. Reducing Health Care Costs by Reducing the Need and Demand for Medical Services. *New England Journal of Medicine* 329:321–325, 1993.

Frommelt, K.H. The Effects of Death Education on Nurses' Attitudes Toward Caring for Terminally Ill Persons and Their Families. *American Journal of Hospice and Palliative Care* 8(5):37–43, 1991.

Fuchs, V.R. *Who Shall Live? Health, Economics, and Social Choice.* New York: Basic Books, 1974.

Gallup, G., and Newport, F. Mirror of America: Fear of Dying. *Gallup Poll Monthly* 304:51–59, 1991.

Ganzini, L., and Lee, M.A. Psychiatry and Assisted Suicide in the United States. *New England Journal of Medicine* 336:1824–1826, 1997.

GAO (U.S. Congress General Accounting Office). *Board and Care Homes: Elderly at Risk From Mishandled Medications.* HRD-92-45. Washington, D.C.: GAO, 1992.

GAO. *Medicare: Reducing Fraud and Abuse Can Save Billions.* HEHS-95-157. Washington, D.C.: GAO, 1995a.

GAO. *Patient Self-Determination Act: Providers Offer Information on Advance Directives but Effectiveness Uncertain.* HEHS-95-135. Washington, D.C.: GAO, 1995b.

Garrett, J.M., Harris, R.P., Norburn, J.K., et al. Life-Sustaining Treatments during Terminal Illness. *Journal of General Internal Medicine* 8:361–368, 1993.

Garrison, R.S. Traditional Patient Care Model Response. *Journal of Dental Education* 57(5):343–345, 1993.

Gavrin, J., and Chapman, C.R. Clinical Management of Dying Patients. *Western Journal of Medicine* 163(3):268–277, 1995.

Gerteis, M., Edgman-Levitan, S., Daley, J., and Delbanco, T.L., eds. *Through the Patient's Eyes: Understanding and Promoting Patient-Centered Care.* San Francisco, 1993.

Gibelman, M. *Who We Are: A Second Look.* Washington, D.C.: National Association of Social Workers Press, 1997.

Gibson, M. Explicit Rationing/The Oregon Proposal. *EBRI Issue Brief* 136:57–59, April 1993.

Gill, T.M., and Feinstein, A.R. A Critical Appraisal of the Quality of Quality-of-Life Measurements. *Journal of the American Medical Association* 272(8):619–629, 1994.

Gilligan, M.A., and Jensen, N. Use of Advance Directives: A Survey in Three Clinics. *Wisconsin Medical Journal* 94(5):239–243, 1995.

Glaser, B.G., and Strauss, A.L. *Awareness of Dying.* Chicago: Aldine Publishing, 1965.

Glaser, B.G., and Strauss, A.L. *Time for Dying.* Chicago: Aldine Publishing, 1968.

Goisis, A., Gorini, M., Ratti, R., and Luliri, P. Application of a WHO Protocol on Medical Therapy for Oncologic Pain in an Internal Medicine Hospital. *Tumori* 5(1):470–472, 1989.

Gold, M., and Wooldridge, J. Surveying Consumer Satisfaction to Assess Managed Care Quality: Current Practices. *Health Care Financing Review* 16(4):155–173, 1995.

Gold, M., Franks, P., and Erickson, P. Assessing the Health of the Nation: The Predictive Validity of a Preference-Based Measure and Self-Rated Health. *Medical Care* 34(2):163–177, 1996.

Gomez, C.F. Hospice and Home Care: Opportunities for Training. In *Care for the Dying: Identification and Promotion of Physician Competency: Educational Resource Document.* Philadelphia: ABIM, 1996.

Gornick, M., McMillan, A., and Lubitz, J. A Longitudinal Perspective on Patterns of Medicare Payments. *Health Affairs* 12(2):140–150, 1993.

Gornick, M.E., Warren, J.L., Eggers, P.W., et al. Thirty Years of Medicare: Impact on the Covered Population. *Health Care Financing Review* 18:179–237, 1996.

Grannemann, T.W. Priority Setting: A Sensible Approach to Medicaid Policy? *Inquiry* 28:300–305, 1991.

Greenfield, S., Kaplan, S.H., and Ware, J.E., Jr. Expanding Patient Involvement in Care: Effects on Patient Outcome. *Annals of Internal Medicine* 102:520–528, 1985.

Groenewoud, J.H., Van der Mass, P.J., Van der Wal, G., et al., Physician-Assisted Death in Psychiatric Practice in the Netherlands. *New England Journal of Medicine* 336:1795–1801, 1997.

Grond, S., Zech, D., Schug, S.A., et al. Validation of World Health Organization Guidelines for Cancer Pain Relief During the Last Days and Hours of Life. *Journal of Pain and Symptom Management* 6:411–422, 1991.

Grond, S., Zech, D., Lynch, J., et al. Validation of World Health Organization Guidelines for Pain Relief in Head and Neck Cancer: A Prospective Study. *Annals of Otology, Rhinology, and Laryngology* 102:342–348, 1993.

Grossman, S.A., Sheidler, V.R., Sedeen, K., et al. Correlation of Patient and Caregiver Ratings of Cancer Pain. *Journal of Pain and Symptom Management* 6(2):53–57, 1991.

Gruenberg, L., Kaganova, E., and Hornbrook, M.C. Improving the AAPCC with Health-Status Measures from the MCBS. *Health Care Financing Review* 17(3):59–76, 1996.

Grumet, G.W. Health Care Rationing through Inconvenience: The Third Party's Secret Weapon. *New England Journal of Medicine* 321(9):607–611, 1989.

Grunfeld, C., and Feingold, K.R. Regulation of Lipid Metabolism by Cytokines during Host Defense. *Nutrition* 12(1):S24–S26, 1996.

Guralnick, J.M., LaCroix, A.Z., Branch, L.G., et al. Morbidity and Disability in Older Persons in the Years Prior to Death. *American Journal of Public Health* 81:443–447, 1991.

Hadley, J. *More Medical Care, Better Health?* Washington, D.C.: The Urban Institute Press, 1982.

Hadley, J., Steinberg, E.P., and Feder, J. Comparison of Uninsured and Privately Insured Hospital Patients: Condition on Admission, Resource Use, and Outcome. *Journal of the American Medical Association* 265:274–279, 1991.

Hadorn, D.C. The Problem of Discrimination in Health Care Priority Setting. *Journal of the American Medical Association* 268(11):1454–1459, 1992.

Hadorn, D.C., and Brook, R.H. The Health Care Resource Allocation Debate: Defining Our Terms. *Journal of the American Medical Association* 266(23):3328–3331, 1991.

Hafferty, F. *Into the Valley: Death and the Socialization of Medical Students.* New Haven and London: Yale University Press, 1991.

Hafner-Eaton, C. Physician Utilization Disparities Between the Uninsured and Insured. *Journal of the American Medical Association* 269(6):787–792, 1993.

Hahn, R.A. *Sickness and Healing: An Anthropological Perspective.* New Haven and London: Yale University Press, 1995.

Hakim, R.B., Teno, J.M., Harrell, F.E., Jr., et al. Factors Associated with Do-Not-Resuscitate Orders: Patients' Preferences, Prognoses, and Physicians' Judgments. *Annals of Internal Medicine* 125(4):284–293, 1996.

Halevy, A., and Brody, B. Brain Death: Reconciling Definitions, Criteria, and Tests. *Annals of Internal Medicine* 119(6):519–525, 1993.

Halevy, A., and Brody, B. A Multi-Institution Collaborative Policy on Medical Futility. *Journal of the American Medical Association* 276(7):571–574, 1996.

Hall, M.A. The Problems with Rule-Based Rationing. *Journal of Medicine and Philosophy* 19(4):315–332, 1994.

Hamel, M.B., Goldman, L., Teno, J., et al. Identification of Comatose Patients at High Risk for Death or Severe Disability. *Journal of the American Medical Association* 273(23):1842–1848, 1995.

Hamel, M.B., Phillips, R.S., et al. Seriously Ill Hospitalized Adults: Do We Spend Less on Older Patients? *Journal of the American Geriatric Society* 44:1043–1048, 1996.

Hammes, B., and Rooney, B. A Community-Wide Project for Advance Directives. Presented at End of Life Health Care in Managed Care Systems Conference. Center for Biomedical Ethics, University of Minnesota, Minneapolis, November 1–2, 1996.

Hansson, L.F., Norheim, O.F., and Ruyter, K.W. Equality, Explicitness, Severity, and Rigidity: The Oregon Plan Evaluated from a Scandinavian Perspective. *Journal of Medicine and Philosophy* 19(4):343–366, 1994.

Harrington, C., and Newcomer, R. Social Health Maintenance Organizations' Service Use and Costs, 1985–89. *Health Care Financing Review* 12(3):37–52, 1991.

Harvard School of Public Health/Boston Globe Poll. *National Attitudes Toward Death and Terminal Illness.* Needham, Massachusetts: KRC Communication Research, October 1991.

Havighurst, C. Prospective Self-Denial: Can Consumers Contract Today to Accept Health Care Rationing Tomorrow? *University of Pennsylvania Law Review* 140(5):1755–1808, 1992.

Havighurst, C. *Health Care Choices: Private Contracts as Instruments of Health Reform.* Washington, D.C.: A.E.I. Press, 1995.

Hawthorne, M.H., and Hixon, M.E. Functional Status, Mood Disturbance and Quality of Life in Patients with Heart Failure. *Progress in Cardiovascular Nursing* 9(1):22–32, 1994.

Hay, M.W. Principle in Building Spiritual Assessment Tools. *American Journal of Hospice Care* 6:25–31, 1989.

Hayllar, J., and Bjarnason, I. NSAIDs, Cox-2 Inhibitors, and the Gut. *The Lancet* 346:512–522, 1995.

HCFA (U.S. DHHS Health Care Financing Administration). *Medicare: A Profile.* Washington, D.C., February 1995.

HCFA. *The Medicare Hospice Manual.* Washington, D.C., 1996a.

HCFA. Trends in Medicare Home Health Agency Utilization and Payment: CYs 1974–94. *Health Care Financing Review* 1996 (Statistical Suppl.):76–77, 1996b.

Henderson, V. *Basic Principles of Nursing Care.* London: International Council of Nurses, 1961.

Hendrickson, W.D., Payer, A.F., Rogers, L.P., and Markus, J.F. The Medical School Curriculum Committee Revisited. *Academic Medicine* 68(3):183–189, 1993.

Hennezel, M. *Intimate Death: How the Dying Teach Us How to Live.* Translated by C.B. Janeway. New York: Alfred A. Knopf, 1997.

Higginson, I. Audit Methods: A Community Schedule. In *Clinical Audit in Palliative Care,* I. Higginson, ed. New York: Radcliffe Medical Press, 1993.

Higginson, I., Priest, P., and McCarthy, M. Are Bereaved Family Members a Valid Proxy for a Patient's Assessment of Dying? *Social Science Medicine* 38(4):553–554, 1994.

Hill, C.S. The Negative Influence of Licensing and Disciplinary Boards and Drug Enforcement Agencies on Pain Treatment with Opioid Analgesics. *Journal of Pharmaceutical Care in Pain & Symptom Control* 1:43–62, 1993.

Hill, T.P. Treating the Dying Patient: The Challenge for Medical Education. *Archives of Internal Medicine* 155:1265–1269, 1995.

Hill, T.P., and Shirley, D. *A Good Death: Taking More Control at the End of Your Life.* Reading, Massachusetts: Addison-Wesley, 1992.

Hing, E., and Bloom, B. Long-Term Care for the Functionally Dependent Elderly. *Advance Data,* No. 104. Hyattsville, Maryland: National Center for Health Statistics, 1990.

Hobbs, F.B., and Damon, B.L. Sixty-Five Plus in the U.S. In *Current Population Reports, Series P234-190.* Washington, D.C.:U.S. Census Bureau, April 1996.

Hodes, R.L. Cancer Patients' Needs and Concerns When Using Narcotic Analgesics. Pp. 91–99 in *Drug Treatment of Cancer Pain in a Drug-Oriented Society,* Vol. 11: *Advances in Pain Research and Therapy,* C.S. Hill, Jr. and W.S. Field, eds. New York: Raven Press, 1989.

Holland, J.C. and Rowland, J.H., eds. *Handbook of Psycho-oncology: Psychological Care of the Patient with Cancer.* New York: Oxford University Press, 1990.

Holst, D. Minnesota Hospice Association: Increasing Access to Hospice. Presented at End of Life Health Care in Managed Care Systems Conference. Center for Biomedical Ethics, University of Minnesota, Minneapolis, November 1–2, 1996.

Holstein, M., and Cole, T.R. Long-Term Care: A Historical Reflection. Pp. 15–34 in *Long-Term Care Decisions: Ethical and Conceptual Dimensions,* L.B. McCullough and N.L. Wilson, eds. Baltimore: Johns Hopkins University Press, 1995.

Hopkins, S.P., and Carroll, R.J. Severity Adjustment Models for CPI. Pp.91–102 in *Clinical Practice Improvement: A New Technology for Developing Cost-Effective Quality Health Care,* Vol. 1, S.D. Horn and D. Hopkins, eds. Washington, D.C.: Faulkner & Gray's Healthcare Information Center, 1994.

Horgan, J. Seeking a Better Way to Die. *Scientific American* 276(5):100–105, May 1997.

Horn, S.D., and Hopkins, D., eds. *Clinical Practice Improvement: A New Technology for Developing Cost-Effective Quality Health Care.* Washington, D.C.: Faulkner & Gray's Healthcare Information Center, 1994.

Hortobagyi, G.N., Theriault, R.L., Porter, L., et al. Efficacy of Pamidronate in Reducing Skeletal Complications in Patients with Breast Cancer and Lytic Bone Metastases. *New England Journal of Medicine* 335(24):1785–1791, 1996.

Hospice News Service. Capitated Payment Looms for Hospice Industry. *Hospice News Service,* Vol. 7 (No. 3) January 1996 [WWW document]. URL www.rbvdnr.com/health/hospice/cap.htm (accessed November, 1996).

Howell, D.A. Special Services for Children. In *Oxford Textbook of Palliative Medicine,* pp. 718–725. D. Doyle, G.W.C. Hanks, and N. MacDonald, eds. Oxford: Oxford University Press, 1993.

Howell, J.D. Lowell T. Coggeshall and American Medical Education: 1901–1987. *Academic Medicine* 67(11):711–718, 1992.

Howell, J.D. *Technology in the Hospital: Transforming Patient Care in the Early Twentieth Century.* Baltimore: Johns Hopkins University Press, 1995.

Howells, K., and Field, D. Fear of Death and Dying Among Medical Students. *Social Science and Medicine* 16:1421–1424, 1982.

Hoy, T. Hospice Chaplaincy in the Caregiving Team. Pp. 177–196 in *Hospice Care: Principles and Practice,* C.A. Corr and D.M. Corr, eds. London: Faber and Faber, 1983.

Hoyer, T. A History of the Medicare Hospice Benefit. In A Good Dying: Shaping Health Care for the Last Months of Life. Briefing book for symposium sponsored by The George Washington University Center to Improve Care of the Dying and the Corcoran Gallery of Art, April 30, 1996.

Hull, R., Ellis, M., and Sargent, V. *Teamwork in Palliative Care.* Oxford: Radcliffe Medical Press, 1989.

Humphrey, D. *Final Exit: The Practicalities of Self-Deliverance and Assisted Suicide for the Dying.* Eugene, Oregon: Hemlock Society, 1991.

Hunt, S.P., Pini, A., and Evan, G. Induction of C-Fos-Like Protein in Spinal Cord Neurons Following Sensory Stimulation. *Nature* 328:632–634, 1987.

Hunter, K.M. Narratives of Dying. In *Summary of Committee Views and Workshop Examining the Feasibility of an Institute of Medicine Study of Dying, Decisionmaking, and Appropriate Care.* IOM Committee for a Feasibility Study on Care at the End of Life, M.J. Field, ed. Washington, D.C.: Institute of Medicine, 1994.

Hunter, K.M., Charon, R., and Coulehan, J.L. The Study of Literature in Medical Education. *Academic Medicine* 70:787–794, 1995.

Hurney, C. Psyche and Cancer: Odyssey of an Old Idea in the Troubled Waters of Modern Science. *Annals of Oncology* 1:6–8, 1990.

Hyman, S.E., and Nestler, E.J. *The Molecular Foundations of Psychiatry.* Washington, D.C.: American Psychiatric Press, 1993.

Iezzoni, L.I. Risk Adjustment for Medical Outcomes Studies. Pp. 83–97 in *Health Care Quality Management for the 21st Century,* M.L. Grady, ed. Rockville, Maryland: Agency for Health Care Policy and Research (ACHPR Pub. No. 92-0056), 1992.

IHI (Institute for Health Care Improvement). Improving Care at the End of Life (brochure). Boston, 1997.

Illich, I. *Medical Nemesis: The Expropriation of Health.* New York: Pantheon, 1976.

Ingham, J. Physical Symptoms. Paper prepared for Conference on Measuring Care at the End of Life, August 27–28, 1996.

Ingham, J., and Portenoy, R. Symptom Assessment. *Hematology/Oncology Clinics of North America* 10:21–39, 1996.

International Association for the Study of Pain, Subcommittee on Taxonomy. Part II: Pain Terms: A Current List with Definitions and Notes on Usage. *Pain* 6:249–252, 1979.

IOM (Institute of Medicine). *Nursing and Nursing Education: Public Policies and Private Actions.* Washington, D.C.: Committee on Nursing and Nursing Education, 1983.

IOM. *Bereavement: Reactions, Consequences, and Care,* M. Osterweiss, F. Solomon, and M. Green, eds. Washington, D.C.: National Academy Press, 1984.

IOM. *Improving the Quality of Care in Nursing Homes.* Washington, D.C.: National Academy Press, 1986.

IOM. *Controlling Costs and Changing Patient Care?: The Role of Utilization Management.* B.H. Gray and M.J. Field, eds. Washington,, D.C.: National Academy Press, 1989.

IOM. *Medicare: A Strategy for Quality Assurance,* K. N. Lohr, ed. Washington, D.C.: National Academy Press, 1990.

IOM. *Mapping the Brain and Its Functions.* C.B. Pechura and J.B. Martin, eds. Washington, D.C.: National Academy Press, 1991.

IOM. *Guidelines for Clinical Practice: From Development to Use,* M.J. Field and K.N. Lohr, eds. Washington, D.C.: National Academy Press, 1992.

IOM. *Access to Health Care in America,* M. Millman, ed. Washington, D.C.: National Academy Press, 1993a.

IOM. *Employment and Health Benefits: A Connection at Risk,* M.J. Field and H.T. Shapiro, eds. Washington, D.C.: National Academy Press, 1993b.

IOM. *Summary of Committee Views and Workshop Examining the Feasibility of an Institute of Medicine Study of Dying, Decisionmaking, and Appropriate Care.* IOM Committee for a Feasibility Study on Care at the End of Life, M.J. Field, ed. Washington, D.C.: Institute of Medicine, 1994a.

IOM. *Real People, Real Problems: An Evaluation of the Long-Term Care Ombudsman Programs of the Older Americans Act,* J. Harris-Wehling, J.C. Feasley, and C.L. Estes, eds. Washington, D.C.: National Academy Press, 1994b.

IOM. *Federal Regulation of Methadone Treatment,* R.A. Rettig and A. Yarmolinsky, eds. Washington, D.C.: National Academy Press, 1995a.

IOM. *Dental Education at the Crossroads: Challenges and Change,* M.J. Field, ed. Washington, D.C.: National Academy Press, 1995b.

IOM. *Setting Priorities in Clinical Practice Guidelines,* M.J. Field, ed. Washington, D.C.: National Academy Press, 1995c.

IOM. *Best at Home: Assuring Quality Long-Term Care in Home and Community-Based Settings,* J.C. Feasley, ed. Washington, D.C.: National Academy Press, 1996a.

IOM. *Improving the Medicare Market: Adding Choices and Protections,* S.B. Jones and M.E. Lewin, eds. Washington, D.C.: National Academy Press, 1996b.

IOM. *Nursing Staff in Hospitals and Nursing Homes: Is It Adequate?,* G.S. Wunderlich, F.A. Sloan, and C.K. Davis, eds. Washington, D.C.: National Academy Press, 1996c.

IOM. *Pathways of Addiction: Opportunities in Drug Abuse Research.* Committee on Opportunities in Drug Abuse Research. Washington, D.C.: National Academy Press, 1996d.

IOM. *Telemedicine: A Guide to Assessing Telecommunications in Health Care,* M.J. Field, ed. Washington, D.C.: National Academy Press, 1996e.

IOM. *Managing Managed Care: Quality Improvement in Behavioral Health,* M. Edmunds, R. Frank, M. Hogan, et al., eds. Washington, D.C.: National Academy Press, 1997.

Jackson, V.P. Breast Cancer. Pp. 53–60 in IOM, *Effectiveness and Outcomes in Health Care,* K.A. Heithoff and K.N. Lohr, eds. Washington, D.C.: National Academy Press, 1990.

Jadad, A.R., and Browman, G.P. The WHO Analgesic Ladder for Cancer Pain Management: Stepping Up the Quality of Its Evaluation. *Journal of the American Medical Association* 274(23):1870–1873, 1995.

Jaffe, J.H. Drug Addiction and Drug Abuse. In *The Pharmacological Basis of Thereapeutics,* 7th Edition, A.G. Gilman, L.S. Goodman, T.W. Rall, and F. Murad, eds., pp. 532–581. New York: Macmillan Publishers, 1985.

Jaskowiak, N.T., and Alexander, H.R. The Pathophysiology of Cancer Cachexia. In *The Oxford Textbook of Palliative Care,* D. Doyle, G.W. Hanks, N. MacDonald, eds. New York: Oxford University Press, 1997.

JCAHO (Joint Commission on Accreditation of Healthcare Organizations). *Complete Accreditation Manual for Long Term Care.* Oakbrook Terrace, Illinois: JCAHO, 1996a.

JCAHO. *1997 Hospital Accreditation Standards.* Oakbrook Terrace, Illinois: JCAHO, 1996b.

Jecker, N.S. Knowing when to Stop. *Hastings Center Report,* 21:5–8, 1991.

Jecker, N.S., and Emanuel, L. Are Acting and Omitting Morally Equivalent? *Journal of the American Geriatric Society,* 43(6):696–701, 1995.

Jecker, N.S., and Pearlman, R.A. Ethical Constraints on Rationing Medical Care by Age. *Journal of the American Geriatric Society* 37(11):1067–1075, 1989.

Jecker, N.S., and Schneiderman, L.J. Futility and Rationing. *American Journal of Medicine.* 92:189–196, 1992.

Jecker, N.S., and Schneiderman, L.J. Is Dying Young Worse than Dying Old? *Gerontologist* 34(1):66–72, 1994.

Jennings, B. Ethical Challenges of Hospice. In A Good Dying: Shaping Health Care for the Last Months of Life. Briefing book for symposium sponsored by The George Washington University Center to Improve Care of the Dying and the Corcoran Gallery of Art, April 30, 1996.

Johnson, J.R., and Temple, R. Food and Drug Administration Requirements for Approval of New Anticancer Drugs. *Cancer Treatment Report* 69:1155–1159, 1985.

Joint International Research Group of the Institute for Bioethics (Netherlands) and the Hastings Center (United States). What Do We Owe the Elderly: Allocating Social and Health Care Resources. *Hastings Center Report* 24 (Suppl.):S1–S12, 1994.

Jones, S. Paradigm Shifts in Medicare Reform. Research Agenda Brief prepared for The George Washington University Health Insurance Reform Project. Washington, D.C.: January 1996a.

Jones, S. Why Not the Best for the Chronically Ill? Research Agenda Brief prepared for The George Washington University Health Insurance Reform Project. Washington, D.C.: January 1996b.

Jonsen, A.R., and Toulmin, S. *The Abuse of Casuistry: A History of Moral Reasoning.* Berkeley, California: University of California Press, 1988.

Joos, S., Reuler, J.B., Powell, J.L, and Hickam, D.H. Outpatients' Attitudes and Understanding Regarding Living Wills. *Journal of General Internal Medicine* 8(5):259–263, 1993.

Joranson, D.E. Are Health-Care Reimbursement Policies a Barrier to Acute and Cancer Pain Management? *Journal of Pain and Symptom Management* 9(4):244–253, 1994.

Joranson, D.E. Intractable Pain Treatment Laws and Regulations. *American Pain Society Bulletin* 5(2):1–3, 15–17, 1995a.

Joranson, D.E. State Medical Board Guidelines for Treatment of Intractable Pain. *American Pain Society Bulletin* 5(3):1–5, 1995b.

Joranson, D.E. State Intractable Pain Policy: Current Status. *American Pain Society Bulletin,* 1997.

Joranson, D.E., and Colleau, S.M. Highlights of the INCB Report. *Cancer Pain Release* 9 (Suppl.), Summer 1996.

Joranson, D.E., and Gilson, A.M. Controlled Substances, Medical Practice, and the Law. In *Psychiatric Practice Under Fire: The Influence of Government, the Media, and Special Interests on Somatic Therapies,* H.I. Schwartz, ed. Washington, D.C.: American Psychiatric Press, 1994a.

Joranson, D.E., and Gilson, A.M. Policy Issues and Imperatives in the Use of Opioids to Treat Pain in Substance Abusers. *Journal of Law, Medicine, & Ethics* 22(3):5–13, 1994b.

Joranson, D.E., Cleeland, C.S., Weissman, D.E., and Gilson, A.M. Opioides for Chronic Cancer and Non-Cancer Pain: A Survey of State Medical Board Members. *Federation Bulletin* 79(4):15–49, 1992.

Kaczorowski, J.M. Spiritual Well-Being and Anxiety in Adults Diagnosed with Cancer. *Hospice Journal* 5:105–116, 1989.

Kahn, K.L., Keeler, E.B., Sherwood, M.J., et al. Comparing Outcomes of Care Before and After Implementation of the DRG-Based Prospective Payment System. *Journal of the American Medical Association* 264(15):1984–1988, 1990.

Kandel, E.R., Schwartz, J.H., and Jessell, T.M. *Principles of Neural Science,* Third Edition. New York: Elsevier, 1991.

Kane, R.A., and Caplan, A.L., eds. *Everyday Ethics: Resolving Dilemmas in Nursing Home Life.* New York: Springer Publishing, 1990.

Kane, R.A., Illston, L.H., Eustis, N.N., and Kane, R.L. *Quality of Home Care: Concept and Measurement.* Minneapolis: University of Minnesota, 1991.

Kane, R.A., and Kane, R.L. *Long-Term Care: Principles, Programs, and Policies.* New York: Springer Publishing, 1987.

Kane, R.A., Kane, R.L., Illston, L.H., and Eustis, N.N. Perspectives on Home Care Quality. *Health Care Financing Review* 16(1):69–89, 1994.

Kane, R.L., Bernstein, L., et al. A Randomized Controlled Trial of Hospice Care. *Lancet* 1:890–894, 1984.

Kaplan, R.M. Value Judgment in the Oregon Medicaid Experiment. *Medical Care* 32(10):975–988, 1994.

Kapp, M.B. Enforcing Patient Preferences: Linking Payment for Medical Care to Informed Consent. *Journal of the American Medical Association* 261(13):1935–1938, 1989.

Karmali, R.A. Historical Perspective and Potential Use of N-3 Fatty Acids in Therapy of Cancer Cachexia. *Nutrition* 12:S2–S4, 1996.

Kass, N.E., Sugarman, J., Faden, R., and Schoch-Spana, M. Trust: The Fragile Foundation of Contemporary Biomedical Research. *Hastings Center Report* 26(5):25–29, 1996.

Kassirer, J.P. Our Stubborn Quest of Diagnostic Certainty. *New England Journal of Medicine* 320:1489–1491, 1989.

Kathol, R.G., Mutgi, A., Williams, J., et al. Diagnosis of Major Depression in Cancer Patients According to Four Sets of Criteria. *American Journal of Psychiatry* 147(8):1021–1024, 1990.

Katz, J. *The Silent World of Doctor and Patient.* New York: Free Press, 1984.

Keizer, B. *Dancing with Mister D: Notes on Life and Death.* New York: Doubleday, 1994.

Kemper, P., and Murtaugh, C.M. Lifetime Use of Nursing Home Care. *New England Journal of Medicine* 324:595–600, 1991.

Kerlinger, F.N. *Foundations of Behavioral Research,* 3d ed. New York: Holt, Rinehart, and Winston, Inc., 1986.

Kidder, D. The Effects of Hospice Coverage on Medicare Expenditures. *Health Services Research* 27:195–217, 1992.

Kimball, L.R., and McCormick, W.C. The Pharmacologic Management of Pain and Discomfort in Persons with AIDS Near the End of Life: Use of Opioid Analgesia in the Hospice Setting. *Journal of Pain and Symptom Management* 11(2):88–94, 1996.

Kingma, R. Revising Death Education. *Nurse Education* 19(5):15–16, 1994.

Klass, P. *A Not Entirely Benign Procedure: Four Years as a Medical Student.* New York: G.P. Putnam's, 1987.

Kleinman, A. Concepts and a Model for the Comparison of Medical Systems as Cultural Systems. *Social Science Medicine* 12: 85–95, 1978.

Kleinman, A., Eisenberg L., and Good, B. Culture, Illness and Care: Clinical Lessons from Anthropologic and Cross-Cultural Research. *Annals of Internal Medicine* 88: 251–258, 1978.

Kliegman, R.M. Bioethical Perspectives for Pediatric Patients. In *Summary of Committee Views and Workshop Examining the Feasibility of an Institute of Medicine Study of Dying, Decisionmaking, and Appropriate Care.* IOM Committee for a Feasibility Study on Care at the End of Life, M.J. Field, ed. Washington, D.C.: Institute of Medicine, 1994.

Knaus, W.A., Draper, E.A., Wagner, D.P., et al. An Evaluation of Outcome from Intensive Care in Major Medical Centers. *Annals of Internal Medicine* 104(3):410–418, 1986.

Knaus, W.A., Wagner, D.P., Draper, E.A., et al. The APACHE III Prognostic Risk System: Risk Prediction of Hospital Mortality for Critically Ill Hospitalized Adults. *Chest* 100:1619–1636, 1991.

Knaus, W.A., Harrell, F.E., Lynn, J., et al. The SUPPORT Prognostic Model: Objective Estimates of Survival for Seriously Ill Hospitalized Adults. *Annals of Internal Medicine* 122(3):191–203, 1995.

Knight, C., Knight, P., et al. Training Our Future Physicians: A Hospice Rotation for Medical Students. *American Journal of Hospice and Palliative Care* January/February:23–28, 1992.

Koenig, B.A. Cultural Diversity in Decisionmaking about Care at the End of Life. In *Summary of Committee Views and Workshop Examining the Feasibility of an Institute of Medicine Study of Dying, Decisionmaking, and Appropriate Care.* IOM Committee for a Feasibility Study on Care at the End of Life, M.J. Field, ed. Washington, D.C.: Institute of Medicine, 1994.

Koenig, B.A., and Gates-Williams, J. Understanding Cultural Difference in Caring for Dying Patients. *Western Journal of Medicine* 163(3):244–249, 1995.

Kosecoff, J., Kahn, K.L., Rogers, W.H., et al. Prospective Payment System and Impairment at Discharge. *Journal of the American Medical Association* 264(15):1980–1983, 1990.

Kübler-Ross, E. *On Death and Dying.* New York: MacMillian, 1969.

Kübler-Ross, E. *Death the Final Stage of Growth.* Englewood Cliffs, New Jersey: Prentice-Hall, 1975.

Kuilboer, M.M., and van der Lei, J. Exploring the Role of a Critiquing System: A Simulation. *Journal of the American Medical Association* accepted for publication.

Lacqueur, T.W. Working paper for *Project on Death in America.* 1995.

Lansky, D. The New Responsibility: Measuring and Reporting on Quality. *Joint Commission Journal on Quality Improvement* 19(12):545–551, 1993.

Lantos, J.D., and Miles, S.H. Autonomy in Adolescent Medicine: A Framework for Decisions About Life-Sustaining Treatment. *Journal of Adolescent Health Care* 10:460–466, 1989.

Larsson, G., and Starrin, B. Relaxation Training as an Integral Part of Caring Activities for Cancer Patients: Effects on Well-Being. *Scandinavian Journal of Caring Sciences* 6:179–185, 1992.

Laviano, A., Renvyle, T., and Yang, Z. From Laboratory to Bedside: New Strategies in the Treatment of Malnutrition in Cancer Patients. *Nutrition* 12:112–122, 1996.

Lebovits, A.H., Lefkowitz, M., McCarthy, D., et al. The Prevalence and Management of Pain in Patients with AIDS: A Review of 134 Cases. *Clinical Journal of Pain* 5(3):245–248, 1989.

Lee, M.A., and Ganzini, L. Depression in the Elderly: Effect on Patient Attitudes Toward Life-Sustaining Treatment. *Chest* 40:983–988, 1990.

Lee, M.A., and Tolle, S.W. Oregon's Assisted Suicide Vote: The Silver Lining (Letter). *Annals of Internal Medicine* 124(2):267–269, 1996.

Leedom, L., Meehan, W.P., Procci, W., and Zeidler, A. Symptoms of Depression in Patients with Type II Diabetes Mellitus. *Psychosomatics* 32(3):280–286, 1991.

Leibson, C.L., Ballard, D.J., Whisnant, J.P., and Melton, L.J., 3d. The Compression of Morbidity Hypothesis: Promise and Pitfalls of Using Record-Linked Data Bases to Assess Secular Trends in Morbidity and Mortality. *Milbank Memorial Fund Quarterly* 70(1):127–154, 1992.

Leigh, J.P., and Fries, J.F. Education, Gender, and the Compression of Morbidity. *International Journal on Aging and Human Development* 39(3):233–246, 1994.

LeRoith, D. Insulin-Like Growth Factors. *New England Journal of Medicine* 336(9):633–640, 1997.

Lester, D. The Collett-Lester Fear of Death Scale. Pp. 45–60 in *Death Anxiety Handbook: Research, Instrumentation, and Application,* R.A. Neimeyer, ed. Washington, D.C.: Taylor & Francis, 1994.

Levin, D.N., Cleeland, C.S., and Dar, R. Public Attitudes Toward Cancer Pain. *Cancer* 56(9):2337–2339, 1985.

Levinsky, N.G. The Purpose of Advance Medical Planning: Autonomy for Patients or Limitation of Care? *New England Journal of Medicine* 385:741–743, 1996.

Levit, K.R., Lazenby, H.C., Sivarajan, L., et al. DataView: National Health Expenditures, 1994. *Health Care Financing Review* 17(3):205–242, 1996.

Lipowski, Z.J. Delirium (Acute Confusional States). *Journal of the American Medical Association* 258:1789–1792, 1987.

Liston, E.H. Education on Death and Dying: A Survey of American Medical Schools. *Journal of Medical Education* 48:577–578, 1973.

Littlefield, C.H., Rodin, G.M., Murrary, M.A., and Craven, J.L. Influence of Functional Impairment and Social Support on Depressive Symptoms in Persons with Diabetes. *Health-Psychology* 9(6):737–749, 1990.

Lo, B. End of Life Care After Termination of SUPPORT. *Hastings Center Review* 25(6 Suppl.):S6–S8, 1995.

Lo, B., MacLeod, G.A., and Saika, G. Patient Attitudes to Discussing Life-Sustaining Treatment. *Archives of Internal Medicine* 146:1613–1615, 1986.

Lohr, K.N., ed. Advances in Health Status Assessment. *Medical Care* 30(5 Suppl.), 1992.

Lohr, K.N., Aaronson, N.K., Alonso, J., et al. Evaluating Quality-of-Life and Health Status Instruments: Development of Scientific Review Criteria. *Clinical Therapeutics* 18(5):979–992, 1996.

Lohr, K.N., Brook, R.H., Kamberg, C.J., et al. Use of Medical Care in the Rand Health Insurance Experiment. Diagnosis- and Service-Specific Analyses in a Randomized Controlled Trial. *Medical Care* 24(Sept. Suppl.):S1–S87, 1986.

Lomas, J. Words without Action: The Production, Dissemination, and Impact of Consensus Recommendations. *Annual Review of Public Health* 12:41–65, 1991.

Lomas, J., Enkin, M., Anderson, G.M., et al. Opinion Leaders vs Audit and Feedback to Implement Practice Guidelines: Delivery After Previous Cesarean Section. *Journal of the American Medical Association* 265:2202–2207, 1991.

Lonetto, R., Mercer, G.W., Fleming, S., et al. Death Anxiety Among University Students in Northern Ireland and Canada. *Journal of Psychology* 104:75–82, 1980.

Loprinzi, C.L., Ellison, N.M., Schaid, D.J., et al. Controlled Trial of Magestrol Acetate for the Treatment of Cancer Anorexia and Cachexia. *Journal of the National Cancer Institute* 82(13):1127–1132, 1990.

Loscalzo, M.J., and Zabora, J.R. Oncology Social Work and Palliative Care in the United States. Unpublished paper provided by M. Loscalzo, 1996.

Lubitz, J.D., and Prihoda, R. The Use and Costs of Medicare Services in the Last Two Years of Life. *Health Care Financing Review* 5:117–131, 1984.

Lubitz, J.D., and Riley, G.F. Trends in Medicare Payments in the Last Year of Life. *New England Journal of Medicine* 328:1092–1096, 1993.

Lubitz, J.D., Beebe, J., and Baker, C. Longevity and Medicare Expenditures. *New England Journal of Medicine* 332(15):999–1003, 1995.

Lundberg, G.D. National Health Care Reform: The Aura of Inevitability Intensifies. *Journal of the American Medical Association* 267:2521–2524, 1992.

Lurie, N., Ward, N.B., Shapiro, M.F., and Brook, R.H. Termination from Medi-Cal: Does It Affect Health? *New England Journal of Medicine* 311(7):480–484, 1984.

Lurie, N., Ward, N.B., Shapiro, M.R., et al. Termination from Medi-Cal: A Follow-Up Study One Year Later. *New England Journal of Medicine* 314(19):1266–1268, 1986.

Lynn, J. Why I Don't Have a Living Will. *Law, Medicine & Health Care* 19(1–2):101–104, 1991.

Lynn, J. Caring at the End of Our Lives. *New England Journal of Medicine* 335(3):201–202, 1996b.

Lynn, J., on behalf of the American Geriatrics Society Ethics Committee. Measuring Care at the End of Life: A Statement of Principles. *Journal of the American Geriatrics Society* 45:526–527, 1997.

Lynn, J., and Cranford, R. *The Persisting Perplexities in the Determination of Death.* Washington, D.C.: Center to Improve Care for the Dying, 1996.

Lynn, J., Harrell, F.E., Jr., Cohn, F., et al. Defining the "Terminally Ill": Insights from SUPPORT. *Duquesne Law Review* 35:311–336, 1996.

Lynn, J., Harrell, F.E., Jr., Cohn, F., et al. Prognoses of Seriously Ill Hospitalized Patients on the Days before Death: Implications for Patient Care and Public Policy. *New Horizons* 5(1):56–71, 1997.

Lynn, J., Teno, J.M., and Harrell, F.E., Jr. Accurate Prognostications of Death: Opportunities and Challenges for Clinicians. *Western Journal of Medicine* 163(3):250–257, 1995.

Lynn, J., Teno, J.M., Phillips, R.S., et al. Perceptions by Family Members of the Dying Experience of Older and Seriously Ill Patients. *Annals of Internal Medicine* 126(2):97–106, 1997.

MacDonald, N. Palliative Care: The Fourth Phase of Cancer Prevention. *Cancer Detection and Prevention* 15:253–255, 1991.

MacDonald, N. Priorities in Education and Research in Palliative Care. *Palliative Medicine* 7(Suppl. 1):65–76, 1993.

MacDonald, N. Educational Strategies for Improving Physician Care of Dying Patients. In *Summary of Committee Views and Workshop Examining the Feasibility of an Institute of Medicine Study of Dying, Decisionmaking, and Appropriate Care.* IOM Committee for a Feasibility Study on Care at the End of Life, M.J. Field, ed. Washington, D.C.: Institute of Medicine, 1994.

MacDonald, N. Suffering and Dying in Cancer Patients: Research Frontiers in Controlling Confusion, Cachexia, and Dyspnea. *Western Journal of Medicine* 163(3):278–286, 1995.

MacDonald, N. Palliative Care in Canada: Some Issues Relevant to Germany. Based on a presentation to the *Griedrich Ebert Stiftung*, Bonn, Germany, October 30, 1996.

MacDonald, N. Survey of Medical Student Exposure to Palliative Care in Canadian Medical Schools, 1996, submitted for publication.

MacLeod, R.D. and Nash, A. Teaching Palliative Care in a General Practice: A Survey of Educational Needs and Preferences. *Journal of Palliative Care* 7:4, 9–12, 1991.

Madan, T.N. Dying with Dignity. *Social Science and Medicine* 35(4):425–432, 1992.

Madara, J., Parkos, C. et al. CI-Secretion in a Model Intestinal Epithelium Induced by a Neutrophil-Derived Secretagogue. *Journal of Clinical Investigation* 89:6, 1938–1944, 1989.

Mahoney, J.J. *Statement Before the IOM Committee on Care at the End of Life on Behalf of the National Hospice Organization.* Washington, D.C., April 29, 1996.

Manning, W.G., Newhouse, J.P., Duan, N., et al. Health Insurance and the Demand for Medical Care: Evidence from a Randomized Experiment. *American Economic Review* 77:251–277, 1987.

Manton, K.G., Corder, L., and Stallard, E. Chronic Disability Trends in Elderly United States Populations: 1982–1994. *Proceedings of the National Academy of Sciences* 94(6):2593–2598, 1997. Retrieved at URL http://www.pnas.org/cgi/content/full/94/6/2593 (accessed 3/24/1997).

Manton, K.G., Stallard, E., and Woodbury, M.A. Home Health and Skilled Nursing Facility Use: 1982–90. *Health Care Financing Review* 16(1):155–186, 1994.

Marcus, W. *Statement Before the IOM Committee on Care at the End of Life.* Irvine, California, November 23, 1996.

Marks, R.M., and Sachar, E.J. Undertreatment of Medical Inpatients with Narcotic Analgesics. *Annals of Internal Medicine* 78(2):173–181, 1973.

Marston, R.Q., and Jones, R.M., eds. Medical Education in Transition. In *Report of the Commission on Medical Education: The Sciences of Medical Practice,* R.Q. Marston and R.M. Jones, eds. Princeton, New Jersey: Robert Wood Johnson Foundation, 1992.

Martinson, I.A. Home Care for Children Dying of Cancer. *Pediatrics* 62(1):108, 1978.

Max, M.B. Improving Outcomes of Analgesic Treatment: Is Education Enough? *Annals of Internal Medicine* 113(11):885–889, 1990.

Max, M.B. *Statement Before the IOM Committee on Care at the End of Life on Behalf of the American Pain Society.* Washington, D.C., April 29, 1996.

Max, M.B., Lynch, S.A., Muir, J., et al. Effects of Desirpamine, Amitriptyline, and Fluoxetine on Pain in Diabetic Neuropathy. *New England Journal of Medicine* 326:1250–1256, 1992.

Mazur, D.J., and Merz, J.F. Patients' Willingness to Accept Life-Sustaining Treatment when the Expected Outcome Is a Diminished Mental Health State: An Exploratory Study. *Journal of the American Geriatric Society* 44:565–568, 1996.

McClam, T. Death Anxiety Before and After Death Education: Negative Results. *Psychological Reports* 46:513–514, 1980.

McClish, D.K., and Powell, S.H. How Well Can Physicians Estimate Mortality in a Medical Intensive Care Unit? *Medical Decisionmaking* 9(2):125–132, 1989.

McCormick, T.R., and Conley, B.J. Patients' Perspectives on Dying and on the Care of Dying Patients. *Western Journal of Medicine* 163(3):236–243, 1995.

McCormick, W., Inui, T., Deyo, R., and Wood, R. Long Term Care Preferences of Hospitalized Patients with AIDS. *Journal of General Internal Medicine* 6:524–528, 1991.

McCue, J.D. The Naturalness of Dying. *Journal of the American Medical Association* 273(13):1039–1043, 1995.

McCullough, L. An Ethical Model for Improving the Patient-Physician Relationship. *Inquiry* 25:454–468, 1988.

McCullough, L.B., and Wilson, N.L., eds. *Long-Term Care Decisions: Ethical and Conceptual Dimensions.* Baltimore: Johns Hopkins University Press, 1995.

McDowell, I., and Newell, C. *Measuring Health: A Guide to Scales and Questionnaires,* 2d Edition. New York: Oxford University Press, 1996.

McMillan, A., et al. Trends and Patterns in Place of Death for Medicare Enrollees. *Health Care Financing Review* 12:1–7, 1990.

McMillan, S.C., and Mahon, M. Measuring Quality of Life in Hospice Patients Using a Newly Developed Hospice Quality of Life Index. *Quality of Life Research* 3:437–447, 1994.

McPherson, K. International Differences in Medical Care Practices. *Health Care Financing Review, 1989 Annual Supplement,* 9–20. 1989.

MDP (Missoula Demonstration Project). *The Quality of Life's End: Progress Report.* Missoula, Montana: November, 1996.

Mechanic, D. Cost Containment and the Quality of Medical Care: Rationing Strategies in an Era of Constrained Resources. *Milbank Memorial Fund Quarterly/Health and Society* 63(3):453–473, 1985.

Medica Foundation. *The 17-Minute Report: Selection Findings from a Statewide and National Survey.* Minneapolis, Minnesota, 1994.

Medica Foundation. *Project DECIDE (Discussion of Evolving Choices In Dying and Ethics): A Roundtable Report to the Community.* Minneapolis, Minnesota, 1996.

Medical Outcomes Trust. Instrument Review Criteria. *Medical Outcomes Trust Bulletin* 3(4):1–4, 1995.

Menzel, P.T. Oregon's Denial: Disabilities and the Quality of Life. *Hastings Center Report* 22(6):21–25, 1992.

Mermann, A.C., Gunn, D.B., and Dickinson, G.E. Learning to Care for the Dying: A Survey of Medical Schools and a Model Course. *Academic Medicine* 66(1):35–38, 1991.

Merriman, M. *Statement Before the IOM Committee on Care at the End of Life on Behalf of the American VITAS Healthcare Corporation of Florida.* Washington, D.C., April 29, 1996.

Meydani, S. N. Effect of (n-3) Polyunsaturated Fatty Acids on Cytokine Production and Their Biologic Function. *Nutrition* 12:S8–S14, 1996.

Meyer, R.A., Campbell, J.N., and Raja, S.N. Peripheral Neural Mechanisms of Nociception. In *Textbook of Pain,* P.D. Wall and R. Melzack, eds., pp. 13–44. Edinburgh: Livingston Churchill, 1994.

Miaskowski, C., Nichols, R., Brody, R., and Synold, T. Assessment of Patient Satisfaction Utilizing the American Pain Society's Quality Assurance Standards on Acute and Cancer-Related Pain. *Journal of Pain System Management* 9:5–11, 1994.

Mikami, M., Tatsumi, K., Kimura, H., et al. Respiration Effect of Synthetic Progestin in Small Doses in Normal Men. *Chest* 96:1073–1075, 1989.

Miles, S.H. Medical Futility. *Law, Medicine, and Health Care* 20(4):310–315, 1992.

Miles, S.H. *Statement Before the IOM Committee on Care at the End of Life on Behalf of the University of Minnesota Center for Biomedical Ethics.* Irvine, California, November 23, 1996.

Miles, S.H., Weber, E.P., and Koepp, R. End-of-Life Treatment in Managed Care: The Potential and the Peril. *Western Journal of Medicine* 163(3):302–305, 1995.

Minnesota Hospice Organization. *Hospice Care: A Physician's Guide.* St. Paul, Minnesota: Minnesota Hospice Organization, 1995.

Mitch, W.E., and Goldberg, A.L. Mechanisms of Muscle Wasting: The Role of the Ubiquitin-Proteasome Pathway. *Mechanisms of Disease* 335(25):1897–1905, 1996.

Moinpour, C.M., Feigl, P., Metch, B., et al. Quality of Life End Points in Cancer Clinical Trials: Review and Recommendations. *Journal of the National Cancer Institute* 81(7):485–495, 1989.

Moldawer, L.L., and Copeland, E.M. Proinflammatory Cytokines, Nutritional Support, and the Cachexia Syndrome: Interactions and Therapeutic Options. *Cancer* 79(9):1828–1839, 1997.

Moldow, G., and Carlsen, M. Development of a Resuscitation Discussion Guide: A Pocket Card for Health Care Professionals. Prepared for Medica Foundation, Project DECIDE. Minneapolis, Minnesota, 1996.

Moons, E.C., and Mackenbach, J.P. Trends in Mortality and Morbidity among the Elderly in The Netherlands, 1970–1989. *Nederlands Tijdschrift der Geneeskunde* 138(29):1466–1472, 1994.

Moore, M.J. Gemcitabine Demonstrates Promising Activity As a Single Agent in the Treatment of Metastatic Transitional Cell in Carcinoma. *Proceedings of the American Society of Clinical Oncology* 15:250, 1996.

Mor, V., and Masterson-Allen, S. *Hospice Care Systems: Structure, Process, Costs, and Outcome.* New York: Springer Publishing, 1987.

Mor, V. Available Data for Studying Dying in America. In *Summary of Committee Views and Workshop Examining the Feasibility of an Institute of Medicine Study of Dying, Decisionmaking, and Appropriate Care.* IOM Committee for a Feasibility Study on Care at the End of Life, M.J. Field, ed. Washington, D.C.: Institute of Medicine, 1994.

Mor, V., and Kidder, D. Cost Savings in Hospice: Final Results of the National Hospice Study. *Health Services Research* 20:407–422, 1985.

Morley, J.E., Kraenzle, D.M., Bible, B., and Bundren, B. Perception of Quality of Life by Nursing Home Residents. *Nursing Home Medicine* 3(8)191–194, 1995.

Morreim, E.H. Stratified Scarcity: Redefining the Standard of Care. *Law, Medicine & Health Care* 17(4):356–367, 1989.

Morrison, R.S. Death: Process or Event? *Science* 173:694–698, 1971.

Morrison, R.S., Morrison, E.W., and Glickman, D.F. Physician Reluctance to Discuss Advance Directives. *Archives of Internal Medicine* 154:2311–2318, 1994.

Morrison, R.S., Olson, E., Mertz, K.R., and Meier, D.E. The Inaccessibility of Advance Directives in Transfer from Ambulatory to Acute Settings. *Journal of the American Medical Assocation* 274:478–482, 1995.

Morrison, R.S., Meier, D.E., and Cassel, C.K. When too Much Is too Little. *New England Journal of Medicine* 335(23):1755–1759, 1996.

Moulin, D.E. Pain in Multiple Sclerosis. *Neurologic Clinics* 7:321–331, 1989.

Murinen, J.M. The Economics of Informal Care: Labor Market Effects in the National Hospice Study. *Medical Care* 24:1007–1017, 1986.

Murphy, D., Murray, A.M., Robinson, B.E., and Campion, E.W. Outcomes of Cardiopulmonary Resuscitation in the Elderly. *Annals of Internal Medicine* 111(3):199–205, 1989.

Murphy, D.J., and Barbour, E.G. GUIDe (Guidelines for the Use of Intensive Care in Denver): A Community Effort to Define Futile and Inappropriate Care. *New Horizons* 2:326–331, 1994.

Murphy, D.J., and Finucane, T.E. New Do-not-Resuscitate Policies: A First Step in Cost Control. *Archives of Internal Medicine* 153:1641–1648, 1993.

Murphy, P. *Statement Before the IOM Committee on Care at the End of Life on Behalf of Marin Home Care.* Irvine, California, November 23, 1996.

Mydan, S. Many Immigrants' Views on Death Are out of the U.S. Mainstream. *N.Y. Times News Service* [WWW document]. URL http://www.lantino.com/heal912.html (accessed 1995).

NAHC (National Association for Home Care). *Basic Statistics about Home Care, 1993.* Washington, D.C.: NAHC, 1993.

Nayfield, S.G., Hailey, B.J., and McCabe, M. *Quality of Life Assessment in Cancer Clinical Trials: Report of the Workshop on Quality of Life Research in Cancer Clinical Trials, July 16–17, 1990.* Bethesda, Maryland: U.S. DHHS, 1991.

NCHS (U.S. DHHS PHS National Center for Health Statistics). *Vital Statistics of the United States, 1980.* Vol. 11, *Mortality,* Part A. DHHS Pub. No. (PHS) 85-1101. Washington, D.C.: U.S. Government Printing Office, 1985.

NCHS. *Vital Statistics of the United States, 1990.* Vol. 11, *Mortality,* Part B. DHHS Pub. No. 94-1102. Washington, D.C.: U.S. Government Printing Office, 1994.

NCHS. *Monthly Vital Statistics Report* 45(3), September 30, 1996.

NCHS. *Advance Data.* No. 280, January 23, 1997.

NCI (U.S. DHHS NIH National Cancer Institute). *Facing Foward: A Guide for Cancer Survivors.* Washington, D.C.: National Institutes of Health, July 1990.

Neimeyer, R.A., and van Brunt, D. Death Anxiety. In *Dying: Facing the Facts,* H. Wass and R.A. Neimeyer, eds. Washington, D.C.: Taylor & Francis, 1995.

Nelson, H.L., and Nelson, J.L. *The Patient in the Family: An Ethics of Medicine and Families.* New York: Routledge, 1995.

Nelson, K.A., Park, K.M., Robinovitz, E., Tsigos, C., and Max, M.B. High-Dose Oral Dextromethorphan in Diabetic Neuropathy Pain and Post Herpetic Neuralgia: A Double-Blind, Placebo Controlled Study. *Neurology, 1996* (in press).

Nessim, S., and Ellis, J. *Cancervive: The Challenge of Life After Cancer.* Boston: Houghton Mifflin, 1991.

Nestler, E.J., Hope, B.T., and Widnell, K.L. Drug Addiction: A Model for the Molecular Basis of Neural Plasticity. *Neuron* 11:995–1006, 1993.

Newhouse, J.P. Patients at Risk: Health Reform and Risk Adjustment. *Health Affairs* 13(1):132–146, 1994.

Newhouse, J.P., and the Insurance Experiment Group. *Free For All?: Lessons from the Rand Health Insurance Experiment.* Cambridge, Massachusetts: Harvard University Press, 1993.

Newhouse, J.P., Manning, W.G., and Keeler, E.B. Adjusting Capitation Rates Using Objective Health Measures and Prior Utilization. *Health Care Financing Review* 10:41–53, 1989.

NHO (National Hospice Organization). *An Analysis of the Cost Savings of the Medicare Hospice Benefit.* NHO Item Code 712901. Miami, Florida: Lewin-VHI, 1995.

NHO. *Hospice Fact Sheet.* Arlington, Virginia: NHO, July 1, 1996a.

NHO. *Press Release: New Findings Address Escalating End-of-Life Debate.* Arlington, Virginia: NHO, October 3, 1996b.

Nightingale, F. *Notes on Nursing: What It Is and What It Is not.* London: Harrison and Sons, 1859.

NIDA (National Institute on Drug Abuse). *National Household Survey on Drug Abuse: Population Estimates 1990.* U.S. Department of Health and Human Services publication ADM 91-1732. Rockville, Maryland: NIDA, 1991.

NIH (National Institutes of Health). Biobehavioral and Pain Research. *NIH Guide* 24(15): 1–9, April 28, 1995.

Non-Small Cell Lung Cancer Collaborative Group. Chemotherapy in Non-Small Cell Lung Cancer: a Meta-Analysis Using Updated Data on Individual Patients from 52 Randomised Clinical Trials. *British Medical Journal* 311:899–909, 1995.

Notzon, F.C., Placek, P.J., and Taffel, S.M. Comparisons of National Cesarean Section Rates. *New England Journal of Medicine* 316:386–389, 1987.

NRC (National Research Council). *The New Americans: Economic, Demographic, and Fiscal Effects of Immigration.* Committee on Population and Committee on National Statistics. J.P. Smith and B. Edmondston, eds. Washington, D.C.: National Academy Press, 1997.

Nuland, S.B. *How We Die: Reflections on Life's Final Chapter.* New York: Alfred A. Knopf, 1994.

Osler, W. *Science and Immortality.* Cambridge: Riverside Press, 1905.

Pallis, C. *ABC of Brain Stem Death.* London: British Medical Journal Publishers, 1983.

Paris, J. Managed Care, Financial Incentives, and Cost Control: Shifts in the Ethical Focus of Health Care Delivery. Presented at End of Life Health Care in Managed Care Systems Conference. Center for Biomedical Ethics, University of Minnesota, Minneapolis, November 1–2, 1996.

Parkin, S. *Statement Before the IOM Committee on Care at the End of Life.* Washington, D.C., April 29, 1996.

Parsons, T. Death in American Society: A Brief Working Paper. *American Behavioral Scientist* May:61–65, 1963.

Paterson, A.H.G., McCloskey, E.V., Ashley, S., et al. Reduction of Skeletal Morbidity and Prevention of Bone Metastases with Oral Clodronate in Women with Recurrent Breast Cancer in the Absence of Skeletal Metastases. *Proceedings of ASCO* 15:104 (Abstract No. 81), 1996.

Patrick, D.L. Finding Health-Related Quality of Life Outcomes Sensitive to Health Care Organization and Delivery. *Medical Care* forthcoming.

Patrick, D.L., and Bergner, M. Measurement of Health Status in the 1990s. *Annual Review of Public Health* 11:165–183, 1990.

Patrick, D.L., and Erickson, P. *Health Status and Health Policy.* New York: Oxford University Press, 1993.

Pattison, E.M. *The Experience of Dying.* Englewood Cliffs, New Jersey: Prentice-Hall, 1977.

Payer, L. *Medicine & Culture: Varieties of Treatment in the United States, England, West Germany, and France.* New York: Henry Holt, 1988.

Pearlman, R.A., Cain, K.C., Patrick, D.L., et al. Insights Pertaining to Patient Assessments of States Worse Than Death. *Journal of Clinical Ethics* 4(1):33–41, 1993.

Pellegrino, E.D. Trust and Distrust in Professional Ethics. Pp. 69–85 in *Ethics, Trust, and the Professions,* E.D. Pellegrino, R.M. Veatch, and J.P. Langan, eds. Washington, D.C.: Georgetown University Press, 1991.

Pellegrino, E.D. The Metamorphosis of Medical Ethics: A 30-Year Retrospective. *Journal of the American Medical Association* 269(9):1158–1162, 1993.

Pellegrino, E.D., and Thomasma, D.C. *For the Patient's Good: The Restoration of Beneficence in Health Care.* New York: Oxford University Press, 1988.

Pepper Commission (U.S. Bipartisan Commission on Comprehensive Health Care). *A Call for Action.* Washington, D.C.: U.S. Government Printing Office, 1990.

Perrin, J.M., Shayne, M.W., and Bloom, S.R. *Home and Community Care for Chronically Ill Children.* New York: Oxford University Press, 1993.

Petersdorf, R.G. Medical Education: The Process, Students, Teachers and Patients. In *Flexner: 75 Years Later. A Current Commentary on Medical Education,* C. Vevier, ed. Lanham, Maryland: University Press of America, 1987.

Pew Health Professions Commission. *Health Professions Education for the Future: Schools in Service to the Nation.* San Francisco: Pew Health Professions Commission, 1993.

PHS (U.S. DHHS Public Health Service). *Health United States, 1995.* Hyattsville, Maryland: PHS Pub. No. 96–1232, 1996.

Plata-Salaman, C.R. Cytokines and Feeding Suppression: And Integrative View Fron Neurologic to Molecular Levels. *Nutrition* 11:674–677, 1995.

Pollack, M.M., Ruttimann, U.E., and Getson, P.R. Accurate Prediction of the Outcome of Pediatric Intensive Care. *New England Journal of Medicine* 316:34–39, 1987.

Pollack, M.M., Patel, K.M., and Ruttimann, U.E. Pediatric End-of-Life Decision Making and the Role for Objective Risk Assessment. In *Summary of Committee Views and Workshop Examining the Feasibility of an Institute of Medicine Study of Dying, Decisionmaking, and Appropriate Care.* IOM Committee for a Feasibility Study on Care at the End of Life, M.J. Field, ed. Washington, D.C.: Institute of Medicine, 1994.

Portenoy, R.K. Chronic Opioid Therapy in Nonmalignant Pain. *Journal of Pain and Symptom Management* 5(1):S46–S62, 1990.

Portenoy, R.K. Opioid Therapy for Chronic Nonmalignant Pain: A Review of the Critical Issues. *Journal of Pain and Symptom Management* 11(4):203–217, 1996.

Portenoy, R.K., and Kanner, R.M., eds. *Pain Management: Theory and Practice.* Philadelphia: F.A. Davis, 1996.

Portenoy, R.K., and Payne, R. Acute and Chronic Pain. Pp. 691–721 in *Substance Abuse: A Comprehensive Textbook,* J.H. Lowinson, P. Ruiz, and R.B. Millman, eds. Baltimore, Maryland: Williams & Wilkins, 1992.

Portenoy, R.K., Thaler, H.T., Kornblith, A.B., et al. Symptom Prevalence, Characteristics and Distress in a Cancer Population. *Quality of Life Research* 3:183–189, 1994.

Porter, J., and Jick, H. In Letter to the Editor. *New England Journal of Medicine* 302(2):123, 1980.

Post, S. Managed Care and End-Stage Dementia. Presented at End of Life Health Care in Managed Care Systems Conference. Center for Biomedical Ethics, University of Minnesota, Minneapolis, November 1–2, 1996.

PPRC (Physician Payment Review Commission). Annual Report to Congress. Washington, D.C., 1988, 1989, 1990, 1991, 1992, 1995, 1996.

President's Commission (President's Commission for the Study of Ethical Problems in Medicine and Biomedical and Behavioral Research). *Defining Death.* Washington, D.C.: U.S. Government Printing Office, 1981.

President's Commission. *Making Health Care Decisions: The Ethical and Legal Implications of Informed Consent in the Patient-Practitioner Relationship.* Vol. 1, *Report,* and Vol. 3, *Studies on the Foundations of Informed Consent.* Washington, D.C.: U.S. Government Printing Office, 1982.

President's Commission. *Deciding to Forego Life-Sustaining Treatment.* Washington, D.C.: U.S. Government Printing Office, 1983.

Pritchard, R., et al., for the SUPPORT Investigators. Regional Variation in the Place of Death. *Journal of General Internal Medicine* 9:146A, 1994.

Prockop, D.J. Basic Science and Clinical Practice. In *Report of the Commission on Medical Education: The Sciences of Medical Practice,* R.Q. Marston and R.M. Jones, eds. Princeton, New Jersey: Robert Wood Johnson Foundation, 1992.

ProPAC (Prospective Payment Assessment Commission). *Medicare and the American Health Care System: Report to the Congress.* Washington, D.C., 1985, 1989, 1991, 1996.

Ptacek, J.T., and Eberhardt, T.L. Breaking Bad News: A Review of the Literature. *Journal of the American Medical Association* 276(6):496–502, 1996.

Puchalski, C. Spirituality and Transcendence. Paper prepared for the Conference on Measuring Care at the End of Life, August 27–28, 1996.

Quill, T. *Death and Dignity: Making Choices and Taking Charge.* New York: W.W. Norton & Company, 1993.

Quill, T. You Promised Me I Wouldn't Die like This!: A Bad Death as a Medical Emergency. *Archives of Internal Medicine* 155(22):1250–1254, 1995.

Rang, H.P., and Urban, L. New Molecules in Analgesia. *British Journal of Anaesthesia* 75(2):145–156, 1995.

Rappaport, W., Prevel, C., Witzke, D., et al. Education about Death and Dying During Surgical Residency. *American Journal of Surgery* 161(6):690–692, 1991.

Rappaport, W., and Witzke, D. Education About Death and Dying During the Clinical Years of Medical School. *Surgery* 113(2):163–165, 1993.

Reagan, M.D. Health Care Rationing: What Does It Mean? *New England Journal of Medicine* 319(17):1149–1151, 1988.

Reed, P.G. Religiousness among Terminally Ill and Healthy Adults. *Research in Nursing and Health* 9:35–41, 1986.

Reed, P.G. Spirituality and Well-Being in Terminally Ill Hospitalized Adults. *Research in Nursing and Health* 10:335–344, 1987.

Reilly, B.M., Magnussen, C.R., Ross, J., et al. Can We Talk?: Inpatient Discussions About Advance Directives in a Community Hospital. *Archives of Internal Medicine* 154:2299–2308, 1994.

Reilly, P. *To Do no Harm: A Journey Through Medical School.* Dover, Massachusetts: Auburn House, 1987.

Reiser, S.J. *Medicine and the Reign of Technology.* New York: Cambridge University Press, 1978.

Reiser, S.J. The Era of the Patient: Using the Experience of Illness in Shaping the Missions of Health Care. *Journal of the American Medical Association* 269(8):1012–1017, 1993.

Relman, A.S. Assessment and Accountability: The Third Revolution in Medical Care. *New England Journal of Medicine* 319(18):1220–1222, 1988.

Rigdon, M.A., and Epting, F.R. Reduction in Death Threat as a Basis for Optimal Functioning. *Death Studies* 9:427–448, 1985.

Riley, G., and Lubitz, J. Longitudinal Patterns of Medicare Use by Cause of Death. *Health Care Financing Review* 11(2):1–12, 1989.

Riley, G., Lubitz, J., Prihoda, R., and Rabey, E. The Use and Costs of Medicare Services by Cause of Death. *Inquiry* 24:233–244, 1987.

Riley, G., Lubitz, J., Prihoda, R., and Stevenson, M.A. Changes in Distribution of Medicare Expenditures among Aged Enrollees, 1969–82. *Health Care Financing Review* 7:53–64, 1986.

Riley, G.F., Potosky, A.L., Lubitz, J.D., and Kessler, L.G. Medicare Payments from Diagnosis to Death for Elderly Cancer Patients by Stage at Diagnosis. *Medical Care* 33(8):828–841, 1995.

Rimer, B., Levy, M.H., Keintz, M.K., et al. Enhancing Cancer Pain Control Regimens Through Patient Education. *Patient Education and Counselling* 10(3):267–277, 1987.

Rinaldi, R.C., Steindler, E.M., Wilford, B.B., and Goodwin, D. Clarification and Standardization of Substance Abuse Terminology. *Journal of the American Medical Association* 259(4):555–557, 1988.

Roach, M.J. Bereavement and Family Burden. Paper prepared for Conference on Measuring Care at the End of Life, August 27–28, 1996.

Robert Wood Johnson Foundation. *Chronic Care in America: A 21st Century Challenge.* Princeton, New Jersey: Robert Wood Johnson Foundation, 1996.

Roos, N.P., Montgomery, P., and Roos, L. Health Care Utilization in the Years Prior to Death. *Milbank Memorial Fund Quarterly* 65(2):231–254, 1987.

Roper, W., Winkenwerder, W., Hackbarth, G., and Krakauer, H. Effectiveness in Health Care: An Initiative to Evaluate and Improve Medical Practice. *New England Journal of Medicine* 319:1197–1202, 1988.

Rosenberg, H.M., Ventura, S.J., and Maurer, J.D. Births and Deaths United States, 1995. *Monthly Vital Statistics Report, Preliminary Data from the Centers for Disease Control and Prevention, National Center for Health Statistics* 45(3) Suppl. 2, October 4, 1996.

Rosenfeld, K.E., Wenger, N.S., et al. Factors Associated with Change in Resuscitation Preference of Seriously Ill Patients. *Archives of Internal Medicine* 156:1558–1564, 1996.

Rosenfeld, B., Breitbart, W., McDonald, M.V., et al. Pain in Ambulatory AIDS Patients. II: Impact of Pain on Psychological Functioning and Quality of Life. *Pain* 68:323–328, 1996.

Ross, M.M., and MacDonald, B. Providing Palliative Care to Older Adults: Context and Challenges. *Journal of Palliative Care* 10(4):5–10, 1994.

Rothman, D.J. *Strangers at the Bedside: A History of How Law and Bioethics Transformed Medical Decision Making.* New York: Basic Books, 1991.

Rothstein, M.A. Genetic Discrimination in Employment and the Americans with Disabilities Act. *Houston Law Review* 29:23–84, 1992.

Roy, R., and Michael, T.A. Survey of Chronic Pain in an Elderly Population. *Canadian Family Physician* 32:513–516, 1986.

Rubenstein, L.B., Kahn, K.L., Reinisch, E.J., et al. Changes in Quality of Care for Five Diseases Measured by Implicit Review, 1981–1986. *Journal of the American Medical Association* 264(15):1974–1979, 1990.

Rubin, H.R., Gandek, B., Rogers, W.H., et al. Patients' Ratings of Outpatient Visits in Different Practice Settings: Results from the Medical Outcomes Study. *Journal of the American Medical Association* 270(7):835–840, 1993.

Sachdeva, R.C., Jefferson, L.S., Coss-Bu, J., and Brody, B.A. Resource Consumption and the Extent of Futile Care Among Patients in a Pediatric Intensive Care Unit Setting. *Journal of Pediatrics* 128:742–747, 1996.

Sachs, G.A. Increasing the Prevalence of Advance Care Planning. *Hastings Center Report* 24(6 Suppl.):S13–S16, 1994.

Sachs, G.A., Stocking, C., and Miles, S. Empowerment of the Older Patient: A Randomized Controlled Trial to Increase Discussion of Use of Advance Directives. *Journal of the American Geriatric Society* 40:269–273, 1992.

Sager, M., Easterlin, D.V., Kindig, D.A., and Anderson, O.W. Changes in the Location of Death After Passage of Medicare's Prospective Payment System. *New England Journal of Medicine* 320(7):433–439, 1989.

Samarel, N. The Dying Process. Pp. 89–116 in *Dying: Facing the Facts,* 3d Edition, H. Wass and R.A. Neimeyer, eds. Washington, D.C.: Taylor & Francis, 1995.

Saunders, C.M., and Sykes, N., eds. *The Management of Terminal Malignant Disease,* 3d Edition. Boston: Edward Arnold, 1993.

Schlesinger, M., and Mechanic, D. Perspectives: Challenges for Managed Competition from Chronic Illness. *Health Affairs* 12(Suppl.):123–137, 1993.

Schmidt, H.G., Machiels-Bongaerts, M., Hermans, H., et al. The Development of Diagnostic Competence: Comparison of a Problem-Based, an Integrated, and a Conventional Medical Curriculum. *Academic Medicine* 71(6)658–664, 1996.

Schmidt, S.A. When You Come into My Room. *Journal of the American Medical Association* 276(7):512, 1996.

Schneiderman, L.J. Should the Institute of Medicine Develop Guidelines for Medical Treatment Decisions in Critically Ill and Dying Patients? In *Summary of Committee Views and Workshop Examining the Feasibility of an Institute of Medicine Study of Dying, Decisionmaking, and Appropriate Care.* IOM Committee for a Feasibility Study on Care at the End of Life, M.J. Field, ed. Washington, D.C.: Institute of Medicine, 1994.

Schneiderman, L.J., Kaplan, R.M., and Pearlman, R.A. Do Physicians' Own Preferences for Life-Sustaining Treatment Influence Their Perceptions of Patients' Preferences? *Journal of Clinical Ethics* 4(1):28–33, 1993.

Schneiderman, L.J., Kronick, R., Kaplan, R.M., et al. Effects of Offering Advance Directives on Medical Treatments and Costs. *Annals of Internal Medicine* 117(7):599–606, 1992.

Schofferman, J., and Brody, R. Pain in Far Advanced AIDS. In *Advances in Pain Research and Therapy,* K.M. Foley, J.J. Bonica, and V. Ventafridda, eds. New York: Raven Press, 1990.

Schroeder, S.A. A Comparison of Western Europe and U.S. University Hospitals: A Case Report from Leuven, West Berlin, Leiden, London, and San Francisco. *Journal of the American Medical Association* 252:240–246, 1984.

Schug, S.A., Zech, D., and Dorr, U. Cancer Pain Management According to WHO Analgesic Guidelines. *Journal of Pain and Symptom Management* 5(1):27–32, 1990.

Schulz, R., Newsom, J., Mittelmark, M., et al. Health Effects of Caregiving. *Annals of Behavioral Medicine* in press, 1997.

Scitovsky, A. The High Cost of Dying: What Do the Data Show? *Milbank Memorial Fund Quarterly/Health and Society* 62(4):591–608, 1984.

Scitovsky, A. Medical Care in the Last Twelve Months of Life: The Relation Between Age, Functional Status, and Medical Care Expenditures. *Milbank Memorial Fund Quarterly* 66(4):640–660, 1988.

Scitovsky, A. The High Cost of Dying Revisited. *Milbank Memorial Fund Quarterly* 72:561–591, 1994.

Scitovsky, A. Age and the Cost of Health Care. Paper presented at the First International Conference on Priorities in Health Care, Stockholm, Sweden, October 13–16, 1996.

Scott, J., and MacDonald, N. Palliative Care Medicine. In *Oxford Textbook of Palliative Medicine,* D. Doyle, G.W. Hanks, and N. MacDonald, eds. New York: Oxford University Press, 1997.

Seale, C., and Cartwright, A. *The Year Before Death.* Aldershot, Hants, England: Ashgate Publishing, 1994.

Sehgal, A.R., Galbraith, A., Chesney, M., et al. How Strictly Do Dialysis Patients Want Their Advance Directives Followed? *Journal of the American Medical Association* 267(1):59–63, 1992.

Sehgal, A.R., Weisheit, C., Miura, Y., et al. Advance Directives and Withdrawal of Dialysis in the United States, Germany, and Japan. *Journal of the American Medical Association* 276(20):1652–1656, 1996.

Seidlitz, L., Duberstein, P.R., Cox, C., and Conwell, Y. Attitudes of Older People Toward Suicide and Assisted Suicide: An Analysis of Gallup Poll Findings. *Journal of the American Geriatric Society* 43(9):993–998, 1995.

Selker, H.P. Systems for Comparing Actual and Predicted Morality Rates: Characteristics to Promote Cooperation in Improving Hospital Care. *Annals of Internal Medicine* 118:820–822, 1993.

Sengstaken, E.A., and King, S.A. The Problems of Pain and Its Detection Among Geriatric Nursing Home Residents. *Journal of American Geriatric Society* 41(5):541–544, 1993.

Sengupta, J.N., Su, X., and Gebhart, G.F. Kappa but not Mu or Delta Opioids Attenuate Responses to Distention of Afferent Fibers Innervating the Rat Colon. *Gastroenterology* 111:968–980, 1996.

Seravalli, E.P. The Dying Patient, the Physician, and the Fear of Death. *New England Journal of Medicine* 319:1728–1730, 1988.

Shapiro, R.S. Liability Issues in the Management of Pain. *Journal of Pain and Symptom Management* 9(3):146–152, 1994a.

Shapiro, R.S. Legal Bases for Control of Analgesic Drugs. *Journal of Pain and Symptom Management* 9(3):153–159, 1994b.

Shaughnessy, P.W., Schlenker, R.E., and Hittle, D.F. Home Health Care Outcomes Under Capitated and Fee-for-Service Payment. *Health Care Financing Review* 16:197–222, 1994.

Sheldon, F. Education and Training for Social Workers in Palliative Care. Pp. 791–799 in *Oxford Textbook of Palliative Medicine.* D. Doyle, G.W.C. Hanks, and N. MacDonald, eds. Oxford: Oxford University Press, 1993.

Shem, S. *The House of God.* New York: R. Marek, 1979.

Shortell, S.M., Gillies, R.R., and Anderson, D.A. The New World of Managed Care: Creating Organized Delivery Systems. *Health Affairs* 13(5):46–64, 1994.

Shortell, S.M., Gillies, R.R., Anderson, D.A., et al. *Remaking Health Care in America: Building Organized Delivery Systems.* San Francisco: Jossey-Bass, 1996.

Sigler, K.A., Guernsey, B.G., Ingrim, N.B., and Buesing, A.A. Effect of a Triplicate Prescription Law on the Prescribing of Schedule II Drugs. *American Journal of Hospital Pharmacy* 41:108–111, 1984.

Singer, P.A., and Lowy, F.H. Rationing, Patient Preferences and Cost of Care at the End of Life. *Archives of Internal Medicine* 152:478–480, 1992.

Singh, G.K., Dochanek, D.K., MacDorman, M.F., et al. Advance Report of Final Mortality Statistics, 1994. *Monthly Vital Statistics Report* 45(3 Suppl.), September 30, 1996.

Skaife, S. Sickness, Health, and the Therapeutic Relationship: Thoughts Arising from the Literature on Art Therapy and Physical Illness. *Inscape* Summer:24–29, 1993.

Smeeding, T., ed. *Should Health Care Be Rationed by Age?* Totawa, NJ: Littlefield, 1987.

Smith, E., Stefanek, M.E., and Joseph, M.V. Spiritual Awareness, Personal Death Perspective and Psychosocial Distress Among Cancer Patients: An Initial Investigation. *Journal of Psychosocial Oncology* 11(3):89–103, 1993.

Smith, M.J., Breitbart, W.S., and Platt, M.M. A Critique of Instruments and Methods to Detect, Diagnose, and Rate Delirium. *Journal of Pain Symptom Management* 10:35–77, 1995.

Snow, C. New Hospice Horizons. *Modern Healthcare* 90–91, 1997.

Sodestrom, L., and Martinson, I. Patients' Spriritual Coping Strategies: A Study of Nurse and Patient Perspectives. *Oncology Nursing Forum* 14(2):41, 1987.

Solomon, M.Z. The Enormity of the Task: The SUPPORT Study and Changing Practice. *Hastings Center Report* 25(6 Suppl.):S28–S32, 1995.

Solomon, M.Z. Educational Methods and Cultural Change. Presentation at Medical Education for Care near the End of Life National Consensus Conference, Washington, D.C., May 16, 1997.

Solomon, M.Z., O'Donnell, L., Jennings, B., et al. Decisions Near the End of Life: Professional Views on Life-Sustaining Treatments. *American Journal of Public Health* 83(1):14–23, 1993.

Sontag, S. *Illness as Metaphor.* New York: Farrar, Strauss, and Giroux, 1978.

Soumerai, S.B., and Avorn, J. Principles of Education Outreach ("Academic Detailing") to Improve Clinical Decision Making. *Journal of the American Medical Association* 263:549–556, 1990.

Soumerai, S.B., Avorn, J., Ross-Degnan, D., and Gormaker, S. Payment Restrictions for Prescription Drugs Under Medicaid: Effects on Therapy, Cost, and Equity. *New England Journal of Medicine* 317(9): 550–555, 1987.

Soumerai, S.B., Ross-Degnan, D., Avorn, J., et al. Effects of Medicaid Drug-Payment Limits on Admission to Hospitals and Nursing Homes. *New England Journal of Medicine* 325(15): 1072–1077, 1991.

Sourkes, B.M. Truth to Life: Art Therapy with Pediatric Oncology Patients and Their Siblings. *Journal of Psychosocial Oncology* 9(2):81–96, 1991.

Speck, P.W. Spiritual Issues in Palliative Care. Pp. 515–525 in *Oxford Textbook of Palliative Medicine,* D. Doyle, G.W.C. Hanks, and N. MacDonald, eds. Oxford: Oxford University Press, 1993.

Spielman, B. Protecting Terminally Ill Patients: The Dilemma of the Deselected Physicians. Presented at End of Life Health Care in Managed Care Systems Conference. Center for Biomedical Ethics, University of Minnesota, Minneapolis, November 1–2, 1996.

Sprung, C.L. Changing Attitudes and Practices in Foregoing Life-Sustaining Treatments. *Journal of the American Medical Association* 263(16):2211–2215, 1990.

Starr, P. *The Social Transformation of American Medicine.* New York: Basic Books, 1982.

Steel, R.K. Analysis of Residency Review Requirements. Paper prepared for Conference on the Education of Physicians about Dying, Hackensack University Medical Center, New Jersey, April 19, 1996.

Steinberg, M.D., Morrison, M.F., Rothchild, E.N., et al. The Role of the Psychiatrist in End-of-Life Treatment Decisions. Pp. 61–69 in *Caring for the Dying: Identification and Promotion of Physician Competency: Educational Resource Document,* Philadelphia: ABIM, 1996.

Stevens, M. Psychological Adaptation of the Dying Child. Pp. 699–707 of *Oxford Textbook of Palliative Medicine,* D. Doyle, G.W.C. Hanks, and N. MacDonald, eds. Oxford: Oxford University Press, 1993.

Stevens, R. *In Sickness and in Wealth: American Hospitals in the Twentieth Century.* New York: Basic Books, 1989.

Stewart, A. *Quality of Life.* Paper prepared for Conference on Measuring Care at the End of Life, August 27–28, 1996.

Storey, P., Hill, H.H., St. Louis, R.H., et al. Subcutaneous Infusions for Control of Cancer Symptoms. *Journal of Pain and Symptom Management* 5(1):33–41, 1990.

Strahan, G.W. An Overview of Nursing Homes and Their Current Residents: Data From the 1995 National Nursing Home Survey. *Advance Data* 280, January 23, 1997.

Strain, J.E. The Treatment of Seriously Disabled Newborns. In *Summary of Committee Views and Workshop Examining the Feasibility of an Institute of Medicine Study of Dying, Decisionmaking, and Appropriate Care.* IOM Committee for a Feasibility Study on Care at the End of Life, M.J. Field, ed. Washington, D.C.: Institute of Medicine, 1994.

Strauss, P.J., Wolf, P., and Shilling, D. *Aging and the Law.* Chicago: Commerce Clearing House, Inc., 1990.

Strickland, A.L., and DeSpelder, L.A. Communicating about Death and Dying. Pp. 37–51 in *A Challenge for Living: Dying, Death, and Bereavement,* I.B. Corless, B.A. Germino, and M.A. Pittman, eds. Boston: Jones and Bartlett, 1995.

Stuart, B., Alexander, C., Arenella, C. et al. *Medical Guidelines for Determining Prognosis in Selected NonCancer Diseases,* 2nd ed. Arlington, Virginia: NHO, 1996.

Sullivan, A. When Plagues End: Notes on the Twilight of an Epidemic. *The New York Times Magazine,* p. 52, November 10, 1996.

Sulmasy, D.P. Managed Care and Managed Death. *Archives of Internal Medicine* 155:243–246, 1995.

Super, A. *Statement Before the IOM Committee on Care at the End of Life on Behalf of Supportive Care of the Dying: A Coalition for Compassionate Care.* Irvine, California, November 23, 1996.

SUPPORT Principal Investigators. A Controlled Trial to Improve Care for Seriously Ill Hospitalized Patients: The Study to Understand Prognoses and Preferences for Outcomes and Risks of Treatments (SUPPORT). *Journal of the American Medical Association* 274:1591–1598, 1995.

Surks, M.I. Generosity of Spirit and Personal Dignity: The Story of Mr. S. Pp. 5–6 in *Caring for the Dying: Identification and Promotion of Physician Competency—Personal Narratives,* Philadelphia: ABIM, 1996.

Swan, J.H., Dewit, S., and Harrington, C. State Medicaid Reimbursement Methods and Rates for Nursing Homes, 1993. Paper prepared for the Department of Housing and Urban Development and the Health Care Financing Administration. Wichita, Kansas: Wichita State University, 1994.

Takahashi, J.S., Pinto, L.H., and Vitaterna, M.H. Forward and Reverse Genetic Approaches to Behavior in the Mouse. *Science* 264:1724–1733, 1994.

Takeda, F. Results of Field-Testing in Japan of WHO Draft Interim Guidelines on Relief of Cancer Pain. *Pain Clinician* 1:83–89, 1986.

Tay, W.K., Shaw, R.J., and Goh, C.R. A Survey of Symptoms in Hospice Patients in Singapore. *Annals of Academic Medicine in Singapore* 23:191–196, 1994.

Tehan, C. *Statement Before the IOM Committee on Care at the End of Life on Behalf of Hospital Home Health Care Agency of California.* Irvine, California, November 23, 1996.

Temkin-Greener, H., Meiners, M., Petty, E.A., and Szydlowski, J.S. The Use and Cost of Health Services prior to Death: A Comparison of the Medicare-Only and the Medicare-Medicaid Elderly Populations. *Milbank Memorial Fund Quarterly* 70(4):679–701, 1992.

Teno, J.M. Consumer Reports and Ratings of Medical Care: Will We Ever Get Satisfaction? Paper prepared for the IOM Conference on Evaluating Health Outcomes for Elderly People in a Changing Health Care Marketplace. Washington, D.C.: June 5, 1996a.

Teno, J.M. Summary of the Conference on Making Toolkit of Instruments to Measure End of Life Care (TIME). Mailed to participants of the Toolkit Conference, 1996b.

Teno, J.M., and Lynn, J. Putting Advance-Care Planning into Action. *Journal of Clinical Ethics* 7(3):100–107, 1996.

Teno, J.M., Lynn, J., et al. Do Advance Directives Save Resources? *Clinical Research* 41:A551 (Abstract), 1993.

Teno, J.M., Lynn, J., Connors, A.F., et al. The Illusion of End-of-Life Resource Savings with Advance Directives. *Journal of the American Geriatrics Society* 45:513–518, 1997.

Teno, J.M., Lynn, J., Phillips, R.S., et al. Do Formal Advance Directives Affect Resuscitation Decisions and the Use of Resources for the Seriously Ill Patient? *Journal of Clinical Ethics* 5(1):23–30, 1994.

Teno, J.M., Lynn, J., Wenger, N., et al. Advance Directives for Seriously Ill Hospitalized Patients: Effectiveness with the Patient Self-Determination Act and the SUPPORT Intervention. *Journal of the American Geriatrics Society* 45:500–507, 1997.

Teno, J.M., Mor, V., and Fleishman, J. Preferences of HIV-infected patients for aggressive versus palliative care (letter to the editor). *New England Journal of Medicine* 324:1140, 1991.

Teno, J.M., Murphy, D., Lynn, J., et al. Prognosis-Based Futility Guidelines: Does Anyone Win? *Journal of the American Geriatrics Society* 42(11):1202–1207, 1994.

Testa, J. Group Systematic Desensitization and Implosive Therapy for Death Anxiety. *Psychological Reports* 48:376–378, 1981.

Thibault, G.E. The Use of Clinical Models for "End of Life" Decision-Making in Critically Ill ICU Patients. In *Summary of Committee Views and Workshop Examining the Feasibility of an Institute of Medicine Study of Dying, Decisionmaking, and Appropriate Care.* IOM Committee for a Feasibility Study on Care at the End of Life, M.J. Field, ed. Washington, D.C.: Institute of Medicine, 1994.

Thomas, T.J., and Ashcraft, M.L.F. Measuring Severity of Illness: Comparison of Inter-rater Reliability Among Severity Methodologies. *Inquiry* 26:483–492, 1989.

Thomas, T.J., and Ashcraft, M.L.F. Measuring Severity of Illness: Comparison of Severity and Severity Systems in Terms of Ability to Explain Variation in Costs. *Inquiry* 28:39–55, 1991.

Thorpe, G. Teaching Palliative Care to United Kingdom Medical Students. *Palliative Medicine* 5(1):6–11, 1991.

Thorpe, G. Enabling More Dying People to Remain at Home. *British Medical Journal* 307:915–918, 1993.

Thorson, J.A., and Powell, F.C. A Revised Death Anxiety Scale. Pp. 3–28 in *Death Anxiety Handbook: Research, Instrumentation, and Application,* R.A. Neimeyer, ed. Washington, D.C.: Taylor & Francis, 1994.

Tinsley, E.S., Baldwin, A.S., Steeves, R.H., et al. Surgeons', Nurses', and Bereaved Families' Attitudes Toward Dying in the Burn Centre. *Burns* 20(1):79–82, 1994.

Todorov, P.T., McDevitt, T.M., Carink, P., et al. Induction of Muscle Protein Degradation and Weight Loss by a Tumor Product. *Cancer Research* 56:1256–1261, 1996.

Tolle, S. Overcoming Obstacles to Compassionate Care of the Dying in Long Term Care. Presentation at Conference on Improving Care near End of Life: Ethical, Legal, and Practical Issues in Long Term Care. Sponsored by Oregon Health Sciences University and Portland State University. Portland, Oregon: May 31, 1996a.

Tolle, S. *Statement Before the IOM Committee on Care at the End of Life on Behalf of the Oregon Health Sciences University Center for Ethics in Health Care.* Irvine, California, November 23, 1996b.

Tolle, S.W., Cooney, T.G., and Hickam, D.H. A Program to Teach Residents Humanistic Skills for Notifying Survivors of a Patient's Death. *Academic Medicine* 64(9):505–506, 1989.

Tores, D., Lemeshow, S., Avrunin, S.J., and Pastides, H. Validation of the Mortality Prediction Model for ICU patients. *Critical Care Medicine* 15:208–213, 1987.

Tosteson, D.C., Adelstein, S.J., and Carver, S.T., eds. *New Pathways to Medical Education: Learning to Learn at Harvard Medical School.* Cambridge, Massachusetts: Harvard University Press, 1994.

Townsend, J. Frank, A.O., Fermont, D., et al. Terminal Cancer Care and Patients' Preference for Place of Death: A Prospective Study. *British Medical Journal* 301:415–417, 1990.

Tu, E.J., and Chen, K. Changes in Active Life Expectancy in Taiwan: Compression or Expansion? *Social Science and Medicine* 39(12):1657–1665, 1994.

Tu, J.V., Pashos, C.L., Naylor, C.D., et al. Use of Cardia Procedures and Outcomes in Elderly Patients with Myocardial Infarction in the United States and Canada. *New England Journal of Medicine* 336:1500–1505, 1997.

Tymchuk, A.J., Ouslander, J.G., Rahbar, B., and Fitten, J. Medical Decisionmaking among Elderly People in Long-Term Care. *Gerontologist* 28:59–63.

UHF (United Hospital Fund). United Hospital Fund Launches $2.2 Million Initiative to Improve Care for Dying Patients (Press Release). *United Hospital Fund: Introduction* [WWW document]. URL http://www.uhfnyc.org:80/intro/prhpci.htm (accessed March 19, 1997).

U.S. Department of Commerce. *Bicentennial Edition Historical Statistics of the United States Colonial Times to 1970,* Part 1. Washington, D.C.: 1975.

Vanderpool, H.Y., ed. *The Ethics of Research Involving Human Subjects: Facing the 21st Century.* Frederick, Maryland: University Publishing Group, Inc., 1996.

Vargo, M. E., and Black, W.F. Psychosocial Correlates of Death Anxiety in a Population of Medical Students. *Psychological Reports* 54:737–738, 1984.

Varricchio, C.G. et al. Introduction. *Journal of the National Cancer Institute Monographs.* 20:vii–viii, 1996.

Veatch, R.M. *Death, Dying, and the Biological Revolution: Our Last Quest for Responsibility.* New Haven, Connecticut: Yale University Press, 1976.

Veatch, R.M., ed. *Life Span Values & Life-Extending Technologies.* San Francisco: Harper & Row, 1979.

Veatch, R.M. DRGs and the Ethical Reallocation of Resources. *Hastings Center Report* 16:32–40, 1986.

Veatch, R.M. The Impending Collapse of the Whole-Brain Definition of Death. *Hastings Center Report* 23(4):18–24, 1993.

Veatch, R.M. Medically Futile Care: The Role of the Physician in Setting Limits. *American Journal of Law & Medicine* 18(1 and 2):15–36).

Veatch, R.M., and Spicer, C.M. Medically Futile Care: The Role of the Physician in Setting Limits. *American Journal of Law and Medicine* 18(1&2):15–36, 1992.

Ventafridda, V., Caraceni, A., and Gamba, A. Field-Testing of the WHO Guidelines for Cancer Pain Relief: Summary Report of Demonstration Projects. In *Proceedings of the Second International Congress on Pain,* Vol. 16, *Advances in Pain Research and Therapy,* K.M. Foley, J.J. Bonica, V. Ventafridda, eds. New York: Raven Press, 1990.

Ventafridda, V., Tamburini, M., Caraceni, A., et al. A Validation Study of the WHO Method for Cancer Pain Relief. *Cancer* 59:851–856, 1987.

Vernon, D.T., and Blake, R.L. Does Problem-Based Learning Work?: A Meta-Analysis of Evaluative Research. *Academic Medicine* 68:550–563, 1993.

Vernon, D.T., and Hosokawa, M.C. Faculty Attitudes and Opinions about Problem-Based Learning. *Academic Medicine* 71(11):1233–1238, 1996.

Virmani, J., Schneiderman, L.J., and Kaplan, R.M. Relationship of Advance Directives to Physician-Patient Communication. *Archives of Internal Medicine* 154:909–913, 1994.

Virnig, B.A., Persily, N.A., Morgan, R.O., et al. Hospice Care in Medicare HMOs and Medicare FFS. Presented at End of Life Health Care in Managed Care Systems Conference. Center for Biomedical Ethics, University of Minnesota, Minneapolis, November 1–2, 1996.

Viste, K.M. *Statement Before the IOM Committee on Care at the End of Life on Behalf of the American Academy of Neurology.* Washington, D.C., April 29, 1996.

Vladeck, B.C. The Economics of End-of-Life Care. Presentation at the Robert Wood Johnson Foundation Conference on "Last Acts: Care and Caring at the End of Life," Crystal City, Virginia, March 12, 1996.

Vladeck, B.C., and Miller, N.A. The Medicare Home Health Initiative. *Health Care Financing Review* 16(1):7–16, 1994.

Vladeck, B.C., Miller, N.A., and Clauser, S.B. The Changing Face of Long-Term Care. *Health Care Financing Review* 14:5–23, 1993.

Volicer, L. *Statement Before the IOM Committee on Care at the End of Life on Behalf of the Alzheimers Association.* Washington, D.C., April 29, 1996.

Von Gunten, C.F. Why I Do What I Do. Pp. 47–48 in *Caring for the Dying: Identification and Promotion of Physician Competency.* Philadelphia, Pennsylvania: ABIM, 1996.

Von Roenn, J.H., Cleeland, C.S., Gonin, R., et al. Physician Attitudes and Practice in Cancer Pain Management: A Survey from the Eastern Cooperative Oncology Group. *Annals of Internal Medicine* 119(2):121–126, 1993.

Wagner, A.M., Baker, M., Campbell, B., et al. Pain Prevalence and Pain Treatments for Residents in Oregon's Long-Term Care Facilities. Prepared for the State of Oregon Senior and Disabled Services Division, Client Care Monitoring Unit, January 1996.

Walker, V.A., Hoskin, P.J., Hanks, G.W., and White, I.D. Evaluation of WHO Analgesic Guidelines for Cancer Pain in a Hospital-Based Palliative Care Unit. *Journal of Pain and Symptom Management* 3:145–150, 1988.

Wall, P.D., and Melzack, R. *Textbook of Pain,* Third Edition. Edinburgh: Churchill-Livingstone, 1994.

Wallston, K.A., Burger, C., Smith, R.A., and Baugher, R.J. Comparing the Quality of Death for Hospice and Non-Hospice Cancer Patients. *Medical Care* 26(2):177–182, 1988.

Ward, S.E., Goldberg, N., Miller-McCauley, V., et al. Patient-Related Barriers to Management of Cancer Pain. *Pain* 52(3):319–324, 1993.

Ward, S.E., and Gordon, D. Application of the American Pain Society Quality Assurance Standards. *Pain* 56:299–306, 1994.

Ward, S.E., and Gordon, D. Patient Satisfaction and Pain Severity as Outcomes in Pain Management: A Longitudinal View of One Setting's Experience. *Journal of Pain and Symptom Management* 11(4):242–251, 1996.

Ware, J.E. Effects of Acquiescent Response Set on Patient Satisfaction Ratings. *Medical Care* 26:327–336, 1978.

Ware, J.E., and Hayes, R.D. Methods for Measuring Patient Satisfaction with Specific Medical Encounters. *Medical Care* 26(4):393–402, 1988.

Ware, J.E., Jr., Bayliss, M.S., Rogers, W.H., et al. Differences in Four-Year Health Outcomes for Elderly and Poor Chronically Ill Patients Treated in HMO and Fee-for-Service Systems: Results from the Medical Outcomes Study. *Journal of the American Medical Association* 276(13):1039–1047, 1996a.

Ware, J.E., Jr., Bayliss, M.S., Rogers, W.H., et al. Elderly and Poor in the Medical Outcomes Study (Letter). *Journal of the American Medical Association* 276(24):1953, 1996b.

Ware, J.E., Jr., Davies, A.R., and Rubin, H.R. Patient's Assessment of Their Care. Pp. 231–247 in *The Quality of Medical Care: Information for Consumers,* Washington, D.C.: Office of Technology Assessment, 1988.

Ware, J.E., Davies-Avery, A., and Stewart, A.L. The Measurement and Meaning of Patient Satisfaction: A Review of the Literature. *Health and Medical Services Review* 1:1–15, 1978.

Wass, H. Concepts of Death: A Developmental Perspective. In *Childhood and Death*, H. Wass and C.A. Corr, eds. Washington: Hemisphere Publishing, 1984.

Wass, H. Death in the Lives of Children and Adolescents. In *Dying: Facing the Facts*. H. Wass and R.A. Neimeyer, eds. Washington, D.C.: Taylor & Francis, 1995.

Wass, H., and Corr, C.A., eds. *Childhood and Death*. Washington: Hemisphere Publishing, 1984.

Wass, H., and Neimeyer, R.A., eds. *Dying: Facing the Facts*. Washington, D.C.: Taylor & Francis, 1995.

Wastila, L.J., and Bishop, C. The Influence of Multiple Copy Prescription Programs on Analgesic Utilization. *Journal of Pharmaceutical Care in Pain and Symptom Control* 4(3):3–19, 1996.

Weeks, W.B., Kofoed, L.L., Wallace, A.E., and Welch, H.G. Advance Directives and the Cost of Terminal Hospitalization. *Archives of Internal Medicine* 154:2077–2083, 1994.

Weissert, W.G. A New Policy Agenda for Home Care. *Health Affairs* Summer:67–77, 1991.

Weissman, D.E., and Haddox, J.D. Opioid Pseudoaddiction: An Iatrogenic Syndrome. *Pain* 36(3):363–366, 1989.

Weissman, D.E., Joranson, D.E., and Hopwood, M.B. Wisconsin Physicians' Knowledge and Attitudes about Opioid Analgesic Regulations. *Wisconsin Medical Journal* 90(12):671–675, 1991.

Wennberg, J.E. Dealing with Medical Practice Variations: A Proposal for Action. *Health Affairs* 3(2):6–32, 1984.

Wennberg, J.E. Unwanted Variations in the Rules of Practice. *Journal of the American Medical Association* 265:1306, 1991.

Wennberg, J.E., and Gittelsohn, A. Small Area Variations in Health Care Delivery. *Science* 142:1102–1108, 1973.

Wennberg, J.E., and Gittelsohn, A. Variations in Medical Care among Small Areas. *Scientific American* 246:120–134, 1982.

Wennberg, J., Mulley, A., Hanley, D., et al. An Assessment of Prostatectomy for Benign Urinary Tract Obstruction. *Journal of the American Medical Association* 259:3027–3030, 1988.

Westman, A.S., and Brackney, B.E. Relationships between Indices of Neuroticism, Attitude toward and Concepts of Death, and Religiosity. *Psychological Reports* 66:1039–1043, 1990.

Wheatley, S.C. *The Politics of Philanthropy: Abraham Flexner and Medical Education*. Madison, Wisconsin: University of Wisconsin Press, 1988.

Wheeler, H.B. Shattuck Lecture: Healing and Heroism. *New England Journal of Medicine* 322:1546, 1990.

White, M., and Fletcher, J. The Patient Self-Determination Act: On Balance, More Help than Hindrance. *Journal of the American Medical Association* 266:410–412, 1991.

WHO (World Health Organization). *Cancer Pain Relief and Palliative Care*. WHO Technical Report Series 804. Geneva: WHO, 1990.

Wiener, J.M. *Rationing in America: Overt and Covert*. Paper presented at Conference on Rationing America's Medical Care: Opening Pandora's Box? The Brookings Institute, Washington, D.C., May 20, 1991.

Wilkinson, A. Physical Functioning. Paper prepared for Conference on Measuring Care at the End of Life, August 27–28, 1996.

Wilson, I.B., and Cleary, P.D. Linking Clinical Variables with Health-Related Quality of Life: A Conceptual Model of Patient Outcomes. *Journal of the American Medical Association* 273(1):59–65, 1995.

Wilson, I.B., and Kaplan, S. Clinical Practice and Patients' Health Status: How Are the Two Related? *Medical Care* 33(1, Suppl.):AS209–AS214, 1995.

Wilson, W.C., Smedira, N.G., Fink, C., et al. Ordering and Administration of Sedatives and Analgesics during the Withholding and Withdrawal of Life Support from Critically Ill Patients. *Journal of the American Medical Association* 267:949–953, 1992.

Winslow, G.R., and Walters, J.W. *Facing Limits: Ethics and Health Care for the Elderly.* Boulder, Colorado: Westview Press, 1992.

Wong, P.T., Reker, G.T., and Glesser, G. Death Attitude Profile—Revised. in *Death Anxiety Handbook: Research, Instrumentation, and Application.* Pp. 121–148, R.A. Neimeyer, ed. Washington, D.C.: Taylor & Francis, 1994.

Woolf, C.J., and Doubell, T.P. The Pathophysiology of Chronic Pain: Increased Sensitivity to Low Threshold Aß-Fibre Inputs. *Current Biology* 4:525–534, 1994.

Yaksh, T.L., and Malmberg, A.B. Central Pharmacology of Nociceptive Transmission, in *Textbook of Pain,* Third Edition, pp. 165–200, P.D. Wall and R. Melzack, eds. Edinburgh: Churchill-Livingstone, 1994.

Yates, J.L., and Glick, H.R. *The Failure of the Patient Self-Determination Act and Advance Medical Directives—and Policy Alternatives for the Right to Die.* Paper prepared for the Annual Meeting of the American Political Science Association, 1995.

Young, M., and Cullen, L. *A Good Death: Conversations with East Londoners.* New York: Routledge, 1996.

Youngner, S.J., and Arnold, R.M. Ethical, Psychosocial, and Public Policy Implications of Procuring Organs from Non-Heart-Beating Cadaver Donors. *Journal of the American Medical Association* 269(21):2769–2774, 1993.

Youngner, S.J., Landefeld, C.S., Coulton, C.J., et al. "Brain Death" and Organ Retrieval: A Cross-Sectional Survey of Knowledge and Concepts among Health Professionals. *Journal of the American Medical Association* 261(15):2205–2210, 1989.

Zampini, K., and Ostroff, J.S. The Post-Treatment Resource Program: Portrait of a Program for Cancer Survivors. *Psycho-oncology* 2:1, 1993.

Zarabozo, C., Taylor, C., and Hicks, J. DataView: Medicare Managed Care: Numbers and Trends. *Health Care Financing Review* 17(3):243–261, 1996.

Zech, D.F.J., et al. Validation of World Health Organization Guidelines for Cancer Pain Relief: A 10-Year Prospective Study. *Pain* 63:65–76, 1995.

Zimmerman, J.M. *Hospice: Complete Care for the Terminally Ill.* Baltimore, Maryland: Urban and Schwarzenberg, 1986.

Zimmerman, J.E., Wagner, D.P., Draper, E.A., and Knaus, W.A. Improving Intensive Care Unit Discharge Decisions: Supplementing Physician Judgment with Predictions of Next Day Risk for Life Support. *Critical Care Medicine* 22(9):1373–1384, 1994.

Appendixes

A

Institute of Medicine Feasibility Study on Care at the End of Life[1] August 1993–February 1994

IOM STUDY COMMITTEE

Christine K. Cassel, M.D.,* *Chair,* Professor of Medicine and Professor of Public Policy Studies, The University of Chicago Medical Center, Chicago, Illinois

Henry J. Aaron, Ph.D.,* Senior Fellow, The Brookings Institution, Washington, D.C.

Robert A. Burt, J.D.,* Alexander M. Bickel Professor of Law, Yale Law School, New Haven, Connecticut

Kathleen M. Foley, M.D.,* The Society of Memorial Sloan-Kettering Cancer Center Chair, Memorial Sloan-Kettering Cancer Center, New York, New York

Robert M. Kliegman, M.D., Professor and Chair of Pediatrics, Medical College of Wisconsin, Milwaukee, Wisconsin

Joanne Lynn,* M.D., Professor of Community and Family Medicine, Dartmouth Medical School, Hanover, New Hampshire

---

[1]The conclusions of this study were reported in *Summary of Committee Views and Workshop Examining the Feasibility of an Institute of Medicine Study of Dying, Decisionmaking, and Appropriate Care* (Washington, D.C.: Division of Health Care Services, February, 1994). Support for this planning study was provided by The Commonwealth Fund.

*Member, Institute of Medicine.

Lawrence Schneiderman, M.D., Professor of Medicine, University of California at San Diego, San Diego, California
George E. Thibault, M.D., Chief of Medicine, Brockton-West Roxbury V.A. Medical Center, W. Roxbury, Massachusetts

STUDY STAFF
DIVISION OF HEALTH CARE SERVICES

Marilyn J. Field, Ph.D., Study Director
Kathleen N. Lohr, Ph.D., Division Director, Health Care Services
Richard D. Rettig, Ph.D., Senior Program Officer
Donna D. Thompson, Project Assistant

WORKSHOP
DYING, DECISIONMAKING, AND APPROPRIATE CARE
National Academy of Sciences • Washington, D.C.
December 2–3, 1993

AGENDA

December 2

1:00 WELCOME, INTRODUCTIONS, AND REVIEW OF
WORKSHOP GOALS

1:15 IMPROVING OUR KNOWLEDGE BASE
Circumstances of Death
Kathleen Foley, M.D., Memorial Sloan-Kettering Cancer Center
Vincent Mor, M.D. (paper only), Brown University
Prognosis
Murray Pollack, M.D., Children's National Medical Center
George Thibault, M.D., Brockton-West Roxbury V.A.
Medical Center
Practitioner Attitudes and Behavior
Christine Cassel, M.D., University of Chicago Medical Center
Discussion

2:45 UNDERSTANDING THE LEGAL AND SOCIAL CONTEXT
Legal Considerations
Robert Burt, J.D., Yale University
James Strain, M.D., Denver, Colorado
Cultural Perspectives
Barbara Koenig, Ph.D., Stanford University Center for
Biomedical Ethics
Kathryn Hunter, Ph.D., Northwestern University
Discussion

4:15 IMPROVING DECISIONMAKING
Educating Physicians
Neil MacDonald, M.D., University of Alberta
Informing Patients and Families
Edwin Cassem, M.D., Massachusetts General Hospital
Developing Practice Guidelines
Lawrence Schneiderman, M.D., University of California at
San Diego
Discussion

6:00   Presentation on SUPPORT Program
        Joan Teno, M.D., and Joanne Lynn, M.D.,
        Dartmouth-Hitchcock Medical Center

December 3

8:00   **ROUNDTABLE DISCUSSION OF PRIORITIES**
        Productive topics and strategies
        Research agenda

10:30   Adjourn Workshop

COMMISSIONED AND COMMITTEE BACKGROUND PAPERS

1. Apparent Impact of Laws Affecting Dying, Decisionmaking and
    Appropriate Care
        Robert A. Burt, J.D.
2. Attitudes of Physicians Toward Caring for the Dying Patient
        Christine Cassel, M.D.
3. Difficult Deliberations about Care at the End of Life
        Edwin Cassem, M.D.
4. Epidemiology of Death: The How, Why, Where and Symptoms of
    Dying
        Kathleen M. Foley, M.D.
5. Narratives of Dying
        Kathryn Montgomery Hunter, Ph.D.
6. Bioethical Perspectives for Pediatric Patients
        Robert M. Kliegman, M.D.
7. Cultural Diversity in Decision-Making about Care at the End of
    Life
        Barbara A. Koenig, Ph.D. (See Appendix E of this report)
8. Educational Strategies for Improving Physician Care of Dying
    Patients
        Neil MacDonald, M.D.
9. Available Data for Studying Dying in America
        Vincent Mor, Ph.D.
10. Pediatric End-of-Life Decision Making and the Role for Objective
    Risk Assessment
        Murray M. Pollack, M.D., Kantilal M. Patel, Ph.D., and
            Urs E. Ruttimann, Ph.D.
11. Should the Institute of Medicine Develop Guidelines for Medical
    Treatment Decisions in Critically Ill and Dying Patients?
        Lawrence J. Schneiderman, M.D.

12. The Treatment of Seriously Disabled Newborns
    James E. Strain, M.D.
13. The Use of Clinical Models for "End of Life" Decision-Making in Critically Ill ICU Patients
    George E. Thibault, M.D. (See Appendix D of this report)

WORKSHOP PARTICIPANTS

Henry J. Aaron, Ph.D.
Senior Fellow
The Brookings Institution
Washington, DC

Linda Blank
Vice President
American Board of Internal
    Medicine
Philadelphia, PA

Robert A. Burt, J.D.
Alexander M. Bickel Professor of
    Law
Yale Law School
New Haven, CT

Christine K. Cassel, M.D.
Professor of Medicine
Professor of Public Policy Studies
The University of Chicago Medical
    Center
Chicago, IL

Edwin H. Cassem, M.D.
Psychiatrist
Massachusetts General Hospital
Boston, MA

Nathan I. Cherny, M.B.B.S.
Pain Fellow
Pain Services, Department of
    Neurology
Memorial Sloan-Kettering Cancer
    Center
New York, NY

Marilyn J. Field, Ph.D.
Senior Program Officer
Institute of Medicine
Washington, DC

Kathleen M. Foley, M.D.
Chief, Pain Services
Department of Neurology
Memorial Sloan-Kettering Cancer
    Center
New York, NY

Carlos Gomez, M.D.
Resident
University of Virginia
Charlottesville, VA

Patrick Hill
Director of Education
Choice in Dying, Inc.
New York, NY

Kathryn Hunter, Ph.D.
Professor of Medicine
Northwestern University
Chicago, IL

Mo Katz
Senior Program Advisor
The Commonwealth Fund
New York, NY

Robert M. Kliegman, M.D.
Professor and Chair of Pediatrics
Medical College of Wisconsin
Milwaukee, WI

Barbara Koenig, Ph.D.
Executive Director
Stanford University Center for
  Biomedical Ethics
Palo Alto, CA

Kathleen Lohr, Ph.D.
Director, Division of Health Care
  Services
Institute of Medicine
Washington, DC

Joanne Lynn, M.D.
Professor of Community and Family
  Medicine
Dartmouth Medical School
Hanover, NH

Neil MacDonald, M.D.
Alberta Council Forum Professor
  of Palliative Medicine
University of Alberta
Edmonton, CANADA

Murray Pollack, M.D.
Associate Director, Pediatric ICU
Children's National Medical Center
Washington, DC

Richard Rettig, Ph.D.
Senior Program Officer
Institute of Medicine
Washington, DC

Lawrence Schneiderman, M.D.
Professor of Medicine
University of California at San
  Diego
La Jolla, CA

Anne A. Scitovsky, M.A.
Senior Staff Scientist, Health
  Economics Department
Palo Alto Medical Foundation
Palo Alto, CA

James E. Strain, M.D.
Denver, CO

William Stubing
President
The Greenwall Foundation
New York, NY

Joan Teno, M.D.
Assistant Professor, Department of
  Community and Family
  Medicine
Dartmouth-Hitchcock Medical
  Center
Hanover, NH

George E. Thibault, M.D.
Chief of Medicine
Brockton-West Roxbury V.A.
  Medical Center
W. Roxbury, MA

Donna D. Thompson
Administrative Assistant
Institute of Medicine
Washington, DC

B

Institute of Medicine
Committee on Care at the End of Life
Public Meetings

PUBLIC HEARING
National Academy of Sciences
Washington, D.C.
APRIL 29, 1996

AGENDA

9:00–9:05   WELCOME
Dr. Christine Cassel

9:05–9:50   **PANEL 1**

American Academy of Pediatrics
Allen Fleischman, M.D., F.A.A.P.
Senior Vice President
New York Academy of Medicine

Alzheimer's Association
Ladislov Volicer, M.D., Ph.D.
Professor of Pharmacology and Psychiatry, Assistant Professor of Medicine
Boston University School of Medicine

American Cancer Society
Mary Simmonds, M.D.
Chair, ACS Advisory Group on Cancer Pain Relief

Agency for HIV/AIDS
Melvin Wilson
Agency Administrator

9:50–10:30   **PANEL 2**

American Alliance of Cancer Pain Initiatives
Kim Calder
MPS Board of Directors
New York State Cancer and AIDS Pain Initiative

American Geriatrics Society
Joseph Fins, M.D.
Vice Chair, Ethics Committee

Gerontological Society of America
Marshall Kapp, J.D., M.P.H.
Director, Office of Geriatric Medicine and Gerontology
Wright State University School of Medicine

10:45–11:45   **PANEL 3**

American Board of Internal Medicine
Linda Blank
Vice President for Clinical Competence and Communications

American Medical Association
Thomas Reardon, M.D.
Vice Chair, Board of Trustees

American Academy of Family Physicians
Bruce Bagley, M.D.
Member, Board of Directors

American Nurses Association
Colleen Scanlon, R.N., J.D.
Director for Ethics and Human Rights

Academy of Hospice Physicians
Ira R. Byock, M.D.
President-Elect

1:00–1:45   **PANEL 4**

American Academy of Neurology
Kenneth M. Viste, Jr., M.D.
President

National Association of Black Social Workers
Iris Carlton-LaNey, Ph.D.
Associate Professor
University of North Carolina Chapel Hill School of Social Work

American Pain Society
Mitchell B. Max, M.D.
Pain Research Clinic
National Institute of Dental Research/National Institutes of Health

1:45–2:30   **PANEL 5**

American Hospital Association
Jonathan T. Lord, M.D.
Senior Advisor for Clinical Affairs

National Hospice Organization
John J. Mahoney
President

American Association of Health Plans
Michael Felder, D.O., M.A.
Chair, Ethics Committee, Community Health Plan

American Association of Homes and Services for the Aging
Stephen Proctor
Chair-Elect

2:30–3:15   **PANEL 6**

VITAS Healthcare Corporation of Florida
Richard B. Fife, M.D.
Vice President for Bioethics and Pastoral Care
Melanie Merriman, M.D.
Director of Outcome Management and Research

Hospice of the Blue Grass
Gretchen Brown, M.S.W.
President and CEO

Washington Home and Hospice
Elizabeth Cobbs, M.D., F.A.C.P.
Medical Director

3:15–4:00   **PANEL 7**

Association of Academic Health Centers
Roger J. Bulger, M.D.
President

American Bar Association Commission on Legal Problems of the Elderly
Charles Sabatino, J.D.
Assistant Director

ADDITIONAL GROUPS SUBMITTING WRITTEN TESTIMONY*

American Association of Retired Persons
American Board of Hospice and Palliative Medicine
American Hospice Foundation
American Medical Directors Association
Choice in Dying
Death with Dignity
The Hospice Nurses Association
International Institute for the Study of Death
The Islamic Medical Association
Kaiser Foundation Health Plan, Inc.
Memorial Sloan-Kettering Cancer Center

---

*100 Groups were invited to submit statements.

PUBLIC MEETING
Arnold and Mabel Beckman Center
National Academy of Sciences
Irvine, California
November 23, 1996

AGENDA

9:00   WELCOME
        Dr. Christine Cassel

9:15–10:45

Supportive Care of the Dying: A Coalition for Compassionate Care
Alicia Super, R.N., B.S.N., O.C.N.
Project Coordinator

Kaiser Permanente of Southern California
Richard Della Penna, M.D.
Regional Elder Care Coordinator

10:45–Noon

Marin (California) Home Care
Patricia Murphy, R.N., M.A.
Director

Hospital Home Health Care Agency of California
Claire Tehan, M.A.
Vice President

Visiting Nurse Associates and Hospice of Northern California
Brad Stuart, M.D.
Medical Director

California Department of Justice
William Marcus, J.D.
Deputy Attorney General
Liaison Counsel, California Board of Pharmacy

City of Hope National Medical Center
Betty Ferrell, Ph.D., F.A.A.N.
Associate Research Scientist

HealthCare Partners Medical Group
Lynne Emma, R.N., M.P.H.
Vice President, Population and Disease Management

2:30–5:00

Washington State Senate Health and Long-Term Care Committee
Donald Sloma
Senior Analyst and Staff Coordinator

Center for Ethics in Health Care, Oregon Health Sciences University
Susan Tolle, M.D., F.A.C.P.
Director

UCLA School of Medicine
Neil Wenger, M.D.
Chair, UCLA Medical Center Ethics Committee

Center for Biomedical Ethics, University of Minnesota
Steven Miles, M.D.
Associate Professor

General discussion

5:00   ADJOURN

C

Examples of Initiatives to Improve
Care at the End of Life[*]

This appendix illustrates the variety of initiatives being undertaken to improve end-of-life care. It is not intended to be comprehensive, and inclusion does not imply endorsement by the Institute of Medicine. A more extensive database is being developed by **Americans for Better Care of the Dying** (202-530-9864) and will be used to facilitate further collaborations and sharing of information. Information for this resource will be appreciated. Initiatives are listed alphabetically by organization.

Alliance for Aging Research
Health Care Costs of the Elderly, Terminally Ill

Contact: Daniel Perry, Executive Director
2021 K Street, NW, Suite 305
Washington, DC 20006
202-293-2856

Research reveals that physician and hospital costs for people in their 80s and 90s are lower than for younger groups. Aggressive technological interventions are more likely to go to people with good functional status and prospects for recovery rather than to older terminally ill people. Despite

---

[*]The committee wishes to express its gratitude to Anne Boling, The George Washington University Center to Improve Care of Dying, for assistance in compiling this appendix.

such scientific evidence, the view of the elderly, terminally ill patient consuming large amounts of resources shortly before he or she dies still pervades our national consciousness. The alliance has examined that view in a recently released study entitled *Seven Deadly Myths: Uncovering the Facts about the High Cost of the Last Year of Life*. This document provides up-to-date data on health care costs during the last year of life in the very old. The study provides an analysis of the most current literature and scientific data available on the topic.

American Academy of Hospice and Palliative Medicine (AAHPM) and American Board of Hospice and Palliative Medicine (ABHPM) Physician Hospice/Palliative Care Training

Contact: Dale Smith, Executive Director
           PO. Box 14288
           Gainesville, Florida 32604-2288
           352-377-8900

The long-term objective of the AAHPM's physician training project is to improve the care of patients with active, progressive, far advanced disease for whom the prognosis is limited and the focus of care is on improving quality of life. To improve the care of terminally ill patients, the Academy is developing a 20-hour curriculum entitled Physician Hospice/Palliative Care Training that promotes physician competence in end-of-life care. The curriculum consists of a series of integrated, clinically-oriented, self-contained, self-instructional modules called UNIPACs that apply adult learning theories and practices to end-of-life care. Each of the approximately 100-page modules follows the recommended format for self-instructional learning and includes behavioral objectives, a pretest, reading material, problems commonly encountered in end-of-life care and suggested interventions, clinical situations for demonstrating knowledge application, a posttest, and references. Several of the UNIPACs also include detachable reference tables that address topics such as oral morphine equivalents, suggested adjuvant drug dosages, causes and treatments for dysphagia and dyspnea, pharmacological treatments for the pain, nausea, and constipation associated with bowel obstruction, and depression assessments.

The UNIPACs are designed for use by practicing physicians, by medical students and residents in academic centers of medicine, and by hospice/ palliative care programs that offer clinical rotations for physicians in training. The curriculum focuses on many of the fundamental elements of end-of-life care identified by the Institute of Medicine, including: 1) effective techniques for assessing and controlling pain and other distressing symptoms, 2) alleviating death-related psychological and spiritual distress, 3) assessing and managing complicated grief reactions, 4) communicating effectively with patients and family members, 5) making ethical decisions, 6) participating on interdisciplinary teams, and 7) cultivating empathy and sensitivity to religious, ethnic, and other differences. The UNIPACs are as follows: 1) The Hospice/Palliative Approach to Caring for the Terminally Ill; 2) Alleviating Psychological and Spiritual Pain in the Terminally Ill; 3) Assessment and Treatment of Pain in the Terminally Ill; 4) Management of Selected Nonpain Symptoms in the Terminally Ill; 5) Caring for the Terminally Ill: Communication and the Interdisciplinary Team Approach; and 6) Ethical and Legal Decision Making When Caring for the Terminally Ill.

The ABHPM has developed a palliative care certification program that includes requirements for licensure, medical specialty certification, clinical and interdisciplinary care experience, and active care of at least 50 terminally ill patients in the last three years. The first certification examination was offered in November 1996.

American Board of Internal Medicine
Project to Improve End-of-Life Patient Care

Contact: Linda Blank
Vice President for Clinical Competence and Communications
American Board of Internal Medicine
510 Walnut Street, Suite 1700
Philadelphia, PA 19106-3699
(215) 446-3500
www.abim.org

In October 1993, the American Board of Internal Medicine (ABIM) began a special project dedicated to improving end-of-life patient care. The fundamental goals of this project were to identify and promote physician competency in the care of dying patients during internal medicine residency and subspecialty fellowship training. Internal medicine program directors were informed about the project and were invited to contribute examples of curricula, conference topics, and educational and experiential activities organized around the care of dying patients and support of family. National meetings and projects of health-related organizations continue to provide a forum for learning from and talking to audiences of physicians, patients, health care professionals, and medical educators. These have included the Association of American Medical Colleges (AAMC), American College of Physicians (ACP), Association of Professors of Medicine (APM), Association of Program Directors in Internal Medicine (APDIM), Clerkship Directors in Internal Medicine (CDIM), International Congress on Palliative Care, and Residency Review Committee for Internal Medicine (RRC-IM).

The ABIM End-of-Life Patient Care Project has created several products including *Caring for the Dying: Identification and Promotion of Physician Competency—Educational Resource Document*, which was developed primarily for program directors and faculty in residency and subspecialty training programs. The companion volume of *Personal Narratives* presents personal stories contributed by physicians that illustrate the special and rewarding connection between doctor and patient in life and in death. Independently developed films, *On the Edge of Being...When Doctors Confront Cancer* and *Notes from the Edge, Diary of Peter Morgan, MD,* created and produced by Ruth Yorkin Drazen, are also provided by ABIM at no cost. Over 30,000 copies of the resource documents have been distributed to training programs, hospices, and nursing homes and at national meetings of various medical organizations. Other products of the project include a set of educational objectives, slide packet, and collection of reprints—all designed for use in educational programs. In addition, a self-assessment survey of internal medicine residents was developed and piloted in 60 representative training programs training over 1600 residents from June 1995 to June 1997 to seek their perceptions. The directors of these programs have also been surveyed. These surveys establish a starting point from which to monitor the project's impact.

Among other steps, the ABIM is encouraging continued development of test items on end-of-life patient care for use on ABIM certification and recertification examinations, the ACP/APM/APDIM in-training examination, and the ACP medical knowledge self-assessment programs. It is also encouraging the American Board of Medical Specialties member boards to include test items on end-of-life patient care on their certification and recertification examinations.

American Medical Association
Program to Train Physicians in End-of-Life Care

Contact: Linda Emanuel, M.D.
            Vice President for Ethics Standards
            American Medical Association
            515 North State Street
            Chicago, IL 60610
            312-464-5619
            www.ama-assn.org

This is a major, profession-wide educational program on how to provide quality advance care planning and comprehensive palliative care. The program combines a top-down approach and a professional grass roots model. The top-down approach provides education at national and regional conferences and workshops and is intended to directly reach about 10 percent of all United States physicians, most of whom will be leaders and role models in their medical communities. To reach the roots of the profession, the program disseminates specially developed continuing medical education materials to *all* direct patient-care physicians in the United States. This program, along with parallel activities already under way at the AMA, will secure endorsement for end-of-life care skills among the leaders and role models in medicine.

This program seeks to educate physicians throughout the country in the practicalities of discussion and completing advance care planning, and in the goals and interdisciplinary clinical skills of palliative care. The program is intended also to promote endorsement of these skills by the leadership and general culture of medicine. The Advance Care Planning activities provide training in practical skills, including role play as well as instruction.

The philosophy of this intervention is that every physician should be able to recognize palliative care needs and either provide them personally, or secure help from an appropriate colleague. Evaluation of the program will occur at predetermined stages. At each step, data will be analyzed, interpreted, and used in a continuous quality improvement approach to insure maximal efficacy of the intervention.

A follow-through program will be designed to consolidate and sustain the intervention effects. It will involve the establishment of a network of centers of expertise that will continue to create the core group of experts who will be the role models and educators of the future. These centers will provide medical school, residency, and fellowship training within integrated programs at health care delivery sites.

Association of Academic Medical Centers
Education of Physicians about Dying

Contact: R. Knight Steel, M.D.
           Hackensack University Medical Center
           30 Prospect
           Hackensack, NJ 07601
           201-996-2503

Despite the changing nature of disease, from acute to chronic, and the aging of the population, much of medicine continues to focus on the three-step sequence of diagnosis, treatment, and cure. Often the medical educational process fosters an attitude of disinterest in managing the care of those who may not be appropriate candidates for "aggressive" intervention. To influence educational policy on the issue of dying, the project will review (1) the requirements of the residency review committees of internal medicine and family practice; (2) the examinations of the primary boards of internal medicine and family practice; and (3) the requirements and examinations for the subspecialties of geriatrics, oncology, and cardiology. The review will determine the extent to which these examinations and training programs are directed to care of the dying, control of pain, and advance directives.

Barnard College
Cross-Cultural Dimensions of Death and Mourning in Relation to Organ Donation

Contact: Lesley A. Sharp, Ph.D.
            Barnard College
            Columbia University
            3009 Broadway
            New York, NY 10027-6598
            212-854-5428

This project is an anthropological investigation into the cross-cultural dimensions of death and mourning, and their specific relevance to professional versus lay attitudes in the context of organ donation and procurement in urban Manhattan. Preliminary research reveals that the donation process alters grieving and may, in fact, prolong and even intensify the period of grief and mourning. The final objective of the anthropological findings of this project will be to suggest future policies and training guidelines for procurement professionals.

Baystate Medical Center
Dialysis Discontinuation: The Decision to Die and the Quality of Dying

Contact: Lewis M. Cohen, M.D.
            759 Chestnut Street
            Springfield, MA 01199
            413-784-3376

A bioethical, psychiatric, and clinical study of the decision by patients to terminate life-sustaining kidney dialysis treatment. Approximately 75 patients with end-stage kidney disease will be observed, interviewed, and evaluated to explore their decisionmaking processes and to examine their quality of death. In a smaller pilot study, Dr. Cohen found that patients and their families usually made the decision to stop treatment because of progressive deterioration, often sought spiritual counseling in making the decision, did not view the decision as being a suicidal act, and did not appear to be unduly influenced by psychiatric disorders such as depression. Seven of 11 patients were judged to have had a "good" death, dying shortly after stopping dialysis without evident physical or psychological suffering.

Colorado Collective for Medical Decisions, Inc.

Contact: Susan Fox Buchanan, J.D.
Executive Director, CCMD
777 Grant Street, Suite 206
Denver, CO 80203
303-832-3002

The Colorado Collective for Medical Decisions (CCMD) is a nonprofit organization and tax-exempt public charity comprised of health care professionals and lay citizens. Its mission is to create clinically sound, community-based guidelines for appropriate end-of-life medical treatment. Draft guidelines are currently being presented to a broad variety of public groups and medical providers in community workshops, clinic interviews, public forums, telephone surveys, and questionnaires. These include recommendations on appropriate end-of-life care, comfort care, shared decision making, cardiopulmonary resuscitation, permanent vegetative state, end-stage dementia, tube feeding, and dialysis.

As a separate phase, CCMD is developing a pilot project to improve medical decisionmaking for patients who are critically ill, permanently unconscious, or debilitated by a progressive and ultimately fatal disease with death expected within one year. The project offers involved parties access to a medical advisory panel, coupled with mediation, as a supplement to existing case conferences and ethics committees. The goal of this project is to contribute to an evolving climate of non-adversarial communication and constructive participation among patients, providers, case managers, and payers. It hopes to minimize poor communication, litigation, and media exposure that can drain and polarize parties.

The pilot project offers two phases to supplement existing ethics committees: mediation and medical review panels. Mediation facilitates non-adversarial communication and resolution among the parties to a conflicted case while the medical review panel makes neutral, non-binding clinical information available to all parties. Innovative aspects of the CCMD pilot project include

- clinical review and mediation outside the treating facility, with the intention of assuring neutral "outside" evaluation;
- clinical review panels constituted as needed from practitioners in

fields of practice unique to each case; there is a pool of variously creden-
tialed physicians rather than a single standing review panel.

• clinical review panels and mediation providing advisory information
and facilitated dialogue, not binding administrative decisionmaking; and

• utilization review, case management, and insurance coverage
issues introduced in a controlled, neutral environment that is intended
to bring resource considerations, as well as clinical information, into
decisionmaking.

Dartmouth College
Multi-Method Research to Understand the Experience of Dying in
Seriously Ill Adults

Contact: Marguerite M. Stevens, Ph.D.
            Associate Professor
            Community and Family Medicine
            Dartmouth College
            7927 Strasenburgh
            Hanover, NH 03755
            603-650-1538

A multi-method, cross-disciplinary analysis will be developed to understand more about the dying experience of seriously ill adults through analyzing patient and family reports of severe pain and developing descriptive
models of "good" and "bad" dying experiences from the viewpoints of the
patient and family. Some of the uniquely detailed database and innovative
methods to be used will be from an already successfully developed pain
intervention database titled, "the Study to Understand Prognoses and Outcomes of Risks of Treatments" (SUPPORT). This database consists of an
innovative method of integrating and summarizing findings via the use of
interview, narrative, and quantitative data. One hundred thirty two cases
will be studied.

Edmonton General Hospital
An Integrated Multidimensional Tool Kit for the Assessment of Terminal
Cancer Patients and Their Families

Contact: Eduardo Bruera, M.D.
            Palliative Care Program
            Grey Nuns Community Health Centre
            1100 Youville Drive West, Room 4324
            Edmonton, Alberta, T6L 5X8 Canada
            403-450-7730

The project will develop a simple, multidimensional kit for the daily or weekly evaluation and follow-up of terminally ill cancer patients and their families. The key component of the kit is an assessment tool for patients to describe their physical and psychological symptoms, cognitive function, spiritual needs, and family support. The tool will enable the health care provider to be aware of these symptoms together with the patient's other vital signs. The design of the kit lends itself to use in the acute, long-term care, home health, or hospice setting.

Episcopal Diocese of Washington
Committee on Medical Ethics

Contact: Cynthia B. Cohen, Ph.D., J.D., Chair
           Committee on Medical Ethics
           PO Box 569
           Garrett Park, MD 20896
           301-942-6077

In the Diocese's project *Are Assisted Suicide and Euthanasia Morally Acceptable for Christians?: Perspectives to Consider*, the Committee on Medical Ethics "addresses the issue of assisted suicide/euthanasia as part of a larger report they are developing entitled, *Toward a Good Christian Death*. They believe that an adequate examination of the morality of assisted suicide and euthanasia requires exploring a whole set of moral and social questions about appropriate and compassionate care near the end of life."

Science has brought tremendous force to bear on the lengthening of life by all possible means in the form of technological advancement. This sometimes leads to a lingering and painful death for loved ones, which has prompted forceful debate about the acceptability of assisted suicide and euthanasia. In this document, the Episcopal Diocese has attempted to provide guidance to its members on the place of these concerns in end-of-life decisionmaking within the boundaries of the Christian faith.

The document examines contemporary factors which have brought the issues of assisted suicide and euthanasia to the forefront of end-of-life discussion. It defines for its constituency the key terms of the debate and discusses the distinction between assisted suicide and euthanasia as well as that between providing adequate pain relief to the dying and assisted suicide/euthanasia. Concluding arguments explore the current debate in detail.

The Fred Friendly Seminar
Before I Die: Medical Care and Personal Choices

Contact: Barbara Margolis
            Seminars, Inc. - WNET
            356 W. 58th St., Room C1035
            New York, NY 10019
            212-560-4944
            www.wnet.org/bid

The Fred Friendly Seminars are an ongoing series of public TV programs exploring important contemporary issues. Invited experts and other panelists engage in a Socratic dialogue to "confront what they would do in complicated situations where the 'right' choice is not clear." In April 1997, *Before I Die: Medical Care and Personal Choices*, funded by the Robert Wood Johnson Foundation, was broadcast nationally. The program's panel of guests confronts a series of hypothetical scenarios dealing with problems of patients and families as they face serious illness, dying, and death. It aimed to illustrate the difficulties of decisionmaking in the context of the current cultural and medical environment.

Concerns addressed in the broadcast included

- why families have such a hard time talking about death;
- whether patients and families expect too much of their physicians;
- how the high financial costs of dying burden patients and their families;
- whether all Americans should be required to clearly state their wishes regarding end-of-life care;
- whether pain at the end of life is necessary and can be alleviated;
- whether medical training related to end of life can be improved;
- why physicians treat patients with aggressive care, despite wishes to the contrary; and
- whether spirituality can be better brought into the dying process.

Videocassettes of the program are available (PBS Video at 1-800-424-7963) along with a companion viewer's guide that includes discussion questions, essays, information about advance planning. A website (www.wnete.org/bid) is intended to encourage ongoing education and dialogue.

Georgetown University St. Francis Center
The School-Based Mourning Group Project: A New Approach to
Assisting Bereaved Inner-City Youth

Contact: Janice L. Krupnick, Ph.D.
                The Georgetown University School of Medicine
                Department of Psychiatry
                3800 Reservoir Road, NW
                Washington, DC 20007
                202-687-1496

The aim of this program is to further develop, evaluate, and disseminate new service delivery programs involving therapies and techniques for further expression of pain and loss for bereaved school-age children in low-income, inner-city public schools who have experienced the death of a parent/parents due to violence, substance abuse, and, increasingly, HIV infection and AIDS.

The George Washington University Center to Improve Care of the Dying

Contact: Joanne Lynn, M.D., Director
                1001 22nd Street, NW, Suite 820
                Washington, DC 20037
                202-467-2222
                www.gwu.edu/~cicd

The Center to Improve Care of the Dying is an interdisciplinary organization engaging in research, advocacy, and education to improve the care of dying patients and those suffering with severely disabling diseases. Center staff encourage the development and realignment of health care funding to engender effective care. The center continues to address spiritual issues and the development of measures of quality of end-of-life services in health care. It was founded on the belief that life under the shadow of death can be rewarding, comfortable, and meaningful for almost all persons—but achieving that goal requires real change in the care system.

For the American Geriatric Society, CICD prepared an amicus brief for U.S. Supreme Court hearings on physician assisted suicide. The brief opposed constitutional recognition of a right to such assistance. The center has also described dying and decisionmaking in seriously ill adults, developed measurement tools for assessing quality of care and to foster development of accountability in care services, and carried out a project to evaluate the treatment of the dying process in medical textbooks.

CICD staff are developing a proposal called *MediCaring*. This project extends the concept of hospice to include a broader population of terminally ill individuals than that which currently benefits from the Medicare hospice program. CICD is responding to a need for comprehensive, supportive, community-based services that meet personal and medical needs, enhance the prioritization of patient autonomy and preferences, provide good symptom management, and ensure family counseling and support. Among other things, *MediCaring* will define financing strategies, recognize the family's role, and identify appropriate limits on medical interventions.

Effective reform will arise from an understanding of how our care system now responds to persons who are dying and from the educated design of improved processes and systems.

City of Hope National Medical Center
HOPE: Homecare Outreach for Palliative Care Education

Contact: Betty R. Ferrell, Ph.D., F.A.A.N.
            Associate Research Scientist
            City of Hope National Medical Center
            1500 E. Duarte Road
            Duarte, CA 91010-3000
            818-359-8111

This is a pilot demonstration to improve the quality of care for patients and families in non-hospice home care agencies through design, implementation, and evaluation of a model education program. The objective is a model program that can be disseminated widely through home care agencies to improve care for terminally ill patients and families. Over two years, a curriculum will be developed to test in five home care agencies that represent various models of home care delivery and provide care to culturally diverse populations.

Institute for Healthcare Improvement
Breakthrough Series Collaboration on Improving Care at the End of Life

Contact: Penny Carver
            Institute for Healthcare Improvement
            135 Francis Street
            Boston, MA 02215
            617-754-4800

Approximately forty health care organizations will be selected to work intensively for 12 months to implement the best available ideas for change and improvement in end-of-life care. The goal will be to achieve rapid, breakthrough change: significant improvement in comfort and satisfaction with reductions in the use of unwanted, non-beneficial, and other wasteful care. IHI will provide process improvement and other information, coaching, and communication strategies. Organizations will provide implementation teams and resource support as well as evaluation and sharing of details of change processes and results.

Areas for improvement include using palliative/supportive care; improving pain management; meeting the needs of families; improving communication among family and health professionals; reducing transitions at the end of life; decisionmaking about treatments; making advance planning work; identifying non-beneficial care; overcoming administrative/legal barriers to optimal care; educating and supporting professionals; promoting multidisciplinary care; and increasing community support for end-of-life care.

Johns Hopkins University
A Problem Solving Approach to Helping Families Care for the Dying Person with Cancer

Contact: Matthew Loscalzo, M.S.W., Director
Oncology Social Work
Johns Hopkins Oncology Center
600 North Wolfe Street
Baltimore, MD 21287
410-955-5668

People who die of cancer and other chronic diseases receive most of their care, during the period just prior to death, from family members who are often unprepared and unskilled in dealing with the complex and demanding tasks they face. This project will develop a program to better prepare family members for caregiving responsibilities. Family caregivers will receive problem solving education, information for solving caregiving problems, and continuing support for their problem solving efforts from health professionals and peers.

Marquette University
Fostering Humane Care of Dying Persons in Nursing Homes

Contact: Sarah A. Wilson, Ph.D., R.N.
PO Box 1881, Clark Hall 319
Milwaukee, WI 53201-1881
414-288-3812

This project will develop an educational program for staff and administrators aimed at improving the care of the dying in nursing homes (long-term care facilities). A qualitative research program will be pursued to identify the difficulties in providing humane care to dying residents in long-term care facilities. The qualitative research will include focus groups consisting of staff and administrators as well as interviews with the family members of recently deceased nursing home residents.

Medicare Rights Center
Initiative for the Terminally Ill on Medicare

Contact: Mary Ann Etiebet, Education Director
          Diane Archer, Executive Director
          Medicare Beneficiaries Defense Fund
          1460 Broadway, 8th Floor
          New York, NY 10036-7393
          212-869-3850

Lack of information about financing options for end-of-life care is a substantial barrier to quality care at the end of life. This initiative will educate consumers, their families, caregivers, professional counselors, and clinicians about Medicare hospice and home health care benefits for the terminally ill in both fee-for-service and HMO settings. The initiative will include an aggressive public relations campaign and consumer guide.

Missoula Demonstration Project, Inc.
The Quality of Life's End

Contact: Ira Byock, M.D., President
          Missoula Demonstration Project, Inc.
          1901 South Higgins Avenue
          Missoula, MT 59801
          406-728-1613

This is a long-term, community-based organization which was created to study and transform the culture and experience of dying, wherein research will be done to define the attitudes, expectations, and experiences related to death and dying in Missoula County, Montana. The results will provide the platform for future interventions and research in the next 15 years focused on bringing quality to life's end.

Mount Sinai Medical Center
National Committee on Financing Care at the End of Life

Contact: Christine K. Cassel, M.D.
           Professor and Chairman, Geriatrics and Adult Development
           Mount Sinai School of Medicine
           Box 1070, One Gustave L. Levy Place
           New York, NY 10029
           212-355-8400

This program, designed as a task force project, is to create a Diagnosis Related Group (DRG) for payment for terminal care services delivered to hospitalized patients and all palliative care. This new code will validate and legitimize the practice of palliative medicine by hospital professionals on behalf of their dying patients, since a reimbursed activity is much more likely to be viewed as an appropriate function for doctors and hospitals.

The National Hospice Organization
Medical Guidelines for Determining Prognosis in Selected Non-Cancer Diseases

Contact: Chris Cody
           The National Hospice Organization
           1901 North Moore Street, Suite 901
           Arlington, VA 22209
           703-294-4421
           www.nho.org

The NHO Standards and Accreditation Committee Medical Guidelines Task Force has developed this document as a guideline for hospice care or for Medicare/Medicaid hospice benefit eligibility for non-cancer patients. Based on medical criteria, the guidelines are designed to aid in identification of patients with a likely survival prognosis of six to twelve months.

General guidelines for determining life expectancy relate to clinical progression of the disease, nutritional status, and patient and family circumstances. In addition, specific criteria are included for heart and pulmonary disease and dementia.

National Prison Hospice Association
Development of Hospice Care in Correctional Facilities

Contact: Elizabeth Craig
            PO Box 941
            Boulder, CO 80306-0941
            303-666-9638
            www.npha.org

NPH provides information to correctional facility professionals on good yet cost-effective care of dying patients. In order to get the message out about the importance of providing compassionate care to dying individuals, NPH produces informational literature, makes presentations, does site visits, promotes inmate volunteer training, and advises in the development of prison hospice programs to promote hospice and similar palliative care programs in local, state, and federal correctional facilities across the country. The promotion effort includes the development of inmate-staffed hospice volunteer programs, development of national prison hospice guidelines, and the creation of a national network for the exchange of information between hospices and prisons.

The Neurologic Institute at Columbia-Presbyterian Medical Center
Palliative Care Decisionmaking and Outcomes in Amyotrophic Lateral Sclerosis

Contact: Lewis P. Rowland, M.D.
            Peregrine L. Murphy, M.Div.
            Dale Lange, M.D.
            Columbia-Presbyterian Medical Center
            710 W. 168th Street, #1311
            New York, NY 10032-2603
            212-305-8551

This project is a longitudinal investigation of the patterns of palliative care in patients with amyotrophic lateral sclerosis (ALS, also known as Lou Gehrig's disease) from diagnosis to death. ALS is an inexorably progressive disease, for which there is no cure. The investigation will examine the relationship between physicians' preferences for and attitudes toward life-sustaining treatment, patients' responses to the options offered, and the medical outcomes. Physicians' attitudes and practices regarding palliative treatment may determine whether patients receive appropriate palliative support and care throughout the course of their illness.

Open Society Institute
Project on Death in America

Contact: Julie A. McCrady
           Project Officer
           Open Society Institute/PDIA
           888 Seventh Avenue
           New York, NY 10106
           212-887-0150
           www.soros.org/death.html

The Faculty Scholars Program

The Faculty Scholars Program of the Project on Death in America supports outstanding clinicians, educators, and researchers in disseminating existing models of good care, developing new models for improving the care of the dying, and creating new approaches to the education of health professionals. One of the goals of the scholars program is to promote the visibility and prestige of clinicians committed to this area of medicine and to enhance their effectiveness as academic leaders, role models, and mentors for future generations of health professionals.

From its inception in July 1994 to the present, the program funded 32 PDIA and six Open Society Institute Soros Faculty Scholars, representing 23 medical schools out of 125 in the United States and 16 in Canada. The awards of $70,000 a year provide scholars with up to three years of support for 60 percent of their time on activities to improve professional practices and education related to end-of-life and bereavement issues.

An illustrative list of scholars and their work follows.

Harvey Max Chochinov, M.D., F.R.C.P.C.
Manitoba Cancer Treatment and Research Foundation, University of Manitoba, Winnipeg, Manitoba
> Research, education, clinical work, and advocacy focused on the psychiatric dimensions of palliative medicine.

Timothy J. Keay, M.D., M.A.–Th., C.A.Q.G.M., F.A.A.F.P.
University of Maryland School of Medicine, Baltimore, Maryland
> Development of a model quality improvement plan with a learner-centered educational program for nursing home physicians that improves the quality of end-of-life nursing home care.

David R. Kuhl, M.D.
University of British Columbia, Palliative Care Program, St. Paul's Hospital, Vancouver, British Columbia
> Development of programs to enhance patient care and physician awareness, based on the results of a study of the emotional, psychological, and spiritual issues surrounding the suffering experienced by people with terminal illnesses.

Marcia Levetown, M.D.
University of Texas Medical Branch at Galveston, Galveston, TX
> Development of a multi-disciplinary curriculum that will focus on inter-disciplinary team building, pain and symptom management, legal and ethical issues in end-of-life care, and the medical professional's own response to helping patients with terminal illnesses and their families.

Michael Lipson, Ph.D.
Columbia College of Physicians and Surgeons and Harlem Hospital, New York, NY
> To develop a skills-based training for health professionals that addresses their personal reconciliation to death and loss.

Susan J. McGarrity, M.D.
Penn. State University Hospital, Milton S. Hershey Medical Center, Hershey, PA
> Establishment of a hospital-based palliative care program to serve Penn State/Hershey Medical Center and its affiliated hospitals.

Walter M. Robinson, M.D., M.P.H.
Harvard Medical School and Children's Hospital, Boston, MA
> An examination of the medical and ethical aspects of end-of-life care for chronically ill children and their families and development of a specialized team of physicians, nurses, and other caregivers to meet their particular needs.

John Lee Shuster, Jr., M.D.
University of Alabama School of Medicine, University of Alabama at Birmingham, Birmingham, AL
> Development of clinical and educational programs focusing on psychiatric issues in terminal care such as anxiety, confusion, and delirium.

Daniel P. Sulmasy, O.F.M., M.D., Ph.D.
Georgetown University Medical Center, Washington, D.C.
   Development of measurements of the quality of care rendered to medical inpatients at the end of life including attention to patient care
   needs and patient and family satisfaction.

Sharon M. Weinstein, M.D.
University of Texas M.D. Anderson Cancer Center, Houston, TX
   Development and implementation of clinical care pathways to im-
   prove the care of dying cancer patients.

Grants Program

   To date, the Grants Program of the Project on Death in America has
supported 81 innovative approaches to understanding and changing the
process of dying and bereavement. Grants have been disbursed in the following areas:

   • the epidemiology, ethnography, and history of dying in the United
States
   • the physical, emotional, spiritual, and existential components in dying and bereavement
      • the contribution of the arts and humanities
      • new service delivery models for the dying and their family and friends
      • educational programs for the public about death and dying
      • educational programs for the health care professions
      • the shaping of governmental and institutional policy

**Oregon Health Sciences University Center for Ethics in Health Care
Research on End-of-Life Care in Oregon**

Contact: Susan W. Tolle, M.D.
           Virginia P. Tilden, R.N., D.N.Sc.
           Oregon Health Sciences University
           3181 SW Sam Jackson Park Rd., L101
           Portland, OR 97201-3098
           503-494-4466

This study compares end-of-life care in the three major settings where death
occurs in Oregon: acute care hospital, nursing homes, and home hospice.
Using death certificates of recently deceased adults, the study will contact
families and providers and collect data on the following key variables re-

lated to the patients and their deaths: (l) advance directives; (2) the extent to which deaths followed advance planning; (3) access to hospice; (4) preference for location of death versus location of actual death; (5) degree of pain and suffering versus effectiveness of comfort care efforts; (6) decisionmaking about level of aggressiveness of treatment; (7) family satisfaction with care and identification of problems; and (8) provider identification of barriers to compassionate care.

The Center is also a locus of continuing medical education activities for the State of Oregon and convened the statewide Task Force to Improve the Care of Terminally Ill Oregonians described later in this appendix.

The Park Ridge Center
Retrieving Spiritual Traditions in End-of-Life Care

Contact: Laurence J. O'Connell, Ph.D., S.T.D.
            211 E. Ontario St., Suite 800
            Chicago, IL 60611-3215
            312-266-2222

This education program is being developed to foster the establishment of structured, supportive environments in which individuals and faith-based communities can draw upon, revitalize, and expand the spiritual and practical resources offered by their religious and cultural traditions for understanding and facing death and dying. The lay ministry program will give participants an opportunity to provide and revitalize spiritual, emotional, and practical support to the dying and their families.

The Pennsylvania State University College of Medicine
McGill University Palliative Care Program
Case Narratives in Palliative Care

Contact: David Barnard, Ph.D.
            Anna Towers, M.D.
            P.O. Box 850
            Hershey, PA 17033-0850
            717-531-8779
            dxb12@psu.edu

The objective is to construct a set of case narratives in palliative care that describe the experiences of dying patients, their families, and health care providers as they interact with each other over the course of the patient's illness and treatment by the palliative care team. The emphasis in each narrative will be the patient's "inner life" or subjective experience and the caregivers' experiences of giving care. The narratives will depict how patients, families, and providers find personal meaning in illness and how personal meanings influence the experience and outcome of care.

Robert Woods Johnson Foundation
Last Acts

Contact: Victoria Weisfeld, M.P.H.
The Robert Wood Johnson Foundation
College Road East
P.O. Box 2316
Princeton, NJ 08543-2316
609-452-8701
www.lastacts.org

Responding to distressing findings from SUPPORT, the largest clinical study ever conducted with dying patients, a coalition of 72 prominent organizations was initiated to improve the quality of care for dying patients in the United States. Former First Lady Rosalynn Carter is the Honorary Chair of Last Acts, a collaboration initially supported by a grant from the Robert Wood Johnson Foundation. The coalition will seek specific reforms aimed at altering the behavior of physicians and other health care providers, payers of care, hospitals and nursing homes, and consumers themselves.

The project began in March 1996 with a conference bringing together leaders from both consumer and health care organizations to explore issues raised by the current end-of-life care system. An outgrowth of this meeting was the formation of six Last Acts Task Forces: The Family, Financing, Workplace, Service Provider, Provider Education, and Palliative Care. Each task force will approach care of the dying from a different perspective. Supporting the task forces are five resource committees covering spirituality, evaluation and outcomes, diversity, standards and guidelines, and communications. The Task Forces will report on their progress at the second Last Acts conference to be held on October 30, 1997.

Sacramento Health Care Decisions
ECHO (Extreme Care, Humane Options)

Contact: Marjorie Ginsberg, Project Director
ECHO
4747 Engle Road
Carmichael, CA 95608
916-484-2485

Community Recommendations for Appropriate, Humane Medical Care for Dying of Irreversibly Ill Patients proposes goals and strategies to be adopted by acute care facilities and providers in northern California's health care system. The document resulted from a multi-year inter-organizational project called Extreme Care, Humane Options (ECHO) under the direction of Sacramento Healthcare Decisions (SHD), a nonprofit, nonpartisan community organization. It is based on the work of multidisciplinary committees composed of local physicians and other health care professionals, and the views and values of local citizens.

The recommendations are predicated on five underlying principles. In summary:

• Patients must have necessary information and opportunity to exercise their right to choose among appropriate treatment alternatives and to refuse treatment offered.

• When cure is no longer possible and death is imminent or a profoundly diminished condition unacceptable to the patient is expected, health care professionals should not recommend procedures that increase patients' pain and suffering.

• The treatment provided by the health care team for those terminally or profoundly, irreversibly ill must be purposefully and conscientiously aimed at meeting the patients' physical, psychological, social, spiritual, and emotional needs in an environment of caring and support.

• The goal of treatment should be improvement of the patient's prognosis, comfort, well-being, or general state of health or maintenance at a level of functioning that constitutes a quality of life satisfactory to the patient. This includes not creating unrealistic expectations about the value of further interventions.

• Though the cost of treatment should not be the primary reason for precluding a treatment option, health care providers and consumers have a duty to be wise stewards of communal resources. Likewise, all must be aware of the financial burdens often borne by patients and families.

Five goals are identified for acute care facilities: develop treatment options responsive to the needs of dying or irreversibly ill patients and their families; identify patients at risk of inappropriate or unwanted medical treatment; improve communication among patients, families, physicians, other health care team members and health care settings to foster informed, timely and mutually satisfactory treatment decisions; assure that the patient/surrogate is the primary decisionmaker in choosing among appropriate treatment options; and support effective processes for preventing and resolving conflicts regarding treatment decisions that respect patient values and the professional integrity of health care providers.

Indicators for offering comfort care are outlined. For instance, comfort care must be an option in the event of persistent vegetative state, minimal cognitive function, irreversible and irreparable organ failure, imminent demise, and if the burdens to the patient of cure-oriented treatment are greater than the medical benefit to the patient.

Roles of other key health care providers are suggested. These include physicians, medical groups, long-term care settings, and health plans and payers. The guidelines identify key elements that could be incorporated into the policies and procedures of healthcare services to improve communication about treatment decisions.

St. Jude Children's Research Hospital
Deciding to End Curative or Life-Sustaining Efforts for Children or Adolescents with Cancer

Contact: Pamela S. Hinds, Ph.D., R.N., C.S.
            Wayne L. Furman, MD
            332 North Lauderdale
            Memphis, TN 38105
            901-495-3679
            pam.hinds@stjude.org

Many health care professionals desire to include the adolescent patient in end-of-life decisionmaking, yet they are reluctant to do so because of a fear that the child may lack sufficient understanding of his or her situation to participate competently. No research-based guidelines exist to help the physician resolve this dilemma. This study will define the factors that pediatric oncology patients, their parents, and health care providers consider when deciding to end curative treatment or life-sustaining efforts. It will also identify the actions of health care providers that contribute to the ability of parents to cope with the death of their child. Guidelines will be developed from the research findings.

Supportive Care of the Dying: A Coalition for Compassionate Care

Contact: Alicia Super, B.S.N., R.N.
            Project Coordinator
            4805 NE Glisan Street, 2E09
            Portland, OR 97213
            503-215-5053, or
            Larry Plutko, Chairperson
            206-464-3392

An interdisciplinary consortium from the Carondelet Health System, Catholic Health Association of the United States, Catholic Health Initiatives, Daughters of Charity National Health System, PeaceHealth, and Providence Health System committed to advancing supportive care and compassionate outreach to persons with life-threatening illness and their families and communities. With support and resources from Catholic health care leaders, administrators, and clinicians, the Supportive Care of the Dying: A Coalition for Compassionate Care (SCD:CCC) is developing comprehensive supportive care delivery models for adaptation to any and all communities in the United States. These models will, initially, be implemented in Catholic health care communities; thereafter, assistance will be offered for implementation within the broader community. It is estimated that this project will be completed in two to three years.

The model of comprehensive supportive care is founded on the moral values and social traditions of Catholic health care. Care of persons with life-threatening illness recognizes the last phase of life as rich and meaningful when multidimensional support for physical, psychosocial, and spiritual suffering are provided not only to the ill person but also to the person's family and the community in which they live. While the dying process is specifically addressed in the comprehensive supportive care model, early assessment and intervention are emphasized as key to achieving goals of relieving pain and minimizing suffering. To this end, the model extends it to non-traditional service areas and beyond the current restraints of hospice.

The initial product of the SCD:CCC is important research into the needs of persons with life-threatening illness, their families, and their communities. The Supportive Care Delivery Model is Catholic health care's compassionate response to this research. This comprehensive model is based upon the actual needs and perceptions of those individuals dealing with life-threatening illness rather than health care providers' assumptions about those needs.

In addition, SCD:CCC is producing the practice guidelines, leadership competency guidelines, educational programs, modules, and teams necessary for successful implementation of the model. All products of the committee shall be piloted in Catholic health systems in selected sites across the nation as determined by SCD:CCC. Products and implementation strategies will be monitored for quality throughout the process. Health care providers, persons with life-threatening illness, families, and community members are active participants in the project due to ongoing outreach from SCD:CCC for input and suggestions.

Task Force to Improve the Care of Terminally Ill Oregonians

Contact: Patrick M. Dunn, M.D.
          Task Force Chair
          Oregon Health Sciences University
          3181 SW Sam Jackson Park Rd., L101
          Portland, OR 97201-3098
          503-494-4466

The task force was convened in January, 1995 by the Oregon Health Sciences University's Center for Ethics in Health Care. Members include state health care professional organizations, state governmental agencies involved in health care, and health systems from the Portland area.

The task force was not designed to develop public policy but rather to act as a resource for those who do. It can tell policy makers what the medical community is doing to improve care for the dying in areas such as pain control and physician-patient-family communication. It can suggest ways in which proposed legislation might help or hinder good care at the end of life. It can provide technical consultation on various aspects of end-of-life care. The task force takes a position of neutrality with respect to physician-assisted suicide.

The Task Force has published a booklet, *The Final Months of Life: A Guide to Oregon Resources*, that is being distributed to all primary care physicians in Oregon.

Task force organizational membership list:

Adventist Medical Center (Portland)
Center for Ethics in Health Care, Oregon Health Sciences University
Department of Veterans Affairs Medical Center (Portland)
Health Law Section, Oregon State Bar
Kaiser Permanente, Northwest
Legacy Health System
National Association of Oncology Social Workers
Oncology Nursing Society, Mt. Hood Chapter
Oregon Alliance of Senior and Health Services
Oregon Association for Home Care
Oregon Association of Hospitals and Health Systems
Oregon Board of Medical Examiners
Oregon Board of Pharmacy
Oregon Health Care Association
Oregon Health Division
Oregon Hospice Association
Oregon Medical Association

Oregon Nurses Association
Oregon Psychiatric Association
Oregon Psychological Association
Oregon Society for Social Work Administrators in Health Care
Oregon State Board of Nursing
Oregon State Pharmacists Association
Sisters of Providence Health System
Tri-County Physician Supervisors Group and State EMS Committee

United Hospital Fund
Hospital Palliative Care Initiative

Contact: Connie Zuckerman, Project Director
           Hospital Palliative Care Initiative
           United Hospital Fund
           350 Fifth Avenue, 23rd Floor
           New York, NY 10118
           212-494-0729
           www.uhfnyc.org/initiat/initiat.htm

The United Hospital Fund's Hospital Palliative Care Initiative is a multi-year, multimillion dollar, 12-hospital research and demonstration initiative with goals to analyze and improve the quality of hospital care for persons near the end of life and to develop new hospital-based palliative care services in New York City hospitals. This initiative seeks to assess and fundamentally change the way hospitals in New York provide care for persons near the end of life and for their families. The initiative blends collaborative analysis and grantmaking to support demonstration projects at five New York City hospitals. Fund staff are directing a rigorous program evaluation and a dissemination strategy involving invitational meetings, conferences, and targeted publications.

The initiative is now in its second phase, following a one-year planning and development phase, in which 12 New York City teaching hospitals, academic medical centers, community hospitals, and municipal hospitals were awarded grants to conduct the research and data collection activities necessary to understand barriers to providing palliative care services and to develop appropriate models of palliative care service delivery within their institutions. In phase II, which began March 1997, 5 of the 12 hospitals were awarded $225,000 grants over a two-year period to implement programs based on the findings from Phase I. The five participating hospitals are:

Beth Israel Medical Center: Creating Medical Leadership
Brooklyn Hospital Center: Building Expertise, Respecting Boundaries
Montefiore Medical Center: Changing Physician Behavior
Mount Sinai Medical Center: Putting Education into Practice
Saint Vincent's Hospital and Medical Center: Raising Consciousness, Integrating Services

To supplement the individual planning projects and the collaborative efforts of grantees working with fund staff, the fund will also conduct its own research activities within these hospitals to further the role of hospital culture and organization as they relate to the delivery of care near the end of life. The fund will publish a report on end-of-life issues in the summer of 1997, drawing heavily on data provided by the hospitals participating in the initiative. It has also used its own grant program to support the work of other experts working in the field. The fund has awarded a one-year grant to support a medical sociologist's study of patterns of end-of-life care and decisionmaking in several NYC hospitals and has awarded another grant to the New York Academy of Medicine to develop an educational program for physicians and other clinicians in palliative care.

University of California—San Diego
A Comparison of Treatments Provided to Terminally Ill Patients in Managed Care and Fee-for-Service Settings

Contact: Lawrence J. Schneiderman, M.D.
Department of Family and Preventive Medicine
9500 Gilman Drive
La Jolla, CA 92093-0622
619-534-4206

The purpose of this study is to measure the effects of managed care on the types and volume of care delivered to the terminally ill. The study focuses on Medicare beneficiaries for two reasons: first, because fee-for-service data are readily available on all Medicare decedents, and second, because large numbers of decedents are enrolled in Medicare. The study seeks to determine whether the medical care delivered to Medicare enrollees in HMOs is any different from the medical care delivered to their fee-for-service counterparts.

University of New Mexico
Project with Hospices

Contact: Walter Forman, M.D., F.A.C.P.
           2100 Ridgecrest Drive, SE
           Albuquerque, NM 87168
           505-272-6082

This is a collaborative project with the hospices in Taos, Santa Fe, Gallup, and Alamogordo to develop a permanent regional educational, training, consulting, and research service in palliative care, including culturally sensitive palliative care.

University of Pittsburgh Medical Center
Evaluating Health Providers' Communication with the Terminally Ill

Contact: Gary Fischer, M.D.
           Assistant Professor of Medicine
           Division of General Internal Medicine
           Montefiore University Hospital, Suite W933
           200 Lothrop Street
           Pittsburgh, PA 15213-2582
           412-692-4857

Over the last ten years, medical educators have identified deficiencies in the care of the terminally ill and developed interventions to correct the problems, yet it is difficult to know if these interventions are improving physicians' interactions with dying patients. This physician-patient communication project will develop a tool for teaching and evaluation purposes. The tool will be used to assess the behavioral skills of health care professionals who care for the terminally ill by using four standardized patient scenarios regarding both giving bad news and eliciting patient preferences.

University of South Florida College of Medicine
Decision to Enter Hospice in the 90s

Contact: Ronald S. Schonwetter, M.D.
           University of South Florida College of Medicine
           Division of Geriatric Medicine
           12901 Bruce B. Downs Blvd., Box 19
           Tampa, FL 33612
           813-877-2200

The purpose of this project is to identify the factors that affect the decision whether to choose palliative/hospice care or to continue with a traditional/curative approach to care for a group of cancer patients with limited life expectancy. Structured interviews will be conducted with cancer patients, their caregivers, and physicians to examine this decision. Interviews will be conducted at The Hospice of Hillsborough, Inc., H. Lee Moffitt Cancer Center and Research Institute, and Tampa General Hospital. Programs should be developed as a result of this study to overcome barriers to receiving hospice care and increase access for terminally ill patients in need of such care.

University of Washington
Assessing Physician Performance in End-of-Life Care

Contact: Paul G. Ramsey, M.D.
Professor and Chair, Department of Medicine
University of Washington, Box 356420
Seattle, WA 98195-6420
206-543-4043

Physicians have a key role in directing care and resources to dying patients. Physicians are in a position to provide support and information to patients and their families as well as facilitate a team approach. Despite increasing interest in improving end-of-life care, no systematic method to assess a physician's performance in this area has been developed.

The evaluation system being developed will be a reliable, valid and comprehensive tool to evaluate physicians' care of dying patients. It will use ratings from peer physicians and nurses, as well as ratings from patients and their primary surrogates (family or close friends) to assess the physician's skills at the end of life.

University of Wisconsin Comprehensive Cancer Center
A Resource Program to Address Barriers to Availability of Opioids for Pain Relief

Contact: David E. Joranson, M.S.S.W., Director
Policy Studies, Pain Research Group, WHO Center
1900 University Ave.
Madison, WI 53705-4013
608-263-7661
www.biostat.wisc.edu/cancer/homepage.html

Although most pain associated with cancer and AIDS for both adults and children can be relieved by the use of opioid analgesics, such as morphine, there are barriers to adequate availability of opioid analgesics for medical use. These barriers include inadequate knowledge of pain physiology, pain management, and pharmacology; exaggerated fear of addiction; legal and regulatory restrictions; uneven health care coverage; lack of funding for health care services; high costs of some opioid medications; lack of opioid policy-related studies; and lack of opioid policy initiatives in the United States and in other countries.

A resource program will be developed to improve the capability of the Pain and Policy Studies Group to provide expert assistance to those seeking to reduce barriers to appropriate use of opioids in the United States and to help develop a cancer pain and palliative care initiative for central and eastern Europe. The center already provides expertise in the area of global pain and opioid availability policy studies and communications, including productions of the WHO newsletter *Cancer Pain Release*. A Resource Guide will be produced and disseminated and a World Wide Web site will be created.

Vermont Ethics Network

Contact: John Campbell, Executive Director
            Arnold Golodetz, M.D.
            Vermont Ethics Network
            City Center—89 Main Street
            Drawer 20
            Montpelier, VT 05620
            802-828-2909

The Vermont Ethics Network is a private, nonprofit educational organization consisting of professional and laypeople throughout Vermont who are interested in medical ethics, and who participate as volunteers in VEN's educational work. The mission is to promote public and professional awareness and understanding of ethical issues in modern health care, and to enhance decisionmaking based on values and principles on both personal and social levels.

Using a grassroots approach, VEN designed the Journey's End Project. They will hold a series of community forums to discuss what Vermonters generally think is the proper distribution of health care resources between hospital care, home care, hospice, and long-term care. The results of the forums will be discussed with health care providers in order to develop practical guidelines for achieving the public's goals. The goals and guidelines will then be presented to policymakers for further discussion and eventual implementation. The group has also published a booklet, *Taking Steps*, which provides a useful information format and worksheet for the public on advance directives.

The Whitmore Foundation
Hospice for the Deaf

Contact: Judith Lauterstein, Ph.D.
            The George Whitmore Foundation
            33 East 38th Street, Suite 3A
            New York, NY 10016
            212-867-6521

When hospitalized, the deaf frequently sustain long periods of social isolation. They cannot communicate with doctors and other hospital staff unless a qualified interpreter is present. Currently, there are no hospice programs actively serving the deaf community. The George Whitmore Foundation, in collaboration with the Jacob Perlow Hospice, will create a program of hospice care for the deaf at the end of life. A key component of this pilot program will be the collection of data from the deaf community about their experiences with end-stage illness.

Additional Internet Sites of Interest

The Compassionate Friends: www.jjt.com
Growth House, Inc.: www.growthhouse.org
The International Work Group on Death, Dying, and Bereavement:
    www.wwdc.com/death/iwg/iwg.html
The Union of American Hebrew Congregations:
    server.huc.edu/rjbackup/uahc/conv/adres/care.html
Health Care Financing Administration: www.hcfa.gov
Agency for Health Care Policy Research: www.ahcpr.gov

D

Prognosis and Clinical Predictive Models for Critically Ill Patients

George E. Thibault, M.D. [*]

The development of clinical predictive models in intensive care units has represented a significant advancement for clinicians, clinical investigators, intensive care unit (ICU) directors, and quality assurance managers. Early classification systems, such as the Killip Class for acute myocardial infarction, the Glasgow Coma Score, and other disease-specific scoring systems, were clinically based, simple, and widely embraced. Over the past decade, more complex models have been developed with the aid of computerized databases and statistical modeling. Knaus' APACHE model, now in its third version, has been the best known of these systems and has been disseminated on a worldwide basis. A similar model has been developed by Pollock for use in Pediatric ICUs (PRISM). Both the APACHE and PRISM models use a consensus-derived scoring system that has subsequently been validated in a variety of settings. Lemeshow and Teres have developed a mortality prediction model (MPM) based on empirical data.

More complex than their predecessors, these systems demonstrate greater precision in classifying patients into risk groups for likelihood of survival. The wide acceptance of these models and their demonstrated ability to accurately place patients in risk strata have led to the hope that these models will be useful to the clinician in making individual patient decisions. Specifically, the hope is expressed that these may enable us to make more

[*]Chief of Medicine, Brockton-West Roxbury Veterans Affairs Medical Center, West Roxbury, Massachusetts. Prepared for the Institute of Medicine Committee for the Feasibility Study on Care at the End of Life. (See Appendix A of this report.)

appropriate and timely decisions regarding the withdrawal or termination of care in critically ill ICU patients. Although it is attractive to use these models to make these difficult decisions on a more rational basis informed by patient risk, we should be cautious in embracing these models for this purpose. This essay will briefly touch on several problems related to this use of these models.

1. There are statistical limitations.

The models produce probability estimates. They are developed and validated on large patient populations. The data and models must be valid and reliable for aggregated groups of patients to satisfy statistical and methodological requirements. They have not been validated for individual patient decisions. For example, a model that predicts a 50 percent mortality for 100 ICU patients may prove to be 100 percent accurate when applied to the next 100 ICU patients viewed as a group, but if the model is used to identify the 50 individual patients who will live and the 50 who will die, it is theoretically possible to misclassify all of the patients and still be 100 percent accurate in aggregate. Among patients with a very high probability (>90 percent) of death, different problems exist. The calibration of the models is most suspect at the extremes of probabilities. The models invariably perform best in the midrange of probabilities and are most useful in that range when used on aggregated patients. Models lack statistical power among very high-risk patients because of the low number of cases in the very high-risk strata. The confidence limits around predictions of very high risk of death are likely to include probabilities that might make both clinicians and family members cautious about discontinuing therapy. In other words, our ability to predict death with sufficient certainty is unlikely to be an achievable goal on statistical grounds alone. The size of the database that would be required for statistical certainty among very high-risk patients is unlikely to ever be achieved within realistic cost and time constraints.

2. The models are inherently imperfect.

The models are in need of constant revision, hence APACHE III. This should give us pause about viewing the most current version of a model as definitive enough to make life or death decisions based on the model alone. These models have a number of potential limitations. Data elements used in the model may be missing or inaccurate. The time at which the variables are captured and their relationships to interventions are also potential sources of bias (see below). The model must be proven to give the same predictive accuracy when applied in different settings and over time (it must be "robust"). An ideal model would also apply to a patient population different from the one upon which it was generated, or at least the patients for whom it is not applicable should be known. Models lack generalizability if they are "overfitted" to the particular population and hence disproportionately reflect outliers or idiosyncratic values in that data set. Models may also fail to distinguish between data elements that represent process of care versus those that more truly represent the patient's condition. Models may also fail to distinguish between the effects of chronic disease compared with those of acute physiological derangement.

3. The model may not adequately account for disease specificity or the effect of intervention.

When APACHE was first developed, it was claimed that the predictive accuracy of this physiological scoring system was independent of disease process. In its third iteration, it is acknowledged that the intercepts are different for different diseases. It is very likely that this is in part true because of the variable effectiveness of interventions in different diseases. One could therefore predict that these relationships could change over time as new interventions are available or understanding of basic pathophysiology improves. Therefore, a given "score" might imply a different prognosis depending on the cause of the physiological derangement (e.g., severe metabolic acidosis due to diabetic ketoacidosis compared with cardiogenic shock).

4. Death is not the only outcome of interest.

The models are used almost exclusively to predict hospital-related death, and this is not the only outcome of interest to clinicians, patients, and families. Different models are likely to be needed to predict functional status, duration and quality of life following an ICU stay, and other outcomes that may be of importance to patients if we are going to use the models to decide when additional care is likely to be warranted or beneficial. Death is obviously the easiest end point to model, but if the models are going to be useful in ICU decisionmaking, we will need other end points to be modeled as well.

5. ICU illness is a dynamic process.

Models that use a single time point, frequently either entry to an intensive care unit or 24 hours later, fail to account for clinical changes over time that are an important part of clinical decisionmaking. Changes in patient clinical status add valuable information to predictive modeling. Several recent model development efforts incorporate this dynamic process (see Chang, 1989, and Lemeshow, 1988). Further developments in time-dependent models may further aid clinicians in using models to make more accurate prognostications.

6. The complexity of the models may make them less credible to clinicians and families.

The less accessible the models, the more they become a "black box." The p values of the current APACHE system are not available in the literature because this is deemed proprietary information by the developers and marketers of this model. Other models are usable only with computer software. These observations do not necessarily make the models less accurate, but they do deny them face validity and credibility with clinicians and families who will be the principal users in making end-of-life decisions.

7. There is a problem in determining the perspective to be taken by the modeler or the user of the model.

Are the models to be judged from the perspective of the individual patient or the perspective of society? If it is society's perspective, then some of the objections about the lack of power and calibration at the extremes may be less of a concern if, overall, the models have good predictive validity. For the physician or family trying to make the best decision possible for an individual patient, however, the performance characteristics of the model for that specific patient are of paramount importance.

All of these objections should not make us nihilistic about the use of models. I believe that the use of these models has furthered our understanding of the relationships between complex illness and outcomes in the ICU. They have refined our language and made more precise our discussions and writings. The models have certainly proven to be extremely useful in making comparisons from one ICU to another and in generating hypotheses about why care may be better and outcomes different in one unit versus another. The models have been helpful for clinical research so that we can be sure that patients are grouped by severity of illness. This is a necessary step in understanding whether observed differences in outcomes are related to structure or process of care as opposed to differences in patient risk. I believe, however, that we are far from achieving the goal of using individual patient level predictors to make difficult and painful decisions regarding which critically ill patients may no longer benefit from intensive care. These clinical predictors are one more piece of information, like any other diagnostic test, to be used in the context of the full clinical picture informed by patient and family preferences. Knowledge of the results of these predictive models and their methodological limits is useful to clinicians in framing the questions about end-of-life decisionmaking for themselves, the other caregivers, patients, and their families. The more accurate the predictive models and the narrower the confidence limits, the more useful they will be. What cutoff point will be the appropriate cutoff point to decide that no more should be done will remain, I believe, an individual decision informed by, but not made exclusively by, these increasingly accurate predictive models.

I am indebted to my colleague, Dr. Jennifer Daley, for her contributions to the ideas in this essay.

REFERENCES

1. Chang, R.W.S. Individual Outcome Prediction Models for Intensive Care Units. *Lancet* 2(8655):143–146, 1989.
2. Daley J., Jencks S., Draper D. et al. Predicting Hospital-Associated mortality for Medicare Patients. *Journal of the American Medical Association* 260(24):3617–3624, 1988.
3. Diamond G.A. Future Imperfect: the Limitations of Clinical Predication Model and the Limits of Clinical Prediction. *Journal of the American College of Cardiology* 14(3):12A–22A, 1989.
4. Iezzoni L.I., Moskowitz M.A. A clinical assessment of Medisgroups. *Journal of the American Medical Association* 260(:31):3159–3163, 1988.
5. Iezzoni L.I. "Black box" medical information systems. A technology needing assessment. *Journal of the American Medical Association* 265(22):3006–3007, 1988.
6. Jancks S.F., Daley J., Draper D., et al. Interpreting hospital mortality date. The role of clinical risk adjustment. *Journal of the American Medical Association* 260(24):3611–3616 1988.
7. Knaus W.A., Draper E.A., Wagner D.P., et al. An evaluation of outcome from intensive care in major medical centers. *Annals of Internal Medicine* 104(3):410–418, 1986.
8. Knaus W.A., Wagner D.P., Draper E.A., Zimmerman J.E., Bergner M., Bastos P.G., et al. The APACHE III prognostic risk system. Risk prediction of hospital mortality for critically ill hospitalized adults. *Chest* 100:1619–1636, 1991.
9. Knaus W.A., Wagner D.P., Zimmerman J.E., Draper E.A. Variations in mortality and length of stay in intensive care units. *Annals of Internal Medicine* 118:753–761, 1993.
10. Lemeshow S., Teres, Avrunin S.J., Pastides H. Predicting the outcome of intensive care patients. *Journal of the American Statistical Association* 83:348–356, 1988.
11. Pollack M.M., Ruttimann U.E., Getson P.R. Accurate prediction of the outcome of pediatric intensive care. *New England Journal of Medicine* 316:134–139, 1987.
12. Pollack M.M., Getson P.R., Ruttimann U.E., Steinhart C.M., Kanter R.K., Katz R.W., et al. Efficiency of intensive care. A comparative analysis of eight pediatric intensive care units. *Journal of the American Medical Association* 258:1481–1486, 1987.
13. Selker H.P. Systems for comparing actual and predicted mortality rates: characteristics to promote cooperation in improving hospital care. *Annals of Internal Medicine* 118:820–822, 1993.
14. Tores D., Lemeshow S., Avrunin S.J., Pastides H. Validation of the mortality prediction model for ICU patients. *Critical Care Medicine* 15:208–213, 1987.
15. Zimmerman J.E., Shorten S.M., Rousseau D.M., Duffy J., et al. Improving intensive care: Observations based on organizational case studies in nine intensive care units. A perspective, multicenter study. *Critical Care Medicine* 21(10):1443–1451, 1993.

E

Cultural Diversity in Decisionmaking About Care at the End of Life

*Barbara A. Koenig, Ph.D.**

INTRODUCTION

The overall goal of this IOM panel is to examine the questions: "What medical care is appropriate at the end of life? Who should decide?" My specific task is to locate these questions within the context of an increasingly diverse U.S. population. This view will of necessity be a fleeting one, providing images of this important terrain from an altitude of 10,000 feet; a quick flyover of issues better studied in-depth at ground level. A detailed examination of the hills and valleys inhabited by Americans from diverse cultural backgrounds is certainly needed; research is currently scant. An IOM study of dying, decisionmaking, and care at the end of life will need to avoid the many obstacles and pitfalls looming in this landscape. Most of the obstacles are camouflaged, hidden in our common sense assumptions about race, ethnicity, and cultural difference and in unexamined assumptions at the core of current bioethics practice. The goal of this paper is to provide a set of signposts for navigating through this terrain. I argue that these signposts are ultimately of more value than an approach that generates a list of "traits" specific to each ethnic group in the United States.

First, I will very briefly discuss how culture is relevant to health care,

---

*Paper prepared by Barbara A. Koenig, Ph.D., Senior Research Scholar and Executive Director, Center for Biomedical Ethics, Stanford University, Palo Alto, California. Prepared for the Institute of Medicine Committee for the Feasibility Study on Care at the End of Life. (See Appendix A of this report.)

363

for the issues surrounding death are but one subset of the general problem of how to take account of culture in the health care system. Next, I will review the key issue of how we talk about and understand cultural difference. What are these categories into which we divide our pluralistic society? I will next address the way in which existing bioethics practices surrounding death have failed to consider cultural difference. The latter topic is the focus of my current research. Using the methodological strategies of medical anthropology, I am studying how California patients from different cultural backgrounds make end-of-life decisions.[1] Implications of cultural diversity on individual decisionmaking and resource allocation will be discussed very briefly. The paper will conclude with recommendations for the IOM panel regarding research, clinical practice, and teaching about cultural diversity and end-of-life decisionmaking.

Although beyond the scope of this brief paper, it is vital to remember that culture is not simply an inconvenient barrier to a rational, scientifically based health care system or a feature of ethnic "others." Deeply embedded cultural values are apparent in the way American medicine has approached the care of the dying, particularly practices that have separated terminal care from mainstream practice, denied the existence of the dying patient, and assumed that death was simply one of many medical problems open to a technological solution (see Callahan, 1993; Muller and Koenig, 1988). Professionals can be usefully thought of as operating within a culture influenced by widespread cultural assumptions and practices as well as by training and experience. There also appears to be a clear line dividing the medical model from the patient's model of death and illness leading to death (Churchill, 1979). And differences in professional culture between nurses and physicians may lead to varying understandings of patients' prognoses, as Anspach has demonstrated for the neonatal intensive care unit (1987). Western European health professionals respond with astonishment when told about the American practice of requiring a "Do Not Resuscitate" order for an elderly person dying in a long-term care facility. Cultural "points of view," based on specific contexts of meaning, do not apply only to patients and families from backgrounds unfamiliar to their health care providers.

In an increasingly plural society, cultural diversity among American health care workers is another important consideration. It would be inappropriate to structure the debate as if providers uniformly express white middle-class culture in opposition to the "ethnic otherness" of patients. Particularly in large urban areas, the diversity of professionals and staff workers in hospitals, nursing homes and long-term care facilities is adding a major area of complexity to decisionmaking about tube feeding, treatment of acute illness, and withdrawal of therapeutic interventions (CAHA, 1993). Many health workers providing direct patient care do not share the assumptions on which current decisionmaking practices are based, such as the importance of respecting patient autonomy.[2]

CULTURE, ILLNESS, AND DEATH

Cultural analysis that reveals patients' understandings of health, illness, suffering, and death is a major concern of medical anthropology (Helman, 1990). Although "culturally sensitive" care has become a politically correct buzzword in health care recently, the use of the culture concept is often remarkably naive. Culture is often treated as a barrier to providing scientific medical care to diverse patients. Rather than recognizing the centrality of culture, "A barely hidden desire to create a 'shopping list' of cultural characteristics is sometimes discernible: Tamils do this, the Cree do that and Guatemalans do the other, in order to systematize and 'tidy up' culture in the same way as are other epidemiologic variables, such as smoking, age, gender, or fertility rates" (Lock, 1993b; p. 139). Culture is to be "overcome" in order to obtain patient compliance.

Most fully developed within the discipline of anthropology, the concept of culture is enormously complex; a full review of definitions is impossible within the scope of this paper. Emphasizing what culture is not is easier and more relevant to the goals of the IOM workshop. It is not a simple "trait," an objective, unchanging variable, located within the individual. Culture does not "determine" behavior under certain specified circumstances. Most importantly, culture is constantly re-created and negotiated within specific social and historical contexts. "Culture is now viewed not merely as a fixed, top-down organization of experience by the symbolic apparatuses of language, aesthetic preference, and mythology; it is also "realized" from the bottom-up in the everyday negotiation of the social world, including the rhythms and processes of interpersonal interactions" (Kleinman and Kleinman, 1991). Seemingly simple (and perhaps simple-minded) calls for "culturally competent care" ignore the dynamic nature of culture. Moreover, in a complex postmodern world, culture can no longer be simply mapped onto geographically isolated ethnic groups (Gupta and Ferguson, 1992). One cannot assume that a patient or family from Southern China will approach decisions about death in a certain culturally specified fashion.

Keeping in mind the warning that culture should not be considered as a simple "predictor" of behavior, it is nonetheless useful to consider how cultural analysis is critical to a full understanding of decisionmaking at life's end. Understandings of how death and the dying process are integrated into the experience of living are useful and can only be obtained by studying actual social processes (see Scheper-Hughes, 1992). Cultural conceptions of the self and personhood, the location of the individual within a social group such as the family, orientation to the future, openness about discussing death, and ideas about what constitutes appropriate behavior by healers are all directly relevant to end-of-life decisions.

In the classic study *Death and Ethnicity,* Kalish and Reynolds document that "ethnic variation is an important factor in attitudes, feelings, beliefs, and expectations that people have regarding death, dying, and bereavement" (1976, p. 49). However, the relationship is not a simple one. The authors continue, "At the same time that our data show substantial ethnic differences, we are also aware that individual differences within ethnic groups are at least as great as, and often much greater than, differences between ethnic groups" (p. 49). Most studies of ethnic difference do not question the assumptions underlying comparisons of this sort. However, a closer look reveals significant hazards in traditional comparative approaches to studying cultural difference.

THINKING ABOUT CATEGORIES:
RACE AND ETHNICITY IN THE U.S. HEALTH SYSTEM

One justification for considering cultural diversity in decisionmaking at the end of life is the enormous demographic change that is transforming the United States. Questions such as "who controls the dying process, what is beneficial treatment for the dying, and how will individuals respond to outcomes data about prognosis?" are being asked within a society that many argue is moving swiftly toward cultural pluralism. Simplistic models of acculturation and assimilation (based on and most applicable to European immigration) have been long abandoned by both historians and social scientists (Glazer and Moynihan, 1963; Lamphere, 1992). In Table E-1, the

TABLE E-1 U.S. Population 1990 and
Percentage Change, 1980–1990

Population Group	U.S. 1990	Change from 1980
African American	12%	13%
Asian and Pacific Islander	3	108
Hispanic origin	9	53
Native American	1	38
White	83	6
All other	4	45
Total	100	10

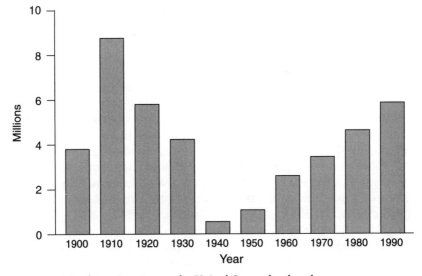

FIGURE E-1 Total immigration to the United States, by decade.

first column presents a summary of U.S. ethnic diversity as of the 1990 census; the second column shows the increase in diversity in U.S. population groups in the 10 years between 1980 and 1990 (Barker, 1992). Figure E-1 demonstrates the increase in (legal) immigration to the United States during this century.[3] In terms of absolute numbers, total immigration will soon equal that of the first decades of the twentieth century; a wave of immigration that fundamentally transformed American society. Bear in mind that the social changes caused by diversity are not uniformly distributed throughout the United States; in 1988, 46 percent of refugees were received by California (Barker, 1992). In many urban and rural counties in California fully one-third of residents are foreign-born, compared with 8 percent nationally (1990 census). However, the salience of cultural diversity is not simply a response to changing demographics. The issues are intricate, deeply political, and have relevance well beyond the realm of health.[4] Debates about appropriate care at the end of life will inevitably become entangled with political struggles about how to recognize "minority" voices in U.S. society.

At first glance, the categories into which we divide ourselves in American society seem self-evident and a feature of nature. In reality, these categories are highly contested politically, changing at least every 10 years when the debate about who "counts" emerges as a new census is planned. The U.S. census categories used to generate the data presented above are the end result of a political debate (featuring arguments about how to count

Hispanic people), which led to Office of Management and Budget Directive 15. This directive regulates the categories used in all federal statistics, including health statistics (OMB, 1978).

Without denying the existence of meaningful differences among groups, it is useful to consider the anthropological view that differences among people are primarily social constructs. Indeed, the traditional distinction between race and ethnicity is based on the notion that biological diversity is not salient in discussing differences among groups; ethnicity or ethnic identity is defined in terms of cultural variation. This was a major change over nineteenth and early twentieth century conceptions of race (or biological variation) as the bedrock of difference. Although the word *race* remains in popular use, there is general agreement that as a scientific classification it is based on outmoded concepts and dubious assumptions about genetic difference" (Barker, 1992, p. 248; see also Lock, 1993a).

Robert Hahn's empirical work with U.S. vital statistics illustrates some of the ambiguity in the way we count and define cultural difference in the United States. Table E-2 presents the results of Hahn's study, comparing the assigned race and ethnicity to U.S. infants at birth and at death one month later (Hahn et al., 1992).[5] The ways in which people define themselves, or are defined by others, are inherently fluid, changing significantly over time. Any attempt to consider issues of difference must include this complexity (CDC, 1993).

The political dangers of accepting social categorization in an uncritical way are best observed by considering such categories in the context of

TABLE E-2 Inconsistencies in Coding of Race and Ethnicity Between Birth and Death in U.S. Infants

Population Group	Discrepancy Birth/Death
African American	4.3%
White	1.2
Japanese	54.1
Chinese	47.6
Hispanic origin	30.3
Total	3.7

SOURCE: Adapted from Hahn et al. (1992).

another society. Sharp has written about the problems of categorization in South Africa.

> To many South Africans it is self-evident, a matter of common sense, that the society consists of different racial and ethnic groups, each of which forms a separate community with its own culture and traditions. It is believed that such groups actually exist objectively in the real world, and that there is nothing anybody can do to change this. . . . We take issue with this notion, arguing that all these groups, and the bases on which they are supposedly constituted, are social and cultural constructions. They are representations, rather than features, of the real world. They comprise the ways in which a portion of South African society tries to tell itself, and others, what that world is like. In other words, they are an interpretation, instead of a mere description of reality. Any interpretation depends on the identity, beliefs, knowledge and interests of the people doing the interpreting, as much as on the characteristics of the objects being interpreted. It follows from this that different races and ethnic groups, unique cultures and traditions, do not exist in any ultimate sense in South Africa, and are real only to the extent that they are the product of a particular worldview. (1988, p. 1)

Programs of research or suggestions for clinical practice that recognize cultural difference (whether defined as race or ethnicity) must be used with extreme caution (see also Sheldon and Parker, 1992; Osborne and Feit, 1992). This is particularly true in the U.S. context because of the significant overlap between categorizations based on race/ethnicity and the economic impoverishment of social class.[6]

CULTURE AND NEW BIOETHICS PRACTICES SURROUNDING DEATH

The timing and manner of death in hospitals and nursing homes are frequently negotiated, dependent on human agency (Slomka, 1992). Death and decisionmaking surrounding the event of death have been a primary focus of the evolving discipline of bioethics over the past 20 to 25 years (Callahan, 1993). Based on philosophical reflection and legal analysis, an array of new bioethics practices have entered into routine clinical care, the most recent being the Patient Self-Determination Act (Lynn and Teno, 1993).

Within the bioethics community, little attention has been paid to questions of ethnic or cultural diversity (for exceptions see Cross and Churchill, 1982; Hahn, 1983). A fundamental, and I would argue problematic, assumption of bioethics discourse has been universality. As Renee Fox has written, "There is a sense in which bioethics has taken its American [Western] societal and cultural attributes for granted, ignoring them in ways that imply that its conception of ethics, its value systems, and its mode of reasoning transcend social and cultural particularities" (1990).

Embedded within the new end-of-life practices are unexamined assumptions that stem from specific Western traditions. Innovations in health care ethics that emphasize advance care planning for death or a patient's "right" to limit or withdraw unwanted therapy appear to presuppose a particular patient. This ideal patient has the following characteristics: (1) a clear understanding of the illness, prognosis, and treatment options that is shared with the members of the health care team; (2) a temporal orientation to the future and desire to maintain "control" into that future; (3) the perception of freedom of choice; (4) willingness to discuss the prospect of death and dying openly; (5) a balance between fatalism and belief in human agency that favors the latter; (6) a religious orientation that minimizes the likelihood of divine intervention (or other "miracles"); and (7) an assumption that the individual, rather than the family or other social group, is the appropriate decisionmaker. Underlying these assumptions—and the innovations in clinical practice, such as the Patient Self-Determination Act, which they have spawned—is a theoretical perspective that I will call, for the sake of simplicity, the "autonomy paradigm." I make the assumption that an emphasis on the principle of autonomy has characterized much bioethics discourse over the past 25 years.[7]

The idealized view of decisionmaking common within bioethics also assumes that health care providers offer real choices to patients at the end of life, rather than simply dictate patients' answers by how information is presented or how scientific facts about prognosis are framed. There is also the (questionable) assumption that patients and providers are equally powerful in the clinical relationship.[8]

Another theme in contemporary bioethics has been the overall relationship of grand-scale ethical theories (like the principle of autonomy) to more mundane matters, such as practical ethical judgments or decisionmaking (Jennings, 1990; Jonsen, 1991; Hoffmaster, 1992). There are many ways to frame this dichotomy; one may speak of the relationship between normative and descriptive inquiry, for example. The two activities yield quite different forms of knowledge. "Theory can be discussed and argued in serene and unspecific terms: read Sidgwick or Rawls, where five hundred pages can go by without a detail of the casuists' 'who, what, when, where, why, and how'?" as Jonsen notes (1991, pp. 14–15). Theory is "very loosely tethered to the ground and can float quite free" (Jonsen, 1991, p. 14). Attention to grand-scale theories precludes attention to the social context of clinical practice.

Empirical or descriptive research in bioethics aims to be grounded, seeking after the "who, what, when, where, why, and how." Recent shifts within academic bioethics have opened the door for empirical work by anthropologists and other social scientists (Marshall, 1992). Attention to cultural diversity is made possible by this theoretical shift of focus.

Nonetheless, philosophical studies of the relevance of cultural difference to bioethics and decisionmaking are in their infancy. Pellegrino et al. (1992) and Veatch (1989) have both edited volumes that catalog the array of religious and cultural perspectives relevant to clinical bioethics. However, these works do not address the issue of potential conflicts in the United States when these myriad traditions collide (Orr et al., 1994). More fundamental is the question of whether an "ethnic perspective" on bioethics is philosophically justifiable, or desirable. African American philosophers express opposing views in a recent volume (Flack and Pellegrino, 1992).

Specific studies of how culturally diverse patients respond to innovations such as advance directives are only beginning to appear.[9] Clinical case reports demonstrate the potential for conflict when patients and providers have conflicting expectations (Meleis and Jonsen, 1983; Muller and Desmond, 1992). Garrett and colleagues have demonstrated that African Americans differ from European Americans in their willingness to complete advance directives and desires about life-sustaining treatment (Garrett et al., 1993). Using survey research to investigate wishes about life-prolonging treatment, Caralis and colleagues found that significantly more African Americans and Hispanics, "wanted their doctors to keep them alive regardless of how ill they were, while more . . . whites agreed to stop life-prolonging treatment under some circumstances" (1993, p. 158).

Although results from surveys asking hypothetical questions about patient preferences have inherent limitations, the findings are intriguing and confirm the importance of political tensions. The probability is high that populations traditionally underserved by the health care system will find it hard to trust that physicians will make decisions in their best interest. Numerous studies have documented the higher morbidity and mortality of U.S. minority populations, as well as lack of access to care (Krieger, 1993; Adler et al., 1993). Empirical evidence documents a lower rate of organ donation by minority groups, perhaps another indication of lack of trust (Kasiske et al., 1991; Kjellstrand, 1988). With the increasing prevalence of managed care, suspicions will mount; economic incentives for the use of life-sustaining interventions will likely be transformed. Mistrust of government programs—and the health professionals seen as government agents— is justified by the historical record (see Jones, 1981, on the Tuskegee syphilis study).

Bioethics research paradigms, because of failure to include analysis of the social context within which end-of-life decisions are made, have failed to account for significant power differentials between patients and providers. My own research demonstrates serious discordance between patient's and family's perceptions of choice regarding end-of-life care for cancer.

INDIVIDUAL CHOICE AND RESEARCH ALLOCATION

Evidence, albeit anecdotal, from ethics committees in California (a state moving toward true cultural pluralism) suggests that the paradigm case brought to committees has changed. Whereas committees were well equipped to deal with cases of clear overtreatment and overuse of resources for a dying patient, the new case consists of a "minority" family demanding further care in the face of health care professionals' definitions of futile treatment.

Current end-of-life decisionmaking practices, based on Western concepts that privilege the individual and individual choice, will inevitably run into difficulties in a society that emphasizes difference. To cite but one example, the state of New Jersey has passed brain death legislation which allows for a religious and cultural exclusion. The statute specifically states that brain death will only be considered the criteria for determining that death has occurred if brain death is acceptable within the patient's or family's religious or cultural tradition. Such legislation raises the specter of families demanding continued treatment of individuals defined by the health care team as dead.

Culturally diverse U.S. populations will vary in their response to practice guidelines and standards based on health services research focusing on measurable outcomes. It is important to move beyond an understanding that blames individuals or rests on the assumption that culture forms a barrier to acceptance of rationally derived scientific facts.

CONCLUSIONS: RECOMMENDATIONS FOR THE IOM STUDY

Based on this very brief overview of key concerns, I would like to make recommendations in the following three areas: (1) developing a research agenda to investigate cultural issues in end-of-life care and decisionmaking, (2) policy change in clinical bioethics practice, and (3) clinical education for health care providers.

Research: First, we need to develop a research agenda that will address how end-of-life decisionmaking is shaped within a particular cultural context. This research will need to be carefully crafted in order to avoid the pitfalls of simplistic and deterministic use of racial, ethnic, or cultural categories. The research needs to be constructed with an eye toward the complexity of power dynamics within the social setting of hospital, clinic, or nursing home. Culture and cultural differences are most effectively studied using the interpretive techniques of the social sciences and humanities. Thus, it will be difficult to integrate research on cultural differences with traditional health services research. However, the rewards of developing new integrative approaches, methods that combine qualitative and quantitative research techniques, will be significant. Only by developing methods sensitive to the complexity of cultural diversity will we be able to avoid the political dangers of recognizing difference in insensitive ways.

Empirical research must address the following key issues: Is information about diagnosis and prognosis openly discussed? If not, how is such information "managed"? How is information about probabalistic outcomes understood? Is death (and its relative likelihood) an appropriate topic for discussion? Is the maintenance of hope, even in the face of bad outcomes, considered essential? How is decisionmaking shared (or delegated) by the individual patient and family? How is the option of quality of life versus quantity of life weighted? Do patients and families trust that health care providers will act in their best interests (within the context of changing reimbursement schemes)? This list undoubtedly needs expansion and refinement.

In addition to empirical research, scholars from bioethics and related disciplines must address fundamental normative issues: What are the implications of respecting cultural or ethnic perspectives in bioethics? How will questions of diversity intersect with questions of justice? When patients and families disagree with providers' assessments of outcomes, how should such disputes be mediated?

Clinical Bioethics Practices: Research results will inform the design and implementation of clinical bioethics practices. Up to now the cultural assumptions underlying existing practices have not been scrutinized. The relevance of these innovations for groups other than middle-class European Americans needs to be addressed. Based on the results of empirical investigation, clinical bioethics policies should be modified. The structure and functioning of institutional ethics committees must be examined to determine if differing perspectives can be heard. The possibility of greater family involvement in decisionmaking must be considered. Legal implications of modifying practices will need to be reviewed since they are likely to be significant.

Education: Clinical education about appropriate end-of-life[10] care must incorporate means of addressing cultural diversity without stereotyping based on preconceived biases or views of particular ethnic groups. This is a challenge since clinicians will desire simple algorithms to help them reduce the enormous complexity of caring for patients from diverse cultural backgrounds. It is impossible to be an expert in every cultural tradition encountered in practice, but it is possible to understand the principal points of variation—conceptions of the person, role of the family, future orientation, communication styles regarding diagnosis and prognosis, and so forth. The most important element of good teaching is emphasizing that patients and families should never be approached as "empty vessels," the bearers of particular cultures.[11] Each patient needs to be approached first as an individual, a lesson which has been central to clinical education and thus does not require a major change of focus or direction.

In this very brief introduction—really an aerial view—of cultural diversity in end-of-life decisionmaking, I have only been able to hint at the most salient issues. In summary, future research, teaching, and practice guidelines should include:

- a sophisticated understanding of culture and health;
- careful use of categorizations based on race, ethnicity, and culture; and
- attention to the cultural assumptions embedded within clinical bioethics practices and their relevance to diverse patient populations.

ADDENDUM

Three Case Narratives

CASE NARRATIVE: George Yengley (All names are pseudonyms.)

Mr. George Yengley is a 59-year-old "Anglo" European American man whose pancreatic cancer was discovered when he collapsed on the street and was taken to the emergency room of the local public hospital. Mr. Yengley's response to his diagnosis and the treatment offered him most closely approximates the idealized patient of the autonomy paradigm. His life story reflects a long-term preoccupation with independence; in fact, he spent most of his adult life as a self-proclaimed loner and only reunited with family (in this instance a niece) when he became ill and was unable to live alone. Even in illness, he remained estranged from his wife and children, and a major worry for him was being burdensome for his niece and her family.

Mr. Yengley was quite open in discussing both diagnosis and the eventual outcome of his cancer. He used the word *cancer* in discussing his illness, avoiding euphemisms. Describing his surgery he stated: "They said that they operated but couldn't get all of it and there was no hope. And you have three months to a year to live. Well, I really think that prediction is wrong, right now. . . . So then you start thinking about your death." Note that although he accepts the overall prognosis, he remains convinced that the timing offered by the physicians is wrong in his case, that he will beat the numbers.

Mr. Yengley's niece was also open in talking about the illness: "I know he has cancer, pancreatic and stomach. And I know at the time he was diagnosed, he had three months to a year to live." Following his initial surgery, the health care team suggested a treatment regimen of radiation therapy and chemotherapy. Mr. Yengley began this treatment course, but stopped all treatment soon thereafter, a course he initiated because of the unpleasant side effects of treatment. Once settled with his niece, he made specific plans for his funeral and began choosing a nursing home/hospice where he could receive end-of-life care, reflecting his desire not to "die at home," which he felt would burden his family.

George Yengley's social worker highlighted the unique elements of his story. "It's interesting because he is such an exceptional guy. He is one of the very few who actually say, 'no, I don't want any more treatment.' . . . He is dealing with his own prognosis and he knows radiation may or may not help. He knew it didn't make him feel good so he stopped. I have a lot of admiration for that. We support his decision." Mr. Yengley's style was much appreciated by the staff, who described him as "strikingly realistic." His oncologist's comments reflect the degree of congruence between Mr. Yengley and the staff. "He very quickly showed himself to be someone who was able to make decisions for himself and not be lost in a sea of emotions."

Embedded within the new end-of-life practices are unexamined assumptions that stem from specific Western traditions. Innovations in health care ethics that emphasize advance care planning for death or a patient's right to limit or withdraw unwanted therapy appear to presuppose a particular patient. This ideal patient has the following characteristics: (1) a clear understanding of the illness, prognosis, and treatment options that is shared with the members of the health care team; (2) a temporal orientation to the future and desire to maintain "control" into that future; (3) the perception of freedom of choice; (4) willingness to discuss the prospect of death and dying openly; (5) a balance between fatalism and belief in human agency that favors the latter and minimizes the likelihood of divine intervention (or other "miracles"); and (6) an assumption that the individual, rather than the family or other social group, is the appropriate decision-maker. Patient George Yengley comes the closest to this ideal patient.

CASE NARRATIVE: Hung Long Lin

Mr. Lin's cancer was diagnosed in China before he immigrated to the United States about one and one-half years ago with his wife and their two sons. The older son attends junior college and speaks English well, always accompanying his monolingual father to the clinic. Since arrival in the United States, Mr. Lin has received treatment for his locally invasive nasopharyngeal cancer, a cancer that has progressed to the point of being immediately life-threatening due to the high likelihood of hemorrhage from major blood vessels in his neck. He has been treated with both radiation therapy and chemotherapy. In addition to conventional oncological treatments, he is taking traditional Chinese medicine.

In contrast to some Chinese patients, Mr. Lin used the word *cancer* (as opposed to *tumor*) in discussing his illness with the Cantonese-speaking interviewer. His son elaborates, "We don't mind saying 'cancer' because we all know that my father has this illness. But we all do our best not to say that. . . . We don't know how long he will live, but we want him to enjoy every day." Other Chinese patients in the study never mentioned the word *cancer* in interviews, using the more neutral Cantonese term for tumor. Yet like Mr. Lin, it was clear they understood the severity of the situation in spite of their hesitancy to openly name the disease.

The professionals caring for Mr. Lin began with the assumption that he must be fully informed. Since Mr. Lin speaks no English, the staff generally rely on Mr. Lin's son to translate. This opens up the possibility of conflicting notions of what constitutes appropriate disclosure. Mr. Lin's son complained, "For us Chinese, we are not used to telling the patient everything, and patients are not used to this either. If you tell them, they can't tolerate it and they will get sicker."

During one visit to the clinic, the physician wanted Mr. Lin's son to explain that chemotherapy had not been effective in his case and that there were no more treatments available. The son was quite distressed. "I did not want to translate this to my father, but the doctor insisted on telling him everything. . . . The doctor found the Chinese-speaking social worker to translate for him and told him everything." When interviewed separately, the oncologist treating Mr. Lin discussed his older son: "He came to every visit and was always clamoring for more chemotherapy for his dad although it was completely unrealistic." In this case, the physician did not succeed in imposing autonomy on the patient over the wishes of the son, who chose to maintain ambiguity and thus hope.

CASE NARRATIVE: Elena Alvarez

Elena Alvarez is a 48-year-old woman who has lived in the United States for many years. Originally from El Salvador, her English is very limited. Before her diagnosis with ovarian cancer, she worked as a child care provider. Her family consists of a brother and her mother; she lives with her elderly mother who has many health problems of her own. Her disease has progressed despite surgery, initial chemotherapy, and a number of attempts at "salvage" chemotherapy.

Elena Alvarez spoke openly about her cancer diagnosis with members of the clinic staff, but maintained a complex silence within her family. For many months she did not name the disease with her elderly mother, preferring to shield her from this information. As her illness progressed, Ms. Alvarez' mother eventually learned that her daughter had cancer. However, the severity of the illness was never addressed. One of the nurses commented, "The other thing that Elena said to us when we had this big meeting was that she has not told her mother the truth about her illness. She can't tell her mother the truth about her illness. So I'm sure they haven't had a real honest conversation about what is going on."

From the point of view of her health care providers, Ms. Alvarez faced many decision points. "However, like many of the other patients in our study, she did not experience any sense of choice. In interviews she stated over and over, "You just have to do the treatment, there isn't an alternative. You get treatment to prolong your life and get well, or you let yourself die." Over a nine-month period, she always "CHOSE" more treatment. During the informed-consent process for entry into the research, we told the patients that we were studying decisionmaking. Some patients, particularly women, found this perplexing and wondered what we were "really studying," since they did not experience their medical care as including decisions. When discussing her "last" drug, tamoxifen, Ms. Alvarez said, "I wait for life. I have the point of view that I am going to be cured. This is going to be my drug. This is going to cure me."

The comments of Elena Alvarez reflect the tension between her beliefs that no choices existed, and the health care team's demands that she make decisions. When asked who was the most important person making decisions about her treatment, Elena answered, "I am," but immediately complained, "Here in this country they don't give you an alternative but to do it alone. . . . In other countries they tell the family and the family has influence. The family decides. Here the patient has to decide for themselves (sic). There is no alternative." She raises two questions: Are there real options, and should the individual patient be shouldered with making decisions alone?

The issue of prognosis was equally complex. Nurse Terry Miller noted, "One of the things that Dr. Ingle and I talked about was, 'when is he going to say that enough is enough,' because this woman is not going to be cured. She is going to die of the disease. Several months ago we sat down with Elena and said, 'it's progressing and we don't know what else we can do for you.' And I asked her at that time, when was she going to know that enough was enough. She told me she would know that when the doctor told her there was nothing left to do." In seeming contradiction to the fundamental assumptions of the autonomy paradigm, Dr. Ingle found it very difficult to discuss the patient's likely prognosis. He explained his frustrations by rehearsing a hypothetical conversation with his patient: "I want to encourage you to keep going with this chemo, but oh, by the way, you're still not going to do well, and you probably only have six months to live. It's kind of hard, and I didn't reiterate that, to tell the truth." The problem is apparent; the doctor is giving the patient mixed messages, and everyone wants someone else to make the hard decisions. Dr. Ingle continued, "She lets me make the decisions for her. In Elena's case I'll tell her what I think is best for her, and I tend to push pretty aggressively with Elena. I'm not willing to just sort of like, let her go." The result is a long delay in acknowledgment that further treatment is futile, a dynamic discussed in many of the background papers written for the IOM workshop.

The situation of Elena Alvarez was complicated by the need for language interpretation. I was able to observe a long and complicated clinical session, involving the patient, the clinical nurse specialist, oncologist, and social worker. A Spanish language interpreter was also present since the encounter was foreseen to be important: would the patient want further salvage chemotherapy for her disease, which had recurred despite numerous interventions (a treatment decision about which she ultimately felt she had no choice)? Although communication is never simple, some elements of failed communication are not overly complex and were evident in the clinical encounter. Throughout the exchange, I noted many instances in which statements by either the patient or one of the team members were simply not translated. The physician was offering chemotherapy, the nurse was reminding the patient that she mustn't wait until it was too late, meaning that she was too ill to travel, if she wanted to return to her native El Salvador. In this cacophonous five-way exchange, it was difficult to determine what "got through" to the patient, who was weeping softly throughout. As discussed earlier, like many patients, Elena appeared to perceive no choice but to follow the physician's option of additional chemotherapy. In later interviews, Dr. Ingle described the patient's prognosis as extremely poor regardless of therapeutic endeavors.

But of most interest was the role of the interpreter in placing the clinical session in a certain cultural context. Toward the end of the interview, the interpreter spoke softly with the patient for some time, not volunteering to translate his own remarks for others in the room. Seemingly distressed by the bluntness of the conversation he had just been translating, he ended the exchange by relating a story to Elena, a story suffused with hope. Once the interpreter had known a person with cancer who was told he would only live for two months, and the person was still alive nine years later! Is the interpreter trying to compensate for the teams' lack of sensitivity to a culturally shared (between patient and translator) need to maintain hope?

In this type of exchange, which voice captures the patient's attention? The role of the white-coated interpreter, who must appear to the patient as a full member of the team, needs further exploration.

ENDNOTES

1.   The study compares cancer patients from European American, Latino, and Chinese American backgrounds. A second study makes a similar cross-cultural/ethnic comparison among patients with end-stage AIDS. Data collection is in process, definitive results from these descriptive studies are not yet available. Preliminary results—three case narratives of patients from diverse cultural backgrounds—were presented at the IOM meeting in December. The case narratives are included here as an appendix. See Koenig et al. (1992), Barnes et al. (1993), and Orona et al. (1994) for preliminary results.

2.   This comment is based on my personal experience serving on ethics committees in long-term care facilities in San Francisco, including On Lok Senior Health Services and Laguna Honda Hospital.

3.   Unpublished table produced by author from census data.

4.   Issues such as immigration, political refugees, ethnic violence, and its relationship to nationalism are all of global and transnational importance. The politics of ethnic difference is one of the central political issues of our time and is crucial in the North/South realignment of world politics. (I thank Arthur Kleinman for reminding me of the scope of these issues.)

5.   Another interpretation is that these discrepancies are caused simply by poor and inaccurate "counting" of differences that are easy to determine. However, there is increasing recognition that the traditional categories used in public health statistics are extremely prob-lematic (see CDC, 1993). This Centers for Disease Control and Prevention report emphasizes that race and ethnicity are social categories, which if misused have serious limitations for understanding variations in health status and potential negative implications for minority populations by reinforcing "stereotyping, mistrust, and racism" (CDC, 1993, p. 13).

6.   A full discussion of the politics of difference as discussed by Charles Taylor (1992) and others is impossible here. A useful example of the dangers of "ghettoization" is a report (January, 1993) in the *New York Times* of Hispanic children, monolingual in English, but nonetheless forced into bilingual education programs in the schools.

7.   I acknowledge that scholars within bioethics have themselves engaged in corrections to this initial tendency to overstress autonomy; thus my intention is not to set up a naive bioethics-equals-autonomy straw man to cut down. In a recent assessment, James Childress (a bioethics founding father) noted, "I come not to bury autonomy, but to praise it. Yet my praise is somewhat muted; for autonomy merits only two cheers, not three" (Childress, 1990, p. 12).

8.   Recent work in bioethics, such as Brody's *The Healer's Power* (1992), has begun to address questions of power in the doctor-patient relationship.

9.   A large empirical study of cultural diversity and advance directives is currently under way at the University of Southern California. Results are not yet available.

10.   I would argue that end-of-life care has been largely neglected in medical education (less so in nursing and other fields). Education is oriented toward action and intervention, not recognizing limits and acknowledging the inevitability of death. Thus more fundamental reform than attention to cultural diversity is called for.

11.   Models based on the work of medical anthropologists like Margaret Lock and Arthur Kleinman are particularly helpful. Teaching about end-of-life care is most likely to be effective if it is integrated within a general approach to cultural diversity in health care.

REFERENCES

Adler, Nancy E., Boyce, W. Thomas, Chesney, Margaret A., et al. 1993. Socioeconomic Inequalities in Health: No Easy Solution. *Journal of the American Medical Association* 269:3140–3145.

Anspach, Renee R. 1987. Prognostic Conflict in Life-and-Death Decisions: The Organization as an Ecology of Knowledge. *Journal of Health and Social Behavior* 28:215–231.

Barker, Judith C. 1992. Cross Cultural Medicine (special issue). *Western Journal of Medicine* 157:248–254.

Barnes, Donelle, Koenig, Barbara A., et al. 1993. "Telling the Truth" about Cancer: The Ambiguity of Prognosis for Culturally Diverse Patients. Paper presented at the Society for Applied Anthropology Annual Meeting, San Antonio, Texas.

Brody, Howard. 1992. The Healer's Power. New Haven, Connecticut: Yale University Press.

California Association of Homes for the Aged. 1993. Inter-Agency Ethics Committee.

Callahan, Daniel. 1993. *The Troubled Dream of Life: Living with Mortality.* New York: Simon & Schuster.

Caralis, PV, et al. 1993. The Influence of Ethnicity and Race on Attitudes toward Advance Directives, Life-Prolonging Treatments and Euthanasia. *Journal of Clinical Ethics* 4:155–165.

Centers for Disease Control and Prevention. 1993. Use of Race and Ethnicity in Public Health Surveillance. *Mortality and Morbidity Weekly Report* 42.

Childress, James F. 1990. The Place of Autonomy in Bioethics. *Hastings Center Report* 20(1):12–17.

Churchill, Larry R. 1979. Interpretations of Dying: Ethical Implications for Patient Care. *Ethics in Science and Medicine* 6:211–222.

Cross, Alan W., and Churchill, Larry R. 1982. Ethical and Cultural Dimensions of Informed Consent: A Case Study and Analysis. *Annals of Internal Medicine* 96:110–113.

Flack, Harley E., and Pellegrino, Edmund D. 1992. *African American Perspective on Bioethics.* Washington, D.C.: Georgetown University Press.

Fox, Renee C. 1990. The Organization, Outlook and Evolution of American Bioethics: From the 1960s into the 1980s. In *Social Science Perspectives on Medical Ethics*, G. Weisz, ed. Dordrecht: Kluwer.

Garrett, J., et al. 1993. Life-Sustaining Treatments During Terminal Illness: Who Wants What? *Journal of General Internal Medicine* 8:361–368.

Glazer, Nathan and Moynihan, Daniel P. 1963. *Beyond the Melting Pot: The Negroes, Puerto Ricans, Jews, Italians and Irish of New York.* Cambridge, Massachusetts: MIT Press.

Gupta, Akhil, and Ferguson, James. 1992. Beyond "Culture:" Space, Identity and the Politics of Difference. *Cultural Anthropology* 7:6–23.

Hahn, Robert. 1983. Culture and Informed Consent. In: *Making Choices. Report of the President's Commission for Ethical Problems in Medicine and Biomedical and Behavioral Research*, pp. 37–62. Washington, D.C.: U.S. Government Printing Office.

Hahn, Robert A., Mulinare, J., and Teutsch, S.M. 1992. Inconsistencies in Coding of Race andEthnicity Between Birth and Death in U.S. Infants. *Journal of the American Medical Association* 267:259–263.

Helman, Cecil. 1990. *Culture, Health, and Illness,* 2d Edition. Boston: Wright.

Hoffmaster, Barry. 1992. Can Ethnography Save the Life of Medical Ethics? *Social Science and Medicine* 35(12):1421–1431.

Jennings, Bruce. 1990. Ethics and Ethnography in Neonatal Intensive Care. In *Social Science Perspectives on Medical Ethics*, G. Weisz, ed. Hingham, Massachusetts: Kluwer, pp. 261–272.

Jones, James. 1981. *Bad Blood: the Scandalous Story of the Tuskegee Experiment.* New York: Free Press.

Jonsen, Albert R. 1991. Of Balloons and Bicycles or the Relationship Between Ethical Theory and Practical Judgment. *Hastings Center Report* 21(5):14–16.

Kalish, Richard A., and Reynolds, David K. 1976. *Death and Ethnicity: A Psychocultural Study.* New York: Baywood (1981 reprint).

Kasiske, B.L. Neylan, J.F., Riggio, R.R., et al. 1991. The Effect of Race on Access and Outcome in Transplantation. *New England Journal of Medicine* 324:302–307.

Kjellstrand, C.M. 1988. Age, Sex, and Race Inequality in Renal Transplantation. *Archives of Internal Medicine* 148:1305–1309.

Kleinman, Arthur. In Press: Anthropology of Bioethics. In *Encyclopedia of Bioethics*, Warren T. Reich, ed. New. York: Macmillan.

Kleinman, Arthur, and Kleinman, Joan. 1991. Suffering and Its Professional Transformation: Toward an Ethnography of Interpersonal Experience. In *Culture, Medicine, Psychiatry* 15:275–301.

Koenig, Barbara A., et al. 1992. Cultural Pluralism and Ethical Decision-Making: Meanings of Autonomy to Patients and Families Facing Life-Threatening Cancer. Paper presented at American Anthropological Association Annual Meeting, San Francisco, California [Under revision for submission.]

Krieger, Nancy. 1993. Analyzing Socioeconomic and Racial/Ethnic Patterns in Health and Health Care. *American Journal of Public Health* 83:1086–1087.

Lamphere, Louise. 1992. *Structuring Diversity: Ethnographic Perspectives on the New Immigration.* Chicago: University of Chicago Press.

Lock, Margaret. 1993a. The Concept of Race: An Ideological Construct. *Transcultural Psychiatric Review* 30:203–227.

Lock, Margaret. 1993b. Education and Self Reflection: Teaching About Culture, Health and Illness. In *Health and Cultures: Exploring the Relationships*, R. Masi, et al., eds. Oakville, Ontario: Mosaic Press.

Lynn, Joanne, and Teno, Joan M. 1993. After the Patient Self-Determination Act: The Need for Empirical Research. *Hastings Center Report* 23:20–24.

Marshall, Patricia. 1992 Anthropology and Bioethics. *Medical Anthropology Quarterly* 6:49–73.

Meleis, Afaf I., and Jonsen, Albert R. 1983. Ethical Crises and Cultural Differences. *Western Journal of Medicine* 138:889–893.

Muller, Jessica H., and Koenig, Barbara A. 1988. On the Boundary of Life and Death: The Definition of Dying by Medical Residents. In *Biomedicine Examined,* Margaret Lock and Deborah Gordon, eds. Boston: Kluwer.

Muller, Jessica H. and Desmond, Brian. 1992. Ethical Dilemmas in a Cross-Cultural Context—A Chinese Example. *Western Journal of Medicine* 157:323–327.

Office of Management and Budget. 1978. Directive No. 15: Race and Ethnic Standards for Federal Statistics and Administrative Reporting. Statistical Policy Handbook. Washington, D.C., U.S. Department of Commerce, Office of Federal Statistical Policy and Standards.

Orona, Celia J., Koenig, Barbara A., and Davis, Anne J. 1994. Cultural Issues in Non-Disclosure. *Cambridge Quarterly for HealthCare Ethics* 3(3).

Orr, Robert D., Marshall, Patricia A., and Osborn, Jamie. 1994. Cross-Cultural Considerations in Clinical Ethics Consultations. (Submitted.)

Osborne, N.G. and Feit, M.D. 1992. The Use of Race in Medical Research. *Journal of the American Medical Research* 267:275–279.

Pellegrino, Edmund D., et al. 1992. *Transcultural Dimensions of Medical Ethics.* Baltimore, Maryland: University Publishing Group.

Scheper-Hughes, Nancy. 1992. *Death without Weeping: The Violence of Everyday Life in Brazil.* Berkeley: University of California Press.

Sharp, John. 1988. Introduction. In *South African Keywords: the Uses and Abuses of Political Concepts.* Cape Town and Johannesburg: David Philip.

Sheldon, T.A., and Parker, H., 1992. Race and Ethnicity in Health Research. *Journal of Public Health Medicine* 14:104–110.

Slomka, Jacqueline. 1992. The Negotiation of Death: Clinical Decision-Making at the End of Life. *Social Science and Medicine* 35:251–259.

Taylor, Charles. 1992. *Multiculturalism and the Politics of Recognition.* Princeton, New Jersey: Princeton University Press.

Veatch, Robert M. 1989. *Cross Cultural Perspectives in Medical Ethics.* Boston: Jones and Bartlett.

F

Measuring Care at the End of Life

Workshop on Toolkit of Instruments to
Measure End-of-Life Care*
Woods Hole, Massachusetts
August 27–28, 1996

AGENDA

August 27

1:30–2:30   **INTRODUCTION AND OVERVIEW**
Joan Teno, M.D.**
Center to Improve Care of the Dying
The George Washington University

2:30–3:00   **What domains should be measured at the end of life?**
Joanne Lynn, M.D.
Director, Center to Improve Care of the Dying
The George Washington University

3:00–4:30   **Presentation and discussion of quality of life and
physical function**
Anita Stewart, Ph.D.
Institute for Health and Aging
University of California, San Francisco

---

*Organized by the Center to Improve Care of the Dying with support from the Nathan
Cummings Foundation.
**Now at Brown University.

Anne Wilkinson, Ph.D.
Center to Improve Care of the Dying
The George Washington University

4:30–6:00   **Presentation and discussion of physical and emotional symptoms**
Jane Ingham, M.D.
Lombardi Cancer Center
Georgetown University

August 28

9:00–10:00   **Presentation and discussion of patient and family satisfaction**
Joan Teno, M.D.

10:00–11:00   **Presentation and discussion of provider skill and continuity and advance care planning**
Molla Donaldson, M.S.
Institute of Medicine

11:00–12:00   **Presentation and discussion of bereavement and family burden**
Barbara Kreling
The George Washington University

Kristen Landrum
Center to Improve Care of the Dying
The George Washington University

1:00–2:00   **Presentation and discussion of spirituality and transcendence**
Barbara Kreling

2:00–3:00   **Next Steps**
Joan Teno, M.D.

PARTICIPANTS

Larry Bergner, M.D.
Vice President for Public Health and Epidimiology
National Opinion Research Center

Ira Byock, M.D.
Director, The Palliative Care Service
President, Missoula Demonstration Project

Carolyn Cocotas
Assistant Vice President, New Measurement Development
National Committee for Quality Assurance

Molla Donaldson, M.S.
Senior Program Officer
Institute of Medicine

Susan Edgman-Levitan
President
The Picker Institute

Linda Emanuel, M.D.
Vice President
American Medical Association

Marilyn Field, Ph.D.
Deputy Director, Health Care Services
Institute of Medicine

Jack Fowler, Ph.D.
Center for Survey Research
University of Massachusetts

Rosemary Gibson
Program Officer
Robert Wood Johnson Foundation

Jane Ingham, M.D.
Director, Palliative Care Program
Lombardi Cancer Center
Georgetown University

Robert Kliegman, M.D.
Chair, Department of Pediatrics
Medical College of Wisconsin

Barbara Kreling
Research Scientist, Division of Research Programs
The George Washington University

Kristen Landrum
Research Assistant, Center to Improve Care of the Dying
The George Washington University

Joanne Lynn, M.D.
Director, Center to Improve Care of the Dying
The George Washington University

Neil MacDonald, M.D.
Director, Cancer Bioethics Program
McGill University

Melanie Merrimen, Ph.D.
Director of Outcomes Measurement
VITAS Healthcare Corporation

Vincent Mor, Ph.D.
Associate Professor of Research
Centers for Long-Term Care Gerontology and Health Care Research
Brown University

Naomi Naierman
President/CEO
American Hospice Foundation

Donald Patrick, Ph.D.
Professor, Department of Health Services
University of Washington

Richard Payne, M.D.
Chief, Pain and Symptom Management Section
M.D. Anderson Cancer Center

Linda Siegenthaler
Center for Primary Care Research
Agency for Health Care Policy and Research

Shoshanna Sofaer, Dr.PH.
Director, Division of Research Programs
The George Washington University

Anita Stewart, Ph.D.
Institute for Health and Aging
University of California, San Francisco

William Stubing
President, Greenwall Foundation

Joan Teno, M.D.
Co-Director, Center to Improve Care of the Dying
The George Washington University

Anne Wilkinson, Ph.D.
Associate Professor of Research
Center to Improve Care of the Dying
The George Washington University

WORKSHOP SUMMARY

Prepared by Joan Teno, M.D., M.S.

Physician-assisted suicide has become an issue of increasing public concern and media attention. A central portion of court cases has focused on individual rights. It has been argued that an important aspect of this debate ought to be how well our hospitals and other health systems care for dying patients. Drs. Melinda Lee and Susan Tolle have noted that the "silver lining" of this debate may be the stimulus for health care institutions to examine the quality of care for dying and seriously ill patients. The aim of this conference was to provide health care institutions with a resource guide (a "toolkit") that would allow them to examine and improve their quality of care for dying patients and their families. With funding support from the Nathan Cummings Foundation and the Robert Wood Johnson Foundation, a multidisciplinary group of 27 persons assembled to review current knowledge about measuring quality of care at the end of life, make recommendations about the use of existing measures, and outline important issues that need urgent work for the vision of the toolkit to go forward.

Deming stated that, "If you don't measure it, you can't improve it." Our ultimate vision for the toolkit was that health care institutions be able to use the toolkit to examine care of the dying, identify opportunities for improvement, and then undertake interventions to improve and enhance the quality of care. The results of this conference represent an early effort to review existing instruments to examine the quality of care for dying persons and their families. This executive summary briefly summarizes the vision for the toolkit and outlines important research and design questions that we encourage both grant funders and researchers to consider in the design of future measures to examine quality of care at the end of life.

Vision for Measures Included in the Toolkit

1. Measures must be clinically meaningful. Clinicians must be convinced that the measure has face validity, that differences are clinically relevant, that the measure detects changes with time, and that a result can raise provider awareness. Measures must also be manageable in their application.

2. The focus of these measures is on the "middle manager" who wants to ask the following questions: "How are we doing in caring for dying patients? What are our strengths? What are our opportunities for improvement?" The ultimate use of these measures will be for quality improvement. In the future, with experience with the measures, development of guide-

lines, and research, the use of these measurements will be extended to inform consumers and purchasers of health care.

3. Such measures must incorporate both the patient and family perspective on the quality of care at the end of life (it should be noted that family is used in the broadest sense, potentially including the patient's partner or other loved ones). The medical record review of people who have died is another important perspective on medical care at the end of life.

4. We urge rapid cycles of improvement in measurement. The first toolkit should quickly become outdated with research and further development of guidelines.

Comment

Limited research to date has been undertaken to examine the quality of care for seriously ill and dying patients. Given this paucity of research, an important first step is to understand the values of both patients and their loved ones. From their unique perspective of this experience, what defines patient- and family-centered medical care? Equally important is descriptive research to examine current knowledge about the quality of care with existing instruments and with the use of qualitative research techniques. Such research should focus not only on the negative, but also on opportunities for growth at the end of life.

In developing measures to guide quality improvement, it is important that measures are clinically meaningful. Clinicians must "buy in" that measures are reflecting important aspects of medical care. If a process of care is measured, there ought to be evidence that the process is related to the valued outcome or that the process is valued as an endpoint based on overwhelming public and professional consensus. Careful attention should be paid to assure that as we define measures, we are also defining standards of care. In developing new measures, we urge that consideration be given to the involvement of national professional organizations and managers in a dialogue such that their views are considered. If the instruments are going to be used, it is important that the measures do not impose unreasonable burdens so that it is realistic to collect reliable and valid information. Involving clinicians and mid-level managers is an important step to assure that instruments are both clinically valid and feasible.

Limited research to date has examined or reported on the degree to which measures are responsive to improvement. Measures must be responsive and eventually measures must be able to discriminate between health care institutions that are and are not delivering quality medical care. It is a realistic goal that measurement tools will be developed that both rate health care institutions on the quality of care and provide consumers with information on deciding which health care plan to select.

Research Priorities and Important Design Questions

There are fundamental details which must be addressed in the design of both surveys and chart review instruments. Some of these details can be resolved with further empirical research (e.g., what do patients really value in end-of-life care?) while other issues will need to be resolved by consensus. Among the key issues that the group identified were the following:

1. What are the proper domains that define quality of care from the patient and family perspective? Are health care institutions accountable for the outcomes in a particular domain?

The work of the American Geriatric Society is an important step in defining the domains of quality medical care at the end of life. It is important that measures reflect patient and family views of what defines quality medical care. An important litmus test is whether there is broad consensus or empirical studies that show that health care institutions ought to be held accountable for those outcomes. Simply stated, is it the prerogative and the capability of the health care system to influence that chosen outcome?

2. What are the proper time periods to assess the quality of care?

Previous research has noted that patients with cancer lose the majority of their function and experience most of their symptoms in the last one to two months of life. Many instruments focus on this sentinel time period. However, diseases other than cancer may not follow this trajectory. Furthermore, concerns with quality of care can occur throughout the patient's illness. Unrelieved pain is problematic at any time period. Different instruments ought to look at important sentinel time periods throughout the illness course to ensure quality medical care.

3. Who is the respondent? What is he or she able to accurately report on?

Nearly one in three patients are unable to be interviewed in the last week of life. To simply disregard their experience would miss important information on the quality of medical care. Yet, a proxy is only able to report on their observations or perceptions of the quality of care. Family members are often more critical and provide an important perspective that can lead to improving the quality of care. Research is needed to understand who can best serve as the respondent. Do you need to use multiple respondents? Such research is needed to design valid instruments.

4. What is the cost-effectiveness of various strategies to get information on the quality of care?

Among the plausible sources of information on the quality of medical care are the medical record, patient, and family interview (both prospective and retrospective interviews after the patient's death). Each have their own costs and limitations regarding accuracy of the data. Additionally, there are various strategies for collecting data which ought to be evaluated (e.g., self-administered, telephone interview, personal interview). Research ought to seek to determine the most cost-effective means to get reliable and valid indicators of quality medical care.

5. How are the respondents' views influenced by the wording and location of the question in the survey?

Research is needed to examine the degree to which the wording and the location of questions influence the respondents' views. For example, does asking questions on symptom data prior to questions on satisfaction influence the patient's response? Total survey design that employs cognitive interviews is important to understand the process undertaken by respondents in answering survey questions. It is only through such efforts that surveys will yield accurate reliable and valid measures.

The above highlights key areas for future consideration in the design of valid and reliable instruments. Measuring the quality of care is the cornerstone to improving and enhancing the quality of care. To that end, the toolkit conference aimed to provide a systemic review of the existing instruments to examine quality of care, make recommendations for promising instruments, create new instruments, and identify a research agenda that focuses on the rapid improvement in measurement of the quality of care at the end of life.

Measurement Tools Suggested as Promising for Further Development and Testing in End-of-Life Care

PHYSICAL SYMPTOMS, compiled and reviewed by Jane Ingham

Verbal Rating Scale (Lasagna, L. Analgesic methodology: A brief history and commentary. *Journal of Clininal Pharmacology* May–June:373–375, 1980).

McGill Short Pain Inventory (Melzack, R. The McGill Pain Questionnaire. In *Pain Measurement and Assessment.* New York: Raven Press, 1983).

Wisconsin Brief Pain Questionnaire (Daut, R.L., Cleeland, C.S., and

Flanery, R.C. Development of the Wisconsin brief pain questionnaire to assess pain in cancer and other diseases. *Pain* 17:197–210, 1983).

Memorial Pain Questionnaire (Fishman, B., Pasteranak, S., Wallenstien, S.L., et al. The memorial pain assessment card: A valid instrument for the evaluation of cancer pain. *Cancer* 60:1151–1158, 1987).

Pain as Assessed in the Medical Outcome Study (Hays, R.D., Nelson, E.C., Rubin, H.R., et al. Further evaluation of the PJHQ scales. *Medical Care* 28: S29–S39, 1990).

Descriptor Differential Scale (Gracely, R.H., and Kwilosz, D.M. The descriptor differential scale: Applying psychophysical principles to clinical pain assessment. *Pain* 35:279–288, 1988).

Integrated Pain Score (Ventrafridda, V., De Conno, F., Di Trapani, P., et al. A new method of pain quantification based on a weekly self-description record of the intensity and duration of pain. In: Bonica J, et al., eds. *Advances in Pain Research and Therapy. vol. 5.* New York: Raven Press, pp. 891–895, 1983).

West Haven-Yale Multidimensional Pain Inventory (Kerns, R.D., Turk, D.C., and Rudy, T.E. The West Haven-Yale multidimensional pain inventory. *Pain* 23:345–356, 1985).

Baseline Dyspnea Index (Mahler, D.A., and Wells, C.K. Evaluation of clinical methods for rating dyspnea. *Chest* 93:580–586, 1988).

Quality of Life in Chronic Lung Disease (Guyatt, G.H., Berman, L.B., Towsend, M. et al. A measure of quality of life for clinical trials in chronic lung disease. *Thorax* 42:773–778, 1987).

Visual analog scale to evaluate fatigue severity (Lee, K.A., Hicks, G., and Nino-Murchia, G. Validity and reliability of a scale to assess fatigue. *Psych Research* 36P:291–298, 1991).

Borg Rating of Dyspnea (Belman, M.J., Brooks, L.R., Ross, D.J., and Mohsenfar, Z. Variability of breathlessness measurement in patients with chronic obstructive pulmonary disease. *Chest* 99:566–571, 1991).

MULTIPLE SYMPTOMS (physical and emotional), compiled and reviewed by Joan Teno

Support Team Assessment Schedule (Butters, E., Higginson, I., George, R., Smits, A., et al. Assessing the symptoms, anxiety and practical needs of HIV/AIDS patients receiving palliative care. *Quality of Life Research* 1:47–51, 1992).

Symptom Distress Scale (McCorkle, R. Development of a symptom distress scale. *Cancer Nursing* 373–378, 1978).

Rotterdam Symptom Checklist (de Haes, J.C., van Kippenberg, F.C., and Neijt, J.P. Measuring psychological and physical symptom distress in cancer patients: Structure and application of the Rotterdam Symptom Checklist. *British Journal of Cancer* 62:1034–1038, 1990).

Edmonton Symptom Assessment System (Bruera, E., Kuehn, N., Miller, M., Selmser, P., and Macmillan, K. The Edmonton Symptom Assessment System (ESAS): A simple method for the assessment of palliative care patients. *Journal of Palliative Care* 7:6–9, 1991).

The Quality of Life Index (Spitzer, W.O., Dobson, A.J., Hall, J., et al. Measuring the quality of life of cancer patients: A concise QL-index for use by physicians. *Journal of Chronic Disease* 34:585–597, 1981).

EORTC QLQ (Anderson, N.K., Ahmedzai, S., Bullinger, M., et al. The European Organization for Research and Treatment of Cancer QOL-C30: A quality of life instrument for use in international trials in oncology. *Journal of the National Cancer Institute* 85:365–376, 1993).

Memorial Symptom Assessment Scale (Portenoy, R.K., Thaler, H.T., Kornblith, A.B., Lepore, J.M., et al. The memorial symptom assessment scale: An instrument for the evaluation of symptom prevalence, characteristics and distress. *European Journal of Cancer* 30A:1326–1336, 1994).

Chronic Respiratory Disease Questionnaire (Guyatt, G.H., Berman, L.B., Townsend, M., Pugsley, S.O., et al. A measure for the quality of life for clinical trials in chronic lung disease. *Thorax* 42:773–778, 1987).

Lung Cancer Symptom Scale (Hollen, P.J., Gralla, J.R., Kris, M.G., and Potanovich, L.M. Quality of life assessment in individuals with lung cancer: Testing the lung cancer symptom scale (LCSS). *European Journal of Cancer* 29A:S52–S58, 1993).

Prostrate Cancer Index Quality of Care In Prostrate Cancer, (UCLA Quality of Life Project. Prostrate Cancer Index, 1996).

Cancer Rehabilitation Evaluation System (Schag, C.A.C., Ganz, P.A., and Heinrich, R.L. Cancer rehabilitation evaluation system-short form (CARES-SF). *Cancer* 68:1406–1413, 1991).

National Hospice Study (Greer 1983, 1988; Reuben, D.B., Mor, V., and Hiris, J. Clinical symptoms and length of survival in patients with terminal cancer. *Archives of Internal Medicine* 148:1586–1591, 1988).

Hospice Quality of Life Index (McMillan, S.C., and Mahon, M. Measuring quality of life in hospice patients using a newly developed hospice quality of life index. *Quality of Life Research.* 3:437–447, 1994).

McGill Quality of Life Questionnaire (Cohen, S.R., Mount, B.M., Strobe, M.G., and Bui, F. The McGill quality of life questionnaire: A measure of quality of life for people with advanced disease. *Palliative Medicine* 9:207–219, 1995).

EORTC QOL-30 (Aaronson, N.K., Ahmedzai, S., Bergman, B., et al. The European organization for research and treatment of cancer QLQ-C30:

A quality-of-life instrument for use in international clinical trials in oncology. *Journal of the National Cancer Institute* 85:365–376, 1993).

VITAS Quality of Life Index (VITAS, Byock, I.R. *Missoula-VITAS Quality of Life index (version 25S).* VITAS Healthcare Corp., 1995).

EMOTIONAL SYMPTOMS, compiled and reviewed by Joan Teno

CES-D Scale (Radloff, S.F. The CES-D Scale: A self-report depression scale for research in the general population. *Applied Psychology Measurement* 1:385–401, 1977).

Mental Health Inventory (Ware, J.E., Jr, Johnston, S.A., Davies-Avery, A, et al. *Conceptualization and Measurement of Health for Adults in the Health Insurance Study. Vol. III. Mental Health.* Santa Monica, CA: Rand Corporation, 1979; Berwick D.M., Murphy J.M., Goldman P.A., et al. Performance of a five-item mental health screening test. *Medical Care* 29:169–176, 1991).

Profile of Mood States (Cella, D.F., Jacobson, P.B., Orlav, E.J., Holland, J.C., et al. A brief POMS measure of distress for cancer patients. *Journal of Chronic Disease* 40:939–942, 1987).

Beck Depression Index (Beck, A.T., Ward, C.H., Mendelson, M., et al. An inventory for measuring depression. *Archives of General Psychiatry* 4:561–571, 1961).

Hospital Anxiety and Depression Scale (Zigmond, A.S., and Snaith, R.P. The hospital anxiety and depression scale. *Acta Psychiatr Scand* 67:361–370, 1983).

Symptom Anxiety and Depression Scale (Bedford, A., Foulds, G.A., and Sheffield, B.F. A new personal disturbance scale (DSSI/SAD). *British Journal of Social and Clinical Psychology* 15:387–394, 1976).

Geriatric Depression Scale (Yesavage, J.A., Brink, T.L., Rose, T.L., et al. Development and validation of a geriatric depression scale: A preliminary report. *Journal of Psychiatric Research* 17:37–43, 1983).

General Health Questionnaire (Goldberg, D.P. *The detection of psychiatric illness by questionnaire.* Oxford University Press: London, 1972).

The Study to Understand Prognoses and Preferences for Outcomes and Risks of Treatments Afterdeath interview (Lynn, J., Teno, J.M., Philips, R.S., and Wu, A.W. Dying experience of older and seriously ill patients: Findings from the SUPPORT and HELP projects. Provisionally accepted, *Annals of Internal Medicine,* 1996).

FUNCTIONAL STATUS MEASURES, compiled and reviewed by Anne Wilkinson

Index of Independence in Activities of Daily Living (ADL) (Katz, S., Ford,

A.B., Moskowitz, R.W., et al. Studies of illness in the aged. The Index of ADL: A standardized measure of biological and psychosocial function. *Journal of the American Medical Association* 185:914–919, 1963).

The Barthel Index (Mahoney, F.I., Wood, O.H., and Barthel, D.W. Rehabilitation of chronically ill patients: The influence of complications on the final goal. *Southern Medical Journal* 51:605–609. 1958).

The Physical Self-Maintenance Scale (Lawton, M.P., and Brody, E. Assessment of older people: Self-maintaining and instrumental activities of daily living. *Gerontologist* 9:179–186, 1969).

A Rapid Disability Rating Scale (Linn, M.W., and Linn, B.S. The Rapid Disability Rating Scale-2. *Journal of the American Geriatrics Society* 30:378–382, 1982).

Stanford Health Assessment Questionnaire (Fries, J.F., Spitz, P.W., and Young, D.Y. The dimensions of health outcomes: The Health Assessment Questionnaire, disability and pain scales. *Journal of Rheumatology* 9:789–793, 1982).

Functional Independence Measure (Hamilton, B.B., Granger, C.V., Sherwin, F.S., et al. *A uniform national data system for rehabilitation outcomes: Analysis and measurement.* Baltimore, Maryland: Paul H. Brookes, 1987).

The PULSES Profile (Moskowitz, E., and McCann, C.B. Classification of disability in the chronically ill and aging. *Journal of Chronic Diseases* 5:342–346, 1957).

The Kenny Self-Care Evaluation (Schoening, H.A., Anderegg, L., Bergstrom, D., et al. Numerical scoring of self-care status of patients. *Archives of Physical and Medical Rehabilitation* 46:689–697, 1965; Schoening, H.A., Iversen, I.A. Numerical scoring of self-care status: A study of the Kenny Self-Care Evaluation. *Archives of Physical and Medical Rehabilitation* 49:221–229, 1968).

The Medical Outcomes Study Physical Functioning Measure (Stewart, A., and Kamberg, C.J. Physical functioning measures. In Stewart, A.L., Ware, J.E. (eds). *Measuring functioning and Well-Being: the Medical Outcomes Study Approach.* Durham, North Carolina: Duke University Press, 1992).

The Functional Status Index (Jette, A.M, and Deniston, O.L. Inter-observer reliability of a functional status assessment instrument. *Journal of Chronic Disease* 31:573–580, 1978; Jette, A.M. Functional capacity evaluation: An empirical approach. *Archives of Physical and Medical Rehabilitation* 61:85–89, 1980).

The Functional Activities Questionnaire (Pfeffer, R.I., Kurosaki,f T.T., Harrach, C.H., et al. Measurement of functional activities in older adults in the community. *Journal of Gerontology* 37:323–329, 1982; Pfeffer, R.I., Kurosaki, T.T., Chance, J.M., et al. Use of the Mental

Function Index in older adults: Reliability, validity, and measurement of change over time. *American Journal of Epidemiology* 120:922–935, 1984).

The Lambeth Disability Screening Questionnaire (Patrick, D.L., Darby, S.C., Green, S., et al. Screening for disability in the inner city. *Journal of Epidemiological Community Health* 35:65–70, 1981).

ATTITUDES, RELIGIOUSNESS, AND SPIRITUALITY, compiled and reviewed by Joan Teno

Attitude Indices

Death Attitude Profile (Gesser, G., et al. Death Attitudes Across The Life Span: Development and Validation of The Death Attitude Profile," *Omega,* 18(2):113–128, 1987).

Life Attitude Profile: A 36-item multidimensional profile developed and tested in a college population and more recently in hospitalized patients and outpatients. This is an excellent instrument for assessing spiritual needs but may need to be modified for a terminally ill population.

McCanse Readiness for Death Instrument (McCanse, R. The McCanse Readiness for Death Instrument: A Reliable and Valid Measure for Hospice Care. *The Hospice Journal* 1995 10(1):15–26, 1995).

Templer's Death Anxiety Scale (Aday, R. Belief in Afterlife and Death Anxiety: Correlates and Comparisons. *Omega,* 18:67–75, 1984).

Purpose in Life Test (PIL) (Crumbaugh, J.C., and Maholick, L.T. *Journal of Clinical Psychology,* 20:200–207, 1964).

The Seeking of Noetic Goals Test (SONG) (Crumbaugh, J., *Journal of Clinical Psychology,* 33(3):900–907, 1977).

Religiousness

Religious Coping Scale (Pargament, K.I. et al. God Help Me: (I): Religious Coping Efforts as Predictors of The Outcomes To Significant Negative Life Events, *American Journal of Community Psyschology,* 18(6): 793–824, 1990).

Religious Orientation Measure (Allport, G.W. and Ross, M.J. Personal Religious Orientation and Prejudice. *Journal of Personality and Social Psychology,* 5(4):432–443, 1967).

Quest Scale (Batson, C.D., and Schoenrade, P.A. Measuring Religion as Quest: 1) Validity Concerns. *Journal for the Scientific Study of Religion,* 30(4):416–429, 1991; Batson, C.D., and Schoenrade, P.A., Measuring Religion as Quest: 2) Reliability Concerns. *Journal for the Scientific Study of Religion,* 30(4):430–447, 1991).

The **Religiousness Scale** (Strayhorn, J.M., et al. A Measure of Religiousness, and Its Relation To Parent and Child Mental Health Variables. *Journal of Community Psychology,* 18:34–43, 1990).

Religious Coping (Koenig, H., et al. Religious Coping and Depression Among Elderly, Hospitalized Medically Ill Men, *American Jounral of Psychiatry,* 149(12):1693–1700. 1990).

Spirituality

Spiritual Well-Being Scale (Paloutzian, R.F., and Ellison, C.W. Loneliness, Spiritual Well-Being and Quality of Life, in Loneliness: A Sourcebook for Current Therapy A Wiley-Interscience Publ. Peplau and Perlman (ed). 1982).

Death Transcendence Scale (van de Creek, L., and Nye, C. Testing The Death Transcendence Scale. *Journal for the Scientific Study of Religion,* 32 (3):279–283, 1993; Hood, R., and Morris, R. Toward a Theory of Death Transcendence. *Journal for the Scientific Study of Religion,* 22(4):353–365, 1983).

Meaning in Life Scale (Warner, S.C., and Williams, J.I. The Meaning In Life Scale: Determining the Reliability and Validity of A Measure. *Journal of Chrons' Disease,* 40(6):503–512, 1987).

Herth Hope Index (van de Creek, L., et al. Where There's Life, There's Hope, and Where There Is Hope, There Is . . . *Journal of Religion and Health,* 33(1):51–59, 1994).

Index of Core Spiritual Experiences (INSPIRIT) (Kass, J. *Journal for the Scientific Study of Religion,* 30(2):203–211, 1991).

Spiritual Perspective Scale (Reed, P. Spirituality and Well-Being In Terminally Ill Hospitalized Adults. *Research in Nursing and Health,* 10:335–344, 1987).

QUALITY OF LIFE, compiled and reviewed by Anita Stewart

McGill Quality of Life Questionnaire (Cohen, S.R., and Mount, B.M. Quality of Life in Terminal Illness: Defining and Measuring Subjective Well-Being in The Dying. *Journal of Palliative Care,* 8(3):40–45, 1992).

Missoula-VITAS Quality of Life Index (Byock, I.R. Missoula-VITAS quality of life index [version 25S]. VITAS Healthcare Corp, 1995).

McMaster Health Index Questionnaire (Chambers, L.W., et al. The McMaster Health Index Questionnaire. *Journal of Rheumatology,* 9:780–784, 1982).

McAdam and Smith Index of Quality of Life (MacAdam, D.B., and Smith, M. An Initial Assessment of Suffering in Terminal Illness. *Palliative Medicine*, 1:37–47, 1987).

QL Index, HIRC-QL, Uniscale QL (Morris, J.N., et al. Last Days: A Study of The Quality of Life of Terminally Ill Cancer Patients. *Journal of Chronic Diseases*, 39(1):47–62, 1986).

Ferrans and Powers Quality of Life Index (Ferrans, C.E., and Powers, M. Quality of Life Index: Development and Psychometric Properties. *Journal of Advances in Nursing Science*, 8(1):15–24, 1985).

The Hospice Index (McMilan, S.C., and Mahon, M., *Quality of Life Resources*, 3:437–447, 1994).

SATISFACTION, compiled and reviewed by Joan Teno

Picker-Commonwealth Survey of Patient Centered Care (Cleary, P.D., Edgman-Levitan, S., Roberts, M., et al. Patients evaluate their hospital care: A national survey. *Health Affairs,* Winter 1991, 254–267).

Satisfaction Survey from Ware and Colleagues (Davies, A.R., Ware, J.E. GHAA's Consumer Satisfaction Survey and User's Manual. Group Health Association of America: Washington, D.C., 1988; Ware, J.E. Effects of acquiescent response set on patient satisfaction ratings. *Medical Care* 16:327, 1978; Tarlov, A.R., Ware, J.E., Greenfield, S., et al. The medical outcomes study: An application of methods for monitoring the results of medical care. *Journal of American Medical Association*, 262:925, 1989; McCusker, J. Development of scales to measure satisfaction and preferences regarding long-term and terminal care. *Medical Care*, 22:476–493, 1984; Kane, R.L., Bernstein, L., Wales, J., et.al. A randomized controlled trial of hospice care. *Lancet*, April:890–894, 1984; Baker, R., Teno, J.M., Wu, A., et al. Family satisfaction with end of life care. Manuscript in preparation. 1996; Westra, B.L., Cullen, L., Brody, D. et al. Development of the Home Care Client Satisfaction Instrument. *Public Health Nursing*, 12:393–399, 1995).

Patient Judgment System (Nelson, E.C., Hays, R.D., Larson, C., et al. The patient judgement system: reliability and validity. QRB, June:185–191, 1989).

FAMCARE (Kristjanson, L.J. Indicators of quality of palliative care from a family perspective. *Journal of Palliative Care*, 2:7–19, 1989; Kristjanson, L.J. Quality of terminal care: Salient indicators identified by families. *Journal of Palliative Care*, 5:21–30 1989; Kristjanson, L.J. Validity and reliability testing of the FAMCARE scale: Measuring family satisfaction with advanced cancer care. *Social Science Medicine*, 36:693–701, 1993).

Need Satisfaction Scale (Dawson, N.J. Need satisfaction in terminal care settings. *Social Science Medicine*, 32:83–87, 1991; Hampe, S. Needs of the grieving spouse in a hospital setting. *Nurs Res*, 24:113–120, 1975).

Unmet Needs of Patients with Cancer (Houts, P.S., Yasko, J.M., Harvey, H.A., et al. Unmet needs of persons with cancer in Pennsylvania during the period of terminal care. *Cancer*, 62:627–634, 1988).

National Hospice Organization Family Satisfaction Survey (National Hospice Organization. Family Satisfaction Survey. 1996).

Satisfaction of Families of Children with Cancer (Barbarin, O.A., Chesler, M.A. Relationships with the medical staff and aspects of satisfaction with care expressed by parents of children with cancer. *Journal of Community Health*, 9:302–313, 1984).

New York Satisfaction of Hospice Survey (Hannan, E.L., O'Donnell, J.F. An evaluation of hospices in the New York State hospice demonstration program. *Inquiry*, 21:338–348, 1984).

Satisfaction with Hospital-Based Home Care (Beck-Friis, B., Stang, P. The family in hospital-based home care with special reference to terminally ill cancer patients. *Journal of Palliative Care*, 9:5–13, 1993).

SUPPORT Surrogate Afterdeath Report on Dying (Baker, R., Teno, J.M., Wu, A., et al. Family satisfaction with end of life care. Manuscript in preparation. 1996).

Cancer Patient Satisfaction with Care (Wiggers, J.H., Donovan, K.O., Redman, S., and Sanson-Fisher, R.W. Cancer patient satisfaction with care. *Cancer*, 1:610–616, 1990).

Medical Interview Satisfaction Scale (Wolf, M.H., Putnam, S.M., James, S.A., et al. The medical interview satisfaction scale: Development of a scale to measure patient perceptions of physician behavior. *Journal of Behavioral Medicine*, 1:391, 1978).

G

Excerpts from *Medical Guidelines for Determining Prognosis in Selected NonCancer Diseases**

GENERAL GUIDELINES FOR DETERMINING PROGNOSIS

The following parameters may be used to help determine whether a patient is appropriate for hospice care and/or for the Medicare/Medicaid Hospice Benefit. These General Guidelines apply to all patients referred to hospice. However, they may be specifically applied to patients who do not fall under any of the specific diagnostic categories for which disease-specific Guidelines have been written. An example might be the elderly debilitated patient whose intake of food and fluid has declined to the point where weight loss has become significant, although no specific disease predominates in the clinical picture.

The patient should meet all of the following criteria:

I. The patient's condition is life-limiting, and the patient and/or family have been informed of this determination.

    A. A "life-limiting condition" may be due to a specific diagnosis, a combination of diseases, or there may be no specific diagnosis defined.

---

*Stuart, B., Alexander, K., Arenella, C. et al. *Medical Guidelines for Determining Prognosis in Selected NonCancer Diseases*, 2d ed. Washington, D.C.: National Hospice Organization, 1996. Used with permsission. NOTE: Citations and references to appendixes have been omitted.

II. The patient and/or family have elected treatment goals directed toward relief of symptoms, rather than cure of the underlying disease.

III. The patient has *either* of the following:

A. Documented clinical progression of disease, which may include:

   1. Progression of the primary disease process as listed in disease-specific criteria, as documented by serial physician assessment, laboratory, radiologic, or other studies.

   2. Multiple Emergency Department visits or inpatient hospitalizations over the prior six months.

   3. For homebound patients receiving home health services, nursing assessment may be documented.

   4. For patients who do not qualify under 1, 2 or 3, a recent decline in functional status may be documented.

      a. Functional decline should be recent, to distinguish patients who are terminal from those with reduced baseline functional status due to chronic illness. Clinical judgment is required for patients with a terminal condition and impaired status due to a different nonterminal disease; e.g., a patient chronically paraplegic from spinal cord injury who is recently diagnosed with cancer.

      b. Diminished function status may be documented by *either*:

         1. Karnofsy Performance Status of less than or equal to 50 percent, or

         2. Dependence in at least three of six Activities of Daily Living.

            "Activities of Daily Living" are:
            i.   bathing
            ii.   dressing
            iii. feeding
            iv.   transfers
            v.   continence of urine and stool
            vi.   ability to ambulate independently to bathroom

B. Documented recent impaired nutritional status related to the terminal process.

1. Unintentional, progressive weight loss of greater than 10 percent over the prior six months.

2. Serum albumin less than 2.5 gm/dl may be a helpful prognostic indicator, but should not be used in isolation from other factors in I–III above.

MEDICAL GUIDELINES FOR DETERMINING PROGNOSIS: DEMENTIA

This section is meant to assist in determining whether a patient with end-stage dementia is appropriate for hospice care and/or eligible for the Medicare/Medicaid Hospice Benefit. Although dementia shortens life independent of culture or ethnicity, prediction of six-month mortality is challenging. Severity of dementia alone correlates with poor survival in studies of institutionalized and outpatients, but patients with very advanced dementia can survive for long periods with meticulous care as long as they do not develop lethal complications. Death usually occurs, in fact, as a result of comorbid conditions.

The term "dementia" refers here to chronic, primary, and progressive cognitive impairment of either the Alzheimer or multi-infarct type. Although most research on prognosis in dementia is done with Alzheimer's patients, the vascular (multi-infarct) dementias appear to progress to death more quickly. These guidelines do *not* refer to acute, potentially reversible, or secondary dementias, i.e., those due to drug intoxication, cancer, AIDS, major stroke, or heart, renal, or liver failure.

I. Functional Assessment Staging

A. Even severely demented patients may have a prognosis of up to two years. Survival time depends on variables such as the incidence of comorbidities and the comprehensiveness of care.

B. The patient should be at or beyond Stage 7 of the Functional Assessment Staging Scale. The factors listed below should be understood explicitly since many patients do not progress in an orderly fashion through the substages of Stage 7.

    C. The patient should show *all* of the following characteristics:

        1. unable to ambulate without assistance.

        This is a critical factor. Recent data indicate that patients who retain the ability to ambulate independently do not tend to die within six months, even if all other criteria for advanced dementia are present.

        2. unable to dress without assistance.

        3. unable to bathe properly.

        4. urinary and fecal incontinence.

           a. occasionally or more frequently, over the past weeks.

           b. reported by knowledgeable informant or caregiver.

        5. unable to speak or communicate meaningfully.

           a. ability to speak is limited to approximately a *half dozen or fewer intelligible and different words*, in the course of an average day or in the course of an intensive interview.

II. Presence of Medical Complications

    A. The presence of medical comorbid conditions of sufficient severity to warrant medical treatment, documented within the past year, *whether or not the decision was made to treat the condition*, decrease survival in advanced dementia.

    B. Comorbid conditions associated with dementia:

        1. aspiration pneumonia.

        2. pyelonephritis or other upper urinary tract infection.

        3. septicemia.

        4. decubitus ulcers, multiple, stage 3–4.

        5. fever recurrent after antibiotics.

C. Difficulty swallowing food or refusal to eat, sufficiently severe that patient cannot maintain sufficient fluid and calorie intake to sustain life, with patient or surrogate refusing tube feedings or parenteral nutritional.

    1. Patients who are receiving tube feedings must have documented impaired nutritional status as indicated by:

        a. unintentional, progressive weight loss of greater than 10 percent over the prior six months.

        b. serum albumin less than 2.5 gm/dl may be a helpful prognostic indicator, but should not be used by itself.

H

American Board of Internal Medicine Clinical Competence in End-of-Life Care*

Components	Core Competencies
Medical Knowledge	Palliative care • Assessment and treatment of psychological distress • Pharmacological and nonpharmacological treatment of pain and other symptoms
Interviewing/Counseling skills	Listening Truth telling Giving bad news Discussing dying as a process Dealing with families of dying patients
Team Approach	Understanding multidisciplinary natures of end-of-life care (physician, nursing staff, social services, palliative care or hospice team, pharmacist, chaplain, patient, patient's family, patient advocate)

---

*American Board of Internal Medicine, *Caring for the Dying: Identification and Promotion of Physician Competency.* Philadelphia, Author, 1996, p. 41. Used with permission.

Symptom Assessment and Management	Communication skills Comfort Use of opioids, sedatives, or adjuvant analgesics, NSAIDs Control of dyspnea AHCPR and WHO guidelines
Professionalism	Altruism Accountability Confidentiality Transference and countertransference Nonabandonment Honoring patients' wishes Respect for colleagues
Humanistic Qualities	Integrity Compassion Sensitivity to patient needs for comfort and dignity Respect Courtesy
Medical Ethics	Advance directives, DNR/DNI orders, Conflicts of interest Futility Physician-assisted suicide Nutrition/hydration Surrogate decisionmaking Double effect

I

Examples of Medical Education Curricula

THE CANADIAN PALLIATIVE CARE CURRICULUM*

Specific Goals of a Palliative Care Curriculum

Attitude

1. To show students that the therapeutic process involves more than diagnosing and attempting to revert an altered pathophysiologic process and that illness is a complex state with physical, emotional, psychosocial, and spiritual elements.

2. To demonstrate the interdisciplinary approach of Palliative Care.

3. To demonstrate preventive steps to avoid physical, psychosocial, and emotional problems.

4. To emphasize that all interventions should be centered on the patient's needs, desires, and beliefs, thus ensuring patient control, whenever possible, of decisions which affect them.

5. To have students identify their own attitudes toward death and to identify and respect family attitudes toward death.

6. To enable students to understand the unit of care, the family,

---

*Copyright 1991 by Dr. Neil MacDonald for The Canadian Committee on Palliative Care Education, used with permission.

through consideration of the family background and the impact of illness upon the family group.

7. To demonstrate how the impact and interpretation of illness depends on personal attitudes by providing examples of harmonizing the Canadian medical model of care with the cultural and spiritual backgrounds of patients and families.

8. To involve students in discussions on ethical aspects of caregiving including euthanasia, resuscitation, truth telling, paternalism, aggressive versus palliative interventional therapy, incompetent patients, fairness in the health care system, and strategies for resolving ethical issues.

Skill

9. To enable students to integrate knowledge from across disciplines and to critically appraise clinical data, diagnostic tests, and the literature in order to assist with decisions to initiate or stop various investigations and therapy.

10. To demonstrate various techniques for communication with patients and families as well as how and why these techniques would be modified based on the personal, educational, and cultural background of the patient and family.

Knowledge

11. To describe the pathophysiology of common distressing symptoms in patients with advanced chronic disease and to suggest appropriate pharmacologic and non-pharmacologic techniques to combat these symptoms.

12. To have students identify various organizational arrangements for delivery of Palliative Care and the relationship of these organizational structures to the existing health care system including the community resources available to patients with advanced illness and their families.

13. To describe the elements of grief reactions and some techniques to prevent the development of pathologic reactions through caring for the patient and bereaved family.

HARVARD UNIVERSITY MEDICAL SCHOOL

Course Description: Living with Life-Threatening Illness—Care Near the End of Life
J. Andrew Billings, M.D., and Susan Block, M.D.

Caring for patients at the end of life is a basic task of doctoring and one for which students receive relatively little preparation and instruction. This course will combine clinical experiences and readings to provide students with the fundamental knowledge, attitudes, and skills necessary in caring for patients near the end of life. The focal learning experience in the course will be the student's relationship with a patient with a life-threatening illness. Opportunities will be offered in small groups for reflection on personal reactions to the patient, the patient's illness, and the dying process and for receiving supervision about working with the patients from a clinician experienced in caring for dying patients. Six or seven structured learning experiences (panel discussions, large group case discussions, seminars, and lectures) addressing topics such as responses to suffering, symptom control, grief and loss, spiritual issues, and ethical dilemmas will also be offered.

Goals and Objectives: Care Near the End of Life

Knowledge Objectives

- Students will learn the basic elements of the hospice philosophy of care.
- Students will understand the impact of inadequately controlled physical and psychological symptoms on quality of life in patients with life-threatening illness.
- Students will learn the most common physical and psychological symptoms that accompany terminal illness.
- Students will explore the roles of ethical principles (e.g. autonomy, beneficence, non-malfeasance) in making decisionmaking near the end of life.
- Students will learn the phenomenology and course of the grieving process and its impact on physical and psychological health.
- Students will learn about different cultural, religious, and spiritual constructs of the meaning of death and the impact on the experience of life-threatening illness.
- Students will gain an understanding of the experience, for patients and families, of a life-threatening illness.

Skill Objectives

- Students will enhance skills in creating a relationship which fosters the disclosure of intimate and sensitive material about responses to illness.
- Students will acquire skills in communicating with patients and their families about desires for care at the end of life.

Attitudinal Objectives

•   Students will enhance their appreciation of how their own feelings about death affect their interactions with patients.

•   Students will enhance their understanding of the meanings of death to physicians within the culture of medicine.

•   Students will gain understanding of physicians' adaptive and mal-adaptive responses to dying patients.

•   Students will gain enhanced appreciation of patients as teachers about the process of illness and the experience of receiving medical care.

February 8–May 23, 1996, Course Readings and Assignments

Readings (in order of assignment; starred readings optional)

Billings J.A. The Doctor and the Dying Patient, in Billings, JA, Stoeckle J. *The Clinical Encounter.* Chicago, Year Book Medical Publisher, 1989, pp. 193–199.

Cassem N.H. The Person Confronting Death, in Nicholi AM. *The New Harvard Guide to Modern Psychiatry.* Cambridge, Harvard University Press, 1988, pp. 728–758.

Quill T.E. Bad News: Delivery, Dialogue, and Dilemmas. *Archives of Internal Medicine,* 151:463–468, 1991.

Weisman A.D. The Coping Process/Coping and Denial (Chapters 3 and 4), in *Coping with Cancer.* New York, McGraw-Hill, 1979, pp. 27–55.

Nuland S. Hope and the Cancer Patient/The Lessons Learned (Chapters 11 and 12), in Nuland S. *How We Die.* New York, Knopf Publishing, 1994, pp. 222–262.

Callahan, D. Nature, Death, and Meaning: Shaping Our End, in *The Troubled Dream of Life.* pp. 157–186.*

Cassel E.J. The Nature of Suffering and the Goals of Medicine. *New England Journal of Medicine,* 306:639–645, 1989.*

Bulkin W, Lukashok H. Rx for Dying: The Case for Hospice. *New England Journal of Medicine,* 318(6):376–378, 1988.

Billings JA. Specialized Care of the Terminally Ill Patient, in *Care: Principles and Practice of Oncology,* vol. 2. Philadelphia, Lippincott, 1989, pp. 2237–2244.

Management of Cancer Pain. Clinical Practice Guideline: U.S. Department of Health and Human Services, Agency for Health Care Policy & Research. Publication no. 94-0592, March 1994.*

Baer K. *Guide to Hospice Care.* Harvard Health Letter Special Supplement. April 1993.*

Broyard A. *Intoxicated by My Illness and Other Writings on Life and Death.* New York, C. Potter, 1992, pp. 33–58.

Trillin A.S. Of Dragons and Garden Peas: A Cancer Patient Talks to Doctors. *N Engl J Med.* 304(12):699–701, 1981.

Frank A. Seeing Through Pain, in *At the Will of the Body.* Boston, Houghton-Mifflin, 1981, pp. 29–35.

Caralis P.V. et al. The Influence of Ethnicity and Race toward Advance Directives, Life-Prolonging Treatments, and Euthanasia. *Journal of Clinical Ethics,* 4(2)155–165, 1993.

Blackhall L.J. et al. Ethnicity and Attitudes Toward Patient Autonomy. *Journal of the American Medical Association,* 274:820–825, 1995.

Carresse J.A., Rodes, L.A. Western Bioethics on the Navajo Reservation. *Journal of the Amercian Medical Association,* 274:826–829, 1995.

Miles SH, August A. Courts, Gender and "the Right to Die". *Law, Medicine and Health Care,* 18(1–2):85–9). 1990*

Zinsser H. *As I Remember Him: The Biography of R.S.* Boston: Little, Brown, 1939, pp. 437–443.*

Lichstein P.R. Terminating the Doctor/Patient Relationship, in Lipkin M, et al. *The Medical Interview: Clinical Care, Education and Research.* New York, Springer-Verlag, 1994, pp. 196–206.

White L.P. The Self-Image of the Physician and the Care of Dying Patients. *Annals of the New York Academy of Sciences,* 164(3):822–831, 1964.

Morrison R.S. et al. Physician Reluctance to Discuss Advance Directives: An Empiric Investigation of Potential Barriers. *Archives of Internal Medicine,* 154:2311–2318, 1994.

Pfeifer M.P. et al. The Discussion of End-of-Life Medical Care by Primary Care Patients and Physicians: A Multicenter Study Using Structured Qualitative Interviews. *Journal of General Internal Medicine,* 9(Feb):82–88, 1994.

Markson LJ et al. Implementing Advance Directives in the Primary Care Setting. *Archives of Internal Medicine,* 154:2321–2327, 1994.*

Weeks WB et al. Advance Directives and the Cost of Terminal Hospitalization. *Archives of Internal Medicine,* 154:2077–2083, 1994.*

Brock, Death and Dying, in *Life-and-Death Decisions in the Clinic.* pp. 144–183.

Quill T. Death and Dignity: A Case for Individualized Decision Making. *New England Journal of Medicine,* 324(10):691–694, 1991.

SUPPORT Principal Investigators. A Controlled Trial to Improve Care for Seriously Ill Hospitalized Patients. *Journal of the American Medical Association,* 274:1591–1598, 1995.

Solomon A. A Death of One's Own. *The New Yorker.* May 22, 1995:54–69.

Evans RW, Orians C.E., Ascher N.L., The Potential Supply of Organ Donors: An Assessment of the Efficiency of Organ Procurement Efforts in the United States. *Journal of the American Medical Association,* 267(2)239–245, 1992.*

Veatch RM. The Shortage of Organs for Transplantation: Where Do We Go From Here? *New England Journal of Medicine,* 325(17):1243–1249, 1991.*

Cain JM, Hammes BJ. Ethics and Pain Management: Respecting Patient Wishes. *Journal of Pain and Symptom Management,* 9(3):160–164, 1994.*

Neuberger J. *Cultural Issues in Palliative Care.* pp. 507–513.

Chekhov, A. *Grief.*

Beattie A. In the White Night. *The New Yorker.* June 4, 1984: 42–43.

Lindemann E. Symptomatology and Management of Acute Grief. *American Journal of Psychiatry,* 101:141–148, 1944.

Osterweis M., et al. Epidemiologic Perspectives on the Health Consequences of Bereavement, in *Bereavement: Reactions, Consequences and Care.* Washington, D.C., National Academy Press, 1984: pp. 15–44.

Ross E.K. Adults' Reactions to Bereavement, in *Bereavement: Reactions, Consequences and Care.* Washington, D.C., National Academy Press, 1984:47–68.

Irvine P. The Attending at the Funeral. *New England Journal of Medicine,* 312(26):1704–1705, 1985.

Moss H. Elegy for My Sister. *New Selected Poems.* New York, Atheneum, 1985.

Billings J.A. On Being a Reluctant Physicians—Strains and Rewards in Caring of Dying at Home, in *Outpatient Management of Advanced Cancer,* Philadelphia, Lippincott, 1985: pp. 309–318.

Course Assignments

Death Awareness Exercise

- First patient visit: Introduction and discussion of patient's current status, how he or she learned about his or her illness, and his or her feelings about his or her current medical situation.
- Second patient visit with special attention to pain and symptom control issues.
- Third patient visit: Focus on cultural issues and desires for care at the end of life.
- Fourth patient visit: Focus on religious and spiritual issues.
- Complete a personal advance directive.
- Fifth patient visit: Spiritual assessment.
- Sixth patient visit: As a volunteer, helping with some aspect of patient's care, saying goodbye.

J

Committee Biographies

CHRISTINE K. CASSEL, M.D., F.A.C.P., is chairman of the Department of Geriatrics and Adult Development of Mount Sinai Medical Center and professor of geriatrics and medicine. She joined Mount Sinai in 1995 after 10 years as chief of general internal medicine at the University of Chicago, where she was also professor of medicine and public policy studies, chief of the Section of General Internal Medicine, director of the Center on Aging, Health and Society, director of the Center for Health Policy Research, and George M. Eisenberg Professor in Geriatrics. Dr. Cassel received an undergraduate degree in humanities at the University of Chicago and her M.D. at the University of Massachusetts in 1976 and took her training in Internal Medicine at Children's Hospital of San Francisco and at the University of California, San Francisco.

Among Dr. Cassel's numerous publications are three textbooks, *Geriatric Medicine: Principles and Practice* (first published by Springer-Verlag in 1984, now in its third edition), *Ethical Dimensions in the Health Professions,* also in its third edition, and *Nuclear Weapons and Nuclear War: A Source Book for Health Professionals.* Dr. Cassel, a member of the Institute of Medicine, is immediate past president of the American College of Physicians.

ROBERT A. BURT, J.D., is Alexander M. Bickel Professor of Law at Yale University. He has been a member of the Institute of Medicine since 1976, having served on the Council of the Institute from 1990–1993 and most recently as a member of the IOM Committee on Xenograft Transplantation: Ethical Issues and Public Policy. He is a member of the Advisory Board of the Project on Death in America, the Open Society Institute, and chair of the Board of Trustees of the Judge David L. Bazelon Center for Mental Health Law. Mr. Burt earned a B.A. from Princeton University, a B.A. in Jurisprudence at Oxford University, as a Fulbright Scholar, and a J.D. from Yale.

MARGARET L. CAMPBELL, R.N., M.S.N., C.S., has managed the palliative care practice at Detroit Receiving Hospital since 1988. From 1974 to 1988, she served in a number of critical care nursing positions including staff nurse, educator, and clinical nurse specialist. Ms. Campbell serves on the Board of Directors of the Medical Ethics Resource Network of Michigan and is a member of the Human Rights/Ethics Committee of the Michigan Nurses Association. She is a faculty member of the Wayne State University College of Nursing. Ms. Campbell lectures, studies, and publishes on end-of-life care and related issues. She has a diploma in nursing from the Henry Ford Hospital School of Nursing and bachelor's and master's degrees from Wayne State University.

ROBERT KLIEGMAN, M.D., is professor and chair of the Department of Pediatrics at the Medical College of Wisconsin and pediatrician in chief at Children's Hospital of Wisconsin. Dr. Kliegman completed his residency training in general pediatrics at Babies' Hospital in New York, New York. He completed neonatology and metabolism fellowships at Case Western Reserve University in Rainbow Babies and Children's Hospital. Dr. Kliegman's interests include neonatal bioethics and prevention of infant mortality and low birth weight. Dr. Kliegman has focused attention on the problems of low-income and medically underserved children. He has been a child advocate working with the American Academy of Pediatrics, municipal, state, and federal governments (Baby Doe, Health Reform), and The George Washington University Health Policy Institute-Packard Foundation Roundtable.

MATTHEW LOSCALZO, M.S.W., is a research associate at the Johns Hopkins University School of Medicine and the director of oncology social work at the Johns Hopkins Oncology Center. He is also the co-director for cancer pain research at the Johns Hopkins Oncology Center. Prior to his appointment at Johns Hopkins in 1993, Mr. Loscalzo provided psychobehavioral and social work services to patients and families as part of the Pain Service and Supportive Care Team at Memorial Sloan-Kettering Cancer Center. At this position, he was a founding member of one of the first supportive care teams in the United States. He has published widely on cancer pain, psychobehavioral interventions, and palliative care. His many national and international presentations reflect his ongoing interest in cancer pain, palliative care, patient and family advocacy, problem-solving therapies, and psychobehavioral interventions. He is the past president of the Association of Oncology Social Work. Mr. Loscalzo received his master's degree at the New York University School of Social Work.

JOANNE LYNN, M.D., M.A., M.S., is a professor of health care sciences and medicine and the director of the Center to Improve Care of the Dying, a multidisciplinary center committed to research, education, and advocacy to improve the care of seriously ill persons at The George Washington University Medical Center. As a geriatrician, Dr. Lynn has served in a variety of clinical positions, including 17 years as medical director for a nursing home and a hospice. A nationally known expert on end-of-life issues, she was assistant director of the President's Commission for the Study of Ethical Problems in Medicine and Biomedical and Behavioral Research and the principal writer of the commission's book, *Deciding to Forego Life-Sustaining Treatment.* Dr. Lynn was also co-director of the Study to Understand Prognoses and Preferences for Outcomes and Risks of Treatments, a 10-year multicenter study examining the process of care for over 10,000 seriously ill or elderly hospitalized patients. Dr. Lynn has served on many boards including the Board of Directors of Concern for Dying, the American Bar Association's Commission on Legal Problems of the Elderly, and the Hastings Center Task Force which wrote *Guidelines for the Termination of Treatment and the Care of the Dying.* Dr. Lynn was elected to membership in the Institute of Medicine in 1996.

NEIL MacDONALD, C.M., M.D., F.R.C.P.(C), F.R.C.P.(Edin), earned his undergraduate degree at the University of Toronto and his medical degree at McGill University, completing postgraduate studies at the Royal Victoria Hospital and Memorial Sloan-Kettering Cancer Center. Dr. MacDonald was director of Edmonton's Cross Cancer Institute (1971–1987) and director of the Division of Oncology for the University of Alberta (1975–1987). He has acted as chief medical oncology examiner for the Royal College of Physicians and Surgeons and has been an active participant in the American Society of Clinical Oncology, the Canadian Oncology Society, and the Canadian Cancer Society. He was named professor of Palliative Medicine and received one of the first Canadian chairs in the field in 1987. He is the editor of the Canadian Palliative Care Curriculum for undergraduate medical education, co-editor of the *Oxford Textbook of Palliative Medicine,* and past president of the newly formed Canadian Society for Palliative Care Physicians. In 1990–1991, Dr. MacDonald worked as a medical officer at the World Health Organization Cancer Palliative Care Unit in Geneva assisting the unit with development of palliative care policies and educational programs. He is currently director of the Cancer Ethics Program within the Center for Bioethics of the Clinical Research Institute of Montreal. He is also a professor within the Department of Oncology, McGill University Palliative Care Division with clinical responsibilities at the Royal Victoria Hospital in Montreal, Canada.

WILLARD G. MANNING, JR., Ph.D., is director of graduate studies, Doctoral Program in Health Services Research, Policy, and Administration at the University of Minnesota. He is also a professor at the Institute for Health Services Research, School of Public Health at the University of Minnesota. From 1988 to 1991, Dr. Manning was a professor in the Department of Health Services Management and Policy, School of Public Health, and Department of Economics of the University of Michigan. He earned his M.A. and Ph.D. degrees at Stanford University. Throughout his career, Dr. Manning's teaching areas have included microeconomics, health economics for public health students, applied economics, industrial organization, and econometrics. He was elected to Institute of Medicine membership in 1995.

DONALD L. PATRICK, Ph.D., M.S.P.H., is professor and director of the Social and Behavioral Sciences Program in the School of Public Health at the University of Washington. He trained in psychology at Northwestern University and received his Ph.D. degree in sociomedical sciences and M.P.H. degree from Columbia University. He has published widely on outcomes measurement, having worked on the assessment of health status and quality of life throughout his career, including applications to chronic illness and disability, health promotion, evaluation research, poverty and underserved populations, and the design and evaluation of advance directives. Dr. Patrick teaches graduate courses and conducts research on costs and outcomes in health and medicine. He is now working on assessment of the quality of dying. He was the inaugural president of the International Society for Quality of Life Research. He is a member of the Institute of Medicine and a Fellow of the Association of Health Services Research.

RICHARD PAYNE, M.D., is professor of neurology and chief of the Pain and Symptom Management Section at the University of Texas, Department of Neuro-Oncology, M.D. Anderson Cancer Center, in Houston, Texas. The Pain and Symptom Management Section is a multidisciplinary program involving over 40 health care professionals. He is also a clinical associate professor in the Department of Physical Medicine and Rehabilitation at Baylor College of Medicine in Houston. A graduate of Yale University and Harvard Medical School, Dr. Payne completed postgraduate training in internal medicine at the Peter Bent Brigham Hospital in Boston and in neurology at the New York Hospital-Cornell University Medical College. In addition, he completed a fellowship in neuro-oncology and pain management at Memorial Sloan-Kettering Cancer Center in New York. He served on the Agency for Health Care Policy and Research panel that developed guidelines for acute pain management, and later co-chaired the expert panel that developed clinical practice guidelines for the management of cancer pain. Dr. Payne has authored or co-authored over 100 peer-reviewed papers, invited reviews, book chapters, and abstracts. He has co-edited one book with Dr. Kathleen M. Foley. Currently, Dr. Payne serves on the editorial board of the *Pain Forum* (the official journal of the American Pain Society) and the *Journal of Pain and Symptom Management.*

GEORGE E. THIBAULT, M.D., graduated summa cum laude from Georgetown University in 1965 and magna cum laude from Harvard Medical School in 1969. He completed his internship and residency in medicine and fellowship in cardiology at Massachusetts General Hospital (MGH). He also trained in cardiology at the National Heart and Lung Institute in Bethesda and at Guys Hospital in London and served as Chief Resident in Medicine, the Medical Practices Evaluation Unit, and as director of the Medical ICU/CCU at the MGH. In 1978, he became the director of the Training Program in Internal Medicine and assistant chief (and subsequently associate chief) of the Department of Medicine, MGH. In 1988, he became chief of the medical services at Brockton/West Roxbury VA Medical Center and vice chairman of medicine at Brigham and Women's Hospital (BWH). Since July of 1995, Dr. Thibault has been the chief medical officer at the BWH and Professor of Medicine at Harvard Medical School. His research has focused on the evaluation of practices and outcomes of medical intensive care units and variations in the use of cardiac technologies. He has also served on numerous committees of national organizations, including the Institute of Medicine, the Department of Veteran Affairs, the National Institutes of Health, and the American College of Physicians. He has been a visiting scholar at both the Institute of Medicine and Harvard's Kennedy School of Government and a visiting professor of medicine at many medical schools in the United States and abroad.

THERESA H. VARNER, M.S.W., M.A., is the director of the Public Policy Institute at the American Association of Retired Persons (AARP). The Institute is AARP's focal point for public policy research and analysis on health, long-term care, economic security, and consumer issues. Before assuming her current position in 1991, she served for several years as the senior coordinator of the Health Policy Team in the Public Policy Institute. She came to AARP from the Alabama Department of Mental Health where she directed the state's largest hospital-based, pre-release program. Ms.

Varner has presented at numerous national conferences and symposia on a variety of health care reform topics. Her publications have focused on health care coverage, consumer information needs, and long-term care. She also oversaw the development of AARP's draft proposal for health care reform, *Health Care America*. Between 1993 and 1995, she served as a consumer representative on the Institute of Medicine's Committee on the Future of Dental Education. She holds two master's degrees from the University of Alabama, one in social work and one in English literature.

Index